Normal and Malignant Cell Growth

Recent Results in Cancer Research

Fortschritte der Krebsforschung

Progrès dans les recherches sur le cancer

17

Edited by

V. G. Allfrey, *New York* · M. Allgöwer, *Chur* · K. H. Bauer, *Heidelberg* · I. Berenblum, *Rehovoth* · F. Bergel, *London* · J. Bernard, *Paris* · W. Bernhard, *Villejuif* N. N. Blokhin, *Moskva* · H. E. Bock, *Tübingen* · P. Bucalossi, *Milano* · A. V. Chaklin, *Moskva* · M. Chorazy, *Gliwice* · G. J. Cunningham, *London* · W. Dameshek, *Boston* M. Dargent, *Lyon* · G. Della Porta, *Milano* · P. Denoix, *Villejuif* · R. Dulbecco, *San Diego* · H. Eagle, *New York* · R. Eker, *Oslo* · P. Grabar, *Paris* · H. Hamperl, *Bonn* R. J. C. Harris, *London* · E. Hecker, *Heidelberg* · R. Herbeuval, *Nancy* · J. Higginson, *Lyon* · W. C. Hueper, *Bethesda* · H. Isliker, *Lausanne* · D. A. Karnofsky, *New York* · J. Kieler, *København* · G. Klein, *Stockholm* · H. Koprowski, *Philadelphia* L. G. Koss, *New York* · G. Martz, *Zürich* · G. Mathé, *Villejuif* · O. Mühlbock, *Amsterdam* · G. T. Pack, *New York* · V. R. Potter, *Madison* · A. B. Sabin, *Cincinnati* L. Sachs, *Rehovoth* · E. A. Saxén, *Helsinki* · W. Szybalski, *Madison* · H. Tagnon, *Bruxelles* · R. M. Taylor, *Toronto* · A. Tissières, *Genève* · E. Uehlinger, *Zürich* R. W. Wissler, *Chicago* · T. Yoshida, *Tokyo* · L. A. Zilber, *Moskva*

Editor in chief
P. Rentchnick, *Genève*

Springer-Verlag New York, Inc. 1969

Recent Results in Cancer Research

Fortschritte der Krebsforschung

Progrès dans les recherches sur le cancer

17

Normal and Malignant Cell Growth

Edited by

R. J. M. Fry, M. L. Griem and W. H. Kirsten

With 85 Figures

Springer-Verlag New York, Inc. 1969

Symposium on Normal and Malignant Cell Growth
The University of Chicago School of Medicine
February 24th and 25th, 1968

Sponsored by the Swiss League against Cancer

ISBN 978-3-642-48265-6   ISBN 978-3-642-48263-2 (eBook)
DOI 10.1007/978-3-642-48263-2

© 1969 by Springer-Verlag New York Inc.
Softcover reprint of the hardcover 1st edition 1969
Library of Congress Card Number 65-6383

Title No. 3632

Contents

Normal Cell Kinetics
Chairman: M. FRY

Normal Cell Kinetics (cont.)
Chairman: L. LAMERTON

Proliferation of Cancer Cells

Chairman: A. M. BRUES

Preface

This volume presents the Proceedings of the University of Chicago's third Cancer Training Grant supported Teaching Symposium. This Symposium received much of its support from grant number T12 CA 08077-02. Most of the planning of the Symposium and most of the local editing of the Proceedings was carried out by Dr. R. J. Michael Fry of the A.E.C. Argonne National Laboratory and by two members of the Advisory Committee of the Cancer Training Grant, Drs. Melvin Griem and Werner Kirsten. They carried the main responsibility for the Symposium.

The subject of the Symposium, "Normal and Malignant Cell Growth," was chosen because, as the Proceedings reflect, it is a rapidly advancing field of endeavor which is of utmost importance to the understanding of the processes of malignant neoplasia. In fact, there is increasing evidence that knowledge of the kinetics of the cancer cell will greatly influence approaches to cancer therapy.

Like the first two of these Teaching Symposia held in 1964 and 1966, this one attracted about 400 students and staff from this medical institution as well as from other medical centers in the Chicago area. The effective interplay of an excellent group of scientists with a lively and responsive audience was evident as they considered together a topic of great current interest in the field of neoplasia. Much of the credit for the smooth organization and implementation of the Symposium must go to Mrs. Brenda K. Pickens who was ably assisted by Mrs. Jean B. Newgard. Mrs. Pickens' contribution to recording, transcribing and editing the Proceedings is also gratefully acknowledged.

As director of the Cancer Training Grant, I also want to express my appreciation for the contributions of the Advisory Committee to this program and specifically to the success of this Symposium. They are as follows:

GEORGE E. BLOCK, Professor of Surgery and Coordinator of Education in Clinical Oncology.

MELVIN L. GRIEM, Associate Professor of Radiology in the A.E.C. Argonne Cancer Research Hospital and Director, Registry of Neoplastic Diseases.

ELWOOD V. JENSEN, American Cancer Society—Charles Hayden Foundation Research Professor of Physiology in the Ben May Laboratory for Cancer Research.

JOSEPH B. KIRSNER, Professor of Medicine and Chief of Gastroenterology.

WERNER H. KIRSTEN, Professor of Pathology and Pediatrics and N.C.I. Career Development Awardee.

JOHN V. PROHASKA, Professor of Surgery.

HENRY RAPPAPORT, Professor of Pathology and Director of Surgical Pathology.

ROBERT W. WISSLER, Ph.D., M.D.,
Director of Cancer Training Grant
Professor and Chairman
Department of Pathology
University of Chicago
Pritzker School of Medicine and
in the A.E.C. Argonne Cancer Research
Hospital

Introduction

The understanding of the proliferation of cells and tissues has proceeded at a rapid pace over the last decade. The one particularly significant accomplishment has been the introduction of labelled DNA precursors and the use of high resolution autoradiography. These techniques have allowed the physiologist and the pathologist to examine many additional parameters in the process of cell proliferation both *in vitro* and *in vivo*. Knowledge of cell proliferation may be useful in improving our methods of treatment of a number of diseases and particularly a number of the human cancers which defy current treatment methods.

The Cancer Training Grant Director at The University of Chicago, with the help of his Advisory Committee, made plans to hold a teaching symposium on the subject of normal and malignant cell growth as part of the annual program of training in oncology at The University of Chicago. The objectives of the conference were to survey the recent accomplishments in this field and to present for the medical students and house staff the newer developments in the cell proliferation kinetics of normal tissues. As with the previous symposia sponsored by this training grant, leading scientists in various aspects of cell proliferation were invited to present general reviews as well as their latest results. In a number of instances the speaker was followed by an invited discussant.

The first day of the symposium, February 24, 1968, was devoted to the understanding of cell proliferation kinetics and was devoted to the general topics related to normal cell proliferation. A discussion followed this first day symposium so that the main speakers could exchange additional information and could answer questions from the audience. This discussion was especially stimulating under the leadership of Dr. Hewson Swift. On February 25, 1968, the participants considered our current knowledge of the proliferation of tumors. The symposium was summarized most ably by Dr. Harvey Patt.

The form of abbreviation for tritiated thymidine still shows the individuality of authors, but as their meaning is clear, no changes have been made. In order to prevent further reduction of figures, some have been placed to make optimal use of page size.

It is felt that the reader will use the table of contents for his guidance and we hope therefore will not miss the presence of an index.

This symposium held at The University of Chicago has stimulated a number of the staff and the graduate and undergraduate students to organize a weekly conference devoted to the discussion of problems related to cell kinetics.

The symposium was supported in part by the Rosa Kuhn Levy Fund, The Chicago Tumor Institute, the Rockefeller Foundation Grant for the Activities in Nuclear Medicine (Pharmacology), and mainly by the Cancer Training Grant of the National Cancer Institute #T12 CA 08077-02.

We are grateful to all who have made this conference possible.

R. J. M. FRY, M. L. GRIEM, and W. H. KIRSTEN

List of Participants

BASERGA, RENATO
Fels Research Institute and
Department of Pathology
Temple University
Philadelphia, Pennsylvania

BERTALANFFY, FELIX D.
Department of Anatomy
University of Manitoba
Winnipeg, Canada

BOND, VICTOR P.
Medical Department
Brookhaven National Laboratory
Upton, New York

BRUES, AUSTIN M.
Division of Biological and
Medical Research
Argonne National Laboratory and
The University of Chicago
Argonne, Illinois

BUCHER, NANCY L. R.
John Collings Warren Laboratories
Huntington Memorial Hospital
Harvard University
Boston, Massachusetts

CLARKSON, BAYARD
Sloan-Kettering Institute for
Cancer Research
New York, New York

DETHLEFSEN, LYLE A.
Department of Radiology
University of Pennsylvania
Philadelphia, Pennsylvania

FRY, R. J. MICHAEL
Division of Biological and
Medical Research
Argonne National Laboratory
Argonne, Illinois

GRISHAM, J. W.
Department of Pathology
Washington University
St. Louis, Missouri

LAJTHA, LASZLO G.
Patterson Research Laboratories
Christie Hospital and Holt Radium
Institute
Manchester, England

LAMERTON, LEONARD F.
Department of Biophysics
Institute of Cancer Research
Surrey, England

LEIGHTON, JOSEPH
Department of Pathology
University of Pittsburgh
Pittsburgh, Pennsylvania

LESHER, SAMUEL W.
Department of Radiology
Allegheny General Hospital
Pittsburgh, Pennsylvania

LIPKIN, MARTIN
Department of Medicine
Cornell University
New York, New York

MAUER, ALVIN M.
Children's Hospital Research
Foundation and
Department of Pediatrics
University of Cincinnati
Cincinnati, Ohio

PATT, HARVEY M.
Laboratory of Radiobiology
University of California
San Francisco, California

PHILIPS, FREDERICK S.
  Pharmacology Division
  Sloan-Kettering Institute
    for Cancer Research
  New York, New York

PRESCOTT, DAVID
  Institute for Developmental Biology
  University of Colorado
  Boulder, Colorado

REISKIN, ALLAN B.
  Division of Biological and Medical
    Research
  Argonne National Laboratory and
  The University of Chicago
  Argonne, Illinois

ROWLEY, DONALD A.
  Department of Pathology
  University of Chicago
  Chicago, Illinois

SANFORD, KATHERINE K.
  Laboratory of Biology
  National Cancer Institute
  National Institutes of Health
  Bethesda, Maryland

SINCLAIR, WARREN K.
  Division of Biological and
    Medical Research
  Argonne National Laboratory
  Argonne, Illinois

SWIFT, HEWSON H.
  Department of Biology
  University of Chicago
  Chicago, Illinois

TALMAGE, DAVID W.
  Departments of Microbiology and
    Medicine
  University of Colorado
  Denver, Colorado

TUBIANA, MAURICE
  Department of Radiation
  Institute Gustave-Roussy
  Villejuif, France

WHITMORE, GORDON
  University of Toronto and
  Ontario Cancer Institute
  Toronto, Canada

Normal and Malignant Cell Growth

General Introduction

Leonard F. Lamerton

Department of Biophysics
Institute of Cancer Research
Surrey, England

This Conference is a very timely one because the subject of cell proliferation and its control in the various tissues of the body is becoming one of the major growing points in biology. Over the last decade, the emphasis in the study of biological control mechanisms has been primarily at the cellular and sub-cellular level and certainly great advances have been made. But to imagine that this approach alone will provide the answers is to forget that the behavior of the cells in organized tissues or, for that matter, individuals in a society, is as much determined by the properties of the particular organization as by the characteristics of the individual units. In the study of the growth of normal and malignant tissues a two-pronged attack is needed—at the cellular level and at the tissue level. In the context of the present Symposium, the first aspect can be defined as the characterization of the cell cycle. It is the study of the changes a cell must pass through between successive divisions, the biochemical processes involved and the various trigger mechanisms through which the control of cell divisions operates. The second aspect is the characterization of the cell proliferative patterns in the various tissues of the body. This will include the relationship between cell division and tissue architecture, the rates at which cells divide and the proportion of cells taking part in proliferation and how the pattern can change under perturbing influences.

Classical Methods. The reason why this subject, which we may call "Cell Population Kinetics," has developed substantially only in the last few years is because the cells of the body are, from a morphological point of view, singularly uninformative about their proliferative state, except for the changes occurring during the process of mitosis itself, which occupies only a relatively small part of the mitotic cycle.

The classical technique for studying cell proliferation was confined, for most cell systems, to a study of the distribution and frequency of mitotic figures. This technique gave, and continues to give, some useful information. It can tell one something about the relationship between cell division and tissue architecture, and if the duration of observable mitosis is known, the gross rate of production of cells can be determined from the ratio Mitotic Index/Mitotic Duration. The reciprocal of this ratio is often known as the "Turnover Time" of the cell population —the time required for the production of a number of cells equal to the number

1

already present. It must be emphasized that the turnover time is not equal to the cell cycle time—that is, the time between successive divisions of a cell—unless all cells are dividing. A major limitation of the mitotic index technique is that no information is given on the proportion of cells present which are taking part in proliferation, the so-called "growth fraction." A low mitotic index can mean either a few cells dividing rapidly or many cells dividing slowly.

Labeling Methods. The breakthrough in the subject came with the opportunity that was provided for a characterization of the cell cycle using labeled DNA precursors and autoradiography. Howard and Pelc (4) were the first to demonstrate, by autoradiographic means, that DNA synthesis occupied only part of the interval between cell division, starting some time after mitosis and being completed some time before the next mitosis. Thus the cell cycle could be divided up into phases as shown in Fig. 1, and this pattern seems to hold for most, if not all, mammalian cells. The designations "G_1" and "G_2" imply no more than "gaps" in the process. The phases of the diagram must certainly not be taken as representing biochemically homogeneous states, or that the progress of cells through them is necessarily continuous. As we shall see in the course of this Symposium, advances in the understanding of the fine structure of the phases of the cell cycle will determine to a large extent advances in the whole subject of cell population kinetics.

However, even this simple division of the cell cycle has allowed the development of a number of important techniques in cell population kinetics. By administering an appropriately labeled DNA precursor—normally tritium-labeled thymidine— followed by high resolution autoradiography one can identify the cells that are in DNA synthesis and provide them with a permanent marker until such time as it is diluted out by successive cell divisions. To determine the "labeling index," which is analogous to the mitotic index, one takes a sample for autoradiography a short time after the administration of tritiated thymidine, normally about one hour, by which time all the precursor will have been taken up by cells or catabolized, and no labeled cells will yet have divided. The labeling index, by itself, allows only determination of tissue turnover time, as does mitotic index. However, so long as one is prepared to wait for the autoradiographic exposure, it has certain advantages

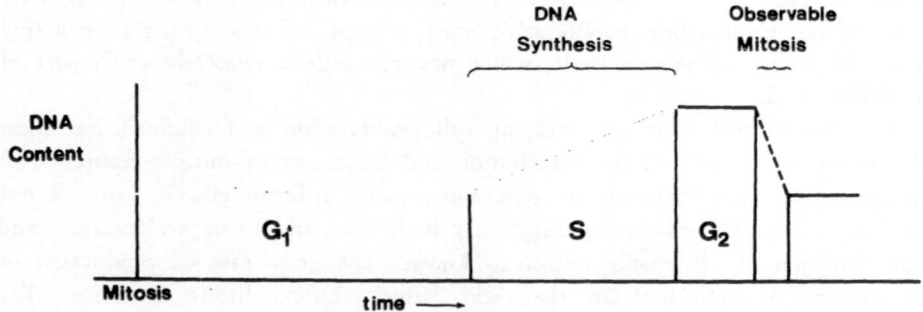

Fig. 1. Diagram of the cell cycle, indicating the sub-divisions formed by the phases of DNA synthesis and mitosis.

over the mitotic index technique, not least that a labeled cell is easily identifiable in all tissues, and cells observed will be in interphase, which is a distinct advantage for recognition when there are various cell types present, as in the bone marrow. Also, since the duration of DNA synthesis is much longer than the duration of mitosis, the labeling index of a tissue will be considerably greater than the mitotic index, unless a metaphase arrest agent such as colchicine is used to increase the number of mitotic figures. Finally, by virtue of the fact that DNA labeling provides a permanent marker, the duration of synthesis can be measured much more precisely and easily than the duration of mitosis.

The labeling technique in cell population kinetics is based on the assumption that the uptake of DNA precursors by the cell will always be followed by cell division. This will not be the case when polyploid cells are being produced, which occurs in certain normal tissues and in some pathological conditions. Also, there is evidence, mainly from work with lower organisms, that metabolic turnover of DNA may occur at any time in the cell cycle. How far this occurs in mammalian cells is still a matter of discussion but Pelc (6) considers that in slowly dividing tissues metabolic turnover of DNA can substantially increase the observed labeling index. This effect, however, would not be serious in the more rapidly dividing tissues of the body.

The application of the labeled DNA method to the measurement of actual cell cycle time and growth fraction depends on its property as a permanent cell marker. There are a number of techniques available, but the one I will describe, that of labeled mitoses, (7), is in common use and will be referred to by a number of speakers at this Symposium. The principle is to administer a labeled DNA precursor, and then at various times afterwards to take samples of the cell population and determine the fraction of mitotic figures which are labeled. Essentially one is labeling a given cohort of cells and watching the passage of this cohort of cells through the window offered by mitosis. For a population of cells all dividing with the same cycle time the fraction of labeled mitosis will vary with time in a regular periodic fashion as shown in Fig. 2 (a), from which the duration of the phases of the cell cycle can be determined. In practice there will always be some spread in the duration of phases of the cell cycle, which will lead to a damping-out of the curve, as shown in Fig. 2 (b). There are now mathematical techniques available (1, 10) whereby information on the distribution of the cell cycle times can be derived from the degree of damping out of the labeled mitoses curves. An example of a labeled mitoses curve, with the derived cell cycle time distribution, is shown in Fig. 3.

If the actual cycle time in a cell population can be determined by the labeled mitoses or other method, and the turnover time from the initial labeling index, then the growth fraction of the population is given by the ratio of cell cycle time to turnover time. However, a practical problem may arise because the labeled mitoses curve is much more sensitive to short cycle times than to long cycle times, and often it will not be possible to distinguish between a nonproliferative fraction and a slowly proliferative fraction in the population.

The difficulties, both practical and theoretical, of measuring long cycle times by

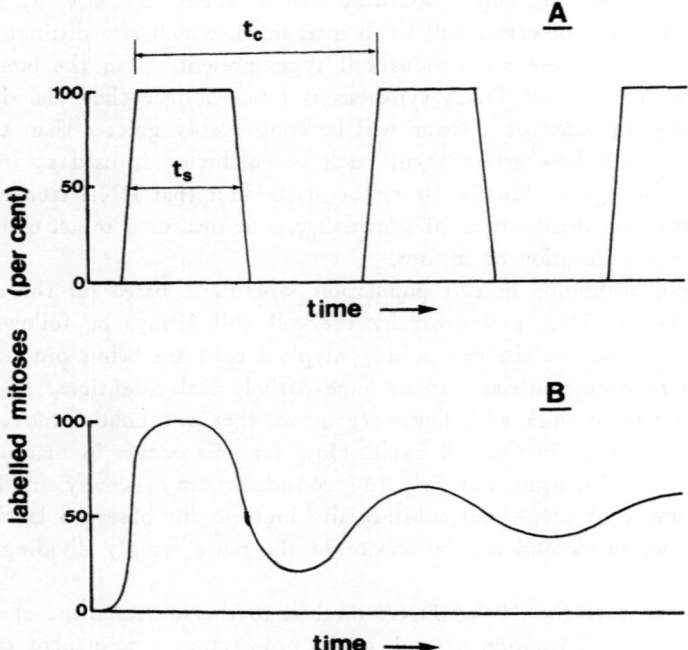

Fig. 2. The form of labeled mitoses curve expected: (a) when cells have identical phasing of the cell cycle; and (b) when there is spread in the phase durations.

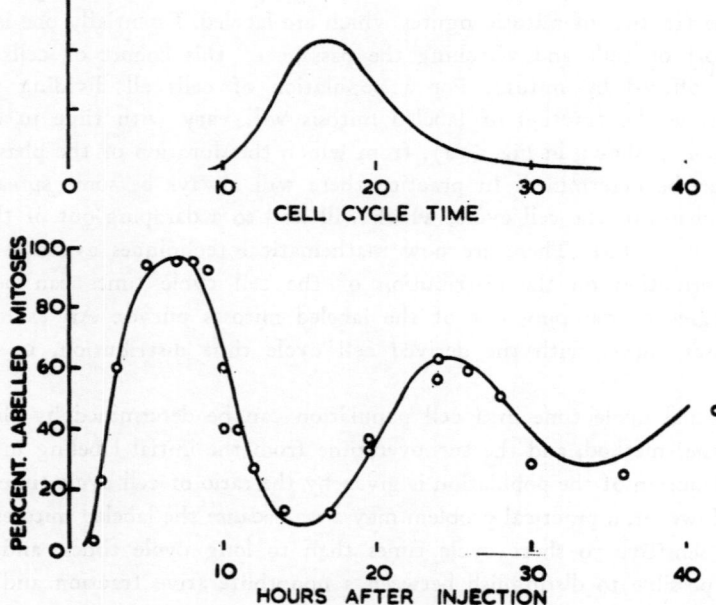

Fig. 3. Experimental labeled mitoses curve for a rat tumor, with derived cell cycle time distribution. (Steel *et al.*, 1966)

the method of labeled mitoses are evident. In the first place a long period of sampling is required if the second peak on the curve is not to be missed—a job suited really only to healthy young Ph.D. students. Also, it would appear that in general a long cycle time is associated with a wide spread in cycle time, so that the second peak may not be very evident.

There are other techniques available for obtaining information on cell cycle time, such as continuous or repeated labeling or measurement of rate of decrease of auto-radiographic grain count due to successive divisions. But they all require serial sampling techniques, which can make studies on experimental animal systems laborious and work on human tissues possible only in very special cases.

Much of the present difficulty would be avoided if we had additional methods for characterizing the proliferative state of a cell population—if the cells could be made to be more informative about their proliferative state. The present position is that a cell in mitosis can be recognized directly and a cell in DNA synthesis by labeling and autoradiography. It is also possible to identify cells in the G_2 stage by appropriate staining and microspectrophotometry, since they will contain double the normal amount of DNA, and this method has been employed in studies of both experimental animal and human cell populations (11, 3). The difficulty is that there is at present no means of determining whether a cell which is not in mitosis, DNA synthesis or G_2 is in the proliferative fraction of the population or not. In other words, there is no direct way of telling whether a cell is in G_1 or out of cycle. If this could be achieved by histochemical or labeling techniques, the study of the cell population kinetics of tissues would be greatly helped. There is another related problem, which is to distinguish, in the nondividing population, those cells which still have proliferative potential from those which are permanently sterile. These are basic problems and will only be solved, if at all, through a much deeper understanding of the biochemistry of the cell cycle.

There are some variations in the techniques of initial labeling index which can be of great value in special circumstances. To determine the initial labeling index of a tissue, it is not necessary to administer the labeled DNA precursor *in vivo*. Fresh tissue, incubated *in vitro*, with a medium containing tritiated thymidine will show a labeling index the same as that *in vivo* (9) since cells in synthesis will continue to synthesize new DNA when placed in a simple culture medium, while at the same time no new cells will enter synthesis. Normally, the incubation has to be carried out under an excess oxygen pressure in order to achieve labeling throughout the specimens. This is proving a most useful technique to use with biopsy specimens of human tumors, since the turnover time, found from the labeling index (together with an assumed or known value for the duration of synthesis), is the potential doubling time of the tissue, assuming no cell loss. A comparison of the potential doubling time and the observed growth rate of a tumor will give the extent of cell loss, by death, exfoliation and other processes, and this can be a most useful piece of information.

Another variant of the technique allows a measurement of the labeling index of cells which cannot be recognized morphologically but which can be studied by functional tests. The stem cells of the haematopoietic system are in this class. We know they exist; we cannot yet recognize them, but we can obtain a measure of their numbers by their capacity to produce red cells. The technique, developed by Becker and his colleagues (2), is to treat the cell population, for instance, bone marrow *in vitro,* with such a high dose of tritiated thymidine that the cells which take it up, *i.e.,* cells in synthesis, are themselves killed by the tritium radiation dose. From a measurement of the loss of stem cell function of the sample one can deduce their labeling index. For obvious reasons this is known as the "thymidine suicide" technique.

You will see, in the course of this Symposium, how these and other techniques, some involving labeling and some not, have been used in the study of the cell proliferation of a variety of normal tissues and cell systems.

Classification of Tissues and Specific Problems. There are various ways in which the tissues of the body may be classified according to their proliferation characteristics. The simplest distinction might seem to be between those tissues in which the cells divide or have a potential for cell division and those in which the cells have lost all capacity for division. This is, in fact, not an easy classification because one can never be certain that a given cell type cannot be made to divide, given the proper stimulus, and advances in molecular biology allow very little in the way of dogmatism concerning the irreversibility of cell differentiation.

The dividing tissues are sometimes classified as either fast renewal or slow renewal tissues. The fast renewal tissues, exemplified by the small intestine, are those in which there is a very rapid turnover of cells, sometimes as rapidly as a day. The slow renewal tissues are those in which the turnover time is long, months or even years. These are exemplified by the liver, the thyroid and skin. This distinction is also not absolute because there is no clear separation between the groups and many of the slow renewal tissues have a remarkable capacity for increasing their rate of cell division under the appropriate stress. This capacity is shared by the liver, the thyroid, the kidney, the salivary glands, the skin, the vascular system and probably a number of other tissues as well. Because of this behavior these tissues are sometimes classed as "conditional renewal" systems.

It has to be recognized that a number of tissues will combine various characteristics. For instance, the red cell system, which Dr. Lajtha will be discussing immediately following this Introduction, comprises a "stem cell" compartment, which has many of the properties of a conditional renewal system, followed by a sequence of proliferating precursors of the erythrocytes, which are dividing very rapidly.

The red cell system has a number of properties which make it very rewarding in a study of cell population kinetics. The first is that the mature product, the red cell, can be serially sampled with little difficulty, and measurements made of cell number, rate of production and life span. Secondly, in addition to the opportunities provided by the use of labeled DNA precursors a great deal of information can be obtained using radioactive iron, since radioactive iron can be regarded, for most practical purposes, as a specific nonexchangeable label for red cells during the course of their production and subsequent functional life. Another very useful property which is the basis of powerful methods of investigation is that, under certain conditions, bone marrow can be transplanted and made to give information on stem cell numbers and properties. However, perhaps the most important point is that a hormone, erythropoietin, has been isolated which appears to play a basic part in the control of red cell production. Thus the opportunity is provided for studying basic control mechanisms, which is the subject of Dr. Lajtha's talk.

The red cell system's one disadvantage from the point of view of studies of cell population kinetics is that, as yet, little is known about the microarchitecture of the system, so that the spatial relationship of the various precursors of the red cell cannot be investigated.

In contrast, the gut provides a system in which the microarchitecture is clearly defined and the small intestine, in particular, has been the subject of many studies. The zone of cell proliferation can be clearly defined and the proliferative characteristics of cells within this zone investigated. Dr. Lesher will be describing the cell population kinetics of the small intestine and the pattern of response to extra demand for cells.

The small intestine illustrates a basic control mechanism found in many normal tissues. Only within a small part of the tissue can cells act as stem cells, that is, continue to divide indefinitely. Outside this zone cells will progress, apparently irreversibly, to become functional and non-dividing. The skin provides another example of this principle, where the basal layer represents the stem cell zone. How far this property of "stemness" is due to the environment in which the cell finds itself and how far to inherited capacity is an interesting and important problem. The classical theory of unequal division of stem cells has not received much support from experimental work. This theory explained the constancy of stem cell numbers in normal tissues as the result of each stem cell division producing one stem cell and one cell that was destined to differentiate. A very elegant autoradiographic experiment of Marques-Pereira and Leblond (5) on mouse oesophagus showed that this was not necessarily so. They found that, following cell division in the basal layer of the tissue, sometimes both daughter cells remained in the basal layer, sometimes both would move out and sometimes one stayed in and one moved out. The simplest explanation was that only the basal layer provided the environment for indefinite cell division and that the cell number of the basal layer was kept constant by cell population pressure. A study of the factors determining "stemness" is not merely of theoretical interest. One of the major characteristics of malignant disease is a breakdown of the normal pattern of cell proliferation because of lack of containment of stem cell activity.

The extent to which cell proliferation and differentiation, as exemplified by specialized function, are opposing factors is a related problem of fundamental interest. In many of the renewal tissues, for instance gut, skin, erythropoietic tissues, specialization is accompanied by loss of proliferative power. However, specialized function does not necessarily remove potential for cell division, as shown by the liver, which is the subject of Dr. Grisham's talk this morning. The liver presents the fascinating situation of highly functional cells where the interval between successive mitoses is normally very long indeed, but can be reduced to a very short interval under demand for extra cells following cell removal or death. This highlights the problem of the conditions under which a cell can remain in a condition of "no cell cycle" but with the capacity for rapid transfer into cycle when required, and the problem of the stage in the cell cycle at which triggering for division occurs. These are general matters that will be discussed by Dr. Prescott in his talk on the regulation of the cell life cycle.

A problem similar to that of the liver and one of great practical significance will be dealt with by Dr. Talmage when he discusses the proliferation of antibody-forming cells. Here increased cell production is stimulated not by cell loss, but by a very specific type of functional demand of the body.

One of the reasons for studying the normal is to understand better the abnormal. The growth and cell proliferation characteristics of cancer will be discussed in to-morrow's sessions, but I think it is important to stress now that, in general, cancer cannot be defined as all-out, uncontrolled proliferation of cells. A high rate of cell proliferation is by no means a general property of cancer—the defect in cancer being essentially lack of control of cell maturation. Also, depending on the type of cancer, there may still be a considerable measure of cell organization present. The successful therapy of cancer by radiation, cytotoxic drugs or other means relies on achieving an adequate differential response between the tumor and normal tissues, which means we have to exploit all possible differences, which will include the differences in cell organization as well as differences in cellular response.

One of the major factors to exploit, by fractionation methods, is the relative repopulation rates of tumor and normal tissue, and this lies very much in the field of interest of this meeting. For many cytotoxic drugs the critical normal tissues will be the gut and the bone marrow, and it is useful that these are two tissues in which available techniques of cell population kinetics are particularly applicable. Dr. Philips will in fact be discussing the susceptibility of intestinal crypt epithelium to anti-tumor agents.

For radiotherapy the problem is somewhat different, since the treatment is much more localized than in the case of cytotoxic drugs. The limitation to the radiation dose that can be given to the tumor will often be set by the response of the skin and vascular system, both tissues with normally a low rate of cell proliferation but with the property of responding dramatically to the appropriate stress. I have already mentioned some of the difficulties of studying the cell population kinetics of slowly dividing tissues, but it is evident that this represents one of the main challenges in our subject, of significance both fundamentally and practically.

References

1. BARRETT, J. C.: A mathematical model of the mitotic cycle and its application to the interpretation of percentage labeled mitoses data. J. Nat. Cancer Inst. **37**, 443–450 (1966).
2. BECKER, A. J., McCULLOUGH, E. A., SIMINOVITCH, C. and TILL, J. E.: The effect of differing demands for blood cell production on DNA synthesis by hemopoietic colony-forming cells of mice. Blood **26**, 296–308 (1965).
3. COOPER, E. H., HALE, A. J. and MILTON, J. D.: The proliferation of infectious mono-nucleosis lymphocytes *in vitro*. Acta. Haematol. **38**, 19–33 (1967).

4. HOWARD, A. and PELC, S. R.: The synthesis of desoxyribonucleic acid in normal and irradiated cells and its relation to chromosome breakage. *In*: Symposium on chromosome breakage. Oliver and Boyd, eds. Heredity 6, 261–273 (1953). Supplement.

5. MARQUES-PEREIRA, J. P. and LEBLOND, C. P.: Mitosis and differentiation in the stratified squamous epithelium of the rat esophagus. Amer. J. Anat. 117, 73–90 (1965).

6. PELC, S. R.: Labeling of DNA and cell division in so-called non-dividing tissues. J. Cell. Biol. 22, 21 (1964).

7. QUASTLER, H. and SHERMAN, F. G.: Cell population kinetics in the intestinal epithelium of the mouse. Exp. Cell. Res. 17, 420–438 (1959).

8. STEEL, G. G., ADAMS, K. and BARRETT, J. C.: Analysis of the cell population kinetics of transplanted tumors of widely-differing growth rate. Brit. J. Cancer 20, 784–800 (1966).

9. STEEL, G. G. and BENSTED, J. P. M.: *In vitro* studies of cell proliferation in tumors. *In*: Critical appraisal of methods and theoretical considerations. Europ. J. Cancer 1, 275–279 (1965).

10. TAKAHASHI, M.: Theoretical basis for cell cycle analysis. *In*: Labeled mitosis wave method. J. Theoret. Biol. 13, 202–211 (1966).

11. WALKER, P. M. B. and RICHARDS, B. M.: Quantitative microscopial techniques for single cells. *In*: The Cell: Biochemistry, Physiology, and Morphology. J. J. Brachet and A. E. Mirsky, eds. Academic Press, New York, vol. 1, 91–138 (1959).

Proliferative Capacity of Hemopoietic Stem Cells

Laszlo G. Lajtha and R. Schofield

Paterson Laboratories
Christie Hospital and Holt Radium Institute
Manchester, England

Until about eight years ago, it was only possible to theorize about the hemopoietic stem cells. Since then, a number of methods have become available which have allowed both quantitative and qualitative studies to be made, and we are beginning to formulate ideas which might give a realistic picture of the properties and nature of the elusive hemopoietic stem cell.

There is no unique definition of the stem cell. It is generally accepted that it is a precursor cell of the morphologically identifiable bone marrow cells: erythroblasts, promyelocytes, megakaryocytes, i.e., it can, given the right stimulus, differentiate. Since the daily requirement for the recognizable bone marrow cells is considerable, and since hemopoiesis in animals treated with acute or chronic cytotoxic regimes (ionizing radiations, cytotoxic chemicals) can recover after relatively severe depletion, the stem cell must possess considerable proliferative capacities. Indeed these two properties: capacity for prolonged (?indefinite) proliferation, and capacity to respond to appropriate stimuli by differentiating into another cell line (or lines) characterize the hemopoietic stem cells.

Methods for Stem Cell Studies

The present methods fall broadly into two categories: those that depend on grafting hemopoietic tissue into suitable recipients, and others in which the degree of hemopoiesis is measured without grafting.

The grafting methods may use a variety of end-points to assess the efficacy of the graft. One end-point is the proportion of irradiated and then grafted animals which survive (20, 25), another is the degree of ^{59}Fe incorporation into RBC 6 to 8 days after grafting (15, 5), or the measurement of splenic uptake of labeled iododeoxyuridine 6 to 8 days after grafting (9). The method which gives the absolute numbers of grafted stem cells is the counting of macroscopically visible splenic colonies, each originating from a single cell (3, 27). While this latter method does measure the absolute numbers of grafted stem cells if the "plating efficiency," i.e., the proportion of injected cells reaching the spleen is determined, all the other methods can measure quantitatively the relative changes in the number of hemopoietic stem cells of the donor animal. It is worth remembering that, so far, splenic colony counting is only possible in the mouse. The other methods are applicable to the rat also. There is little information on the use of these methods in other mammals.

The second group of methods, those not dependent on grafting, can be divided into methods using erythropoietin and those dependent on autorepopulation of the hemopoietic tissue. The erythropoietin methods utilize the re-establishment of erythropoiesis in the polycythemic animal by an injected dose of the humoral factor erythropoietin (12) or by restarting erythropoietin production in the starved and refed mouse (22).

The autorepopulation assay depends on the amount of erythropoiesis (assessed by ^{59}Fe incorporation into RBC) or the number of splenic colonies produced in an animal which had been irradiated while a part of the hemopoietic tissue was shielded (23). In this case repopulation is effected by cells migrating from the shielded area and seeding into the other previously irradiated parts of hemopoietic sites (13, 14). The splenic colonies thus produced are called auto- or endo-colonies as opposed to the "exo" colonies produced by grafting.

These methods do not necessarily measure the same thing. The grafting methods undoubtedly measure the repopulating or colonizing capacity of the grafted sample, the colonizing or colony forming cell (CF) of Till and McCulloch (27). The erythropoietin assay can measure the number of cells which can respond to it by differentiating into erythroblasts (ERC = erythropoietin responsive cell) and the autorepopulating method measures the rate at which repopulating cells can colonize other hemopoietic sites.

Growth Rate Studies

After grafting, *e.g.*, bone marrow cells into irradiated recipients, the spleen can be periodically sampled by killing groups of animals and assaying the number of colony forming units (CFU) in these spleens. Such investigation indicated that after a lag of about 2 days the number of CFU increases logarithmically with a doubling time of about 25 hours (19). It is interesting to note that during the first 24 to 48 hours after grafting there is not only a growth lag, but also an apparent decrease in the number of CFU in the spleen.

Similarly, after a single dose of whole-body irradiation with 400 rad the regrowth of CFU in the spleen follows an exponential line with a doubling time of about 28 hours (26).

These data indicate that CFU growth in the spleen, either after grafting or after a significant depopulation (by 400 rad whole-body irradiation), occurs at a doubling rate of about 25 to 28 hours. There is also clear evidence that this growth results in a significant over-shoot above normal values (26) by a factor of about 4.

The growth of the CFU in the spleen and in the femur may not, however, occur at the same rate after grafting. Comparing the number of CFU in the femur and in the spleen after 900 rad followed by a graft of 10^6 bone marrow cells, Playfair and Cole (21) found that while in the spleen the growth rate is as described earlier by the Toronto workers (19, 26), *i.e.*, doubling at a rate of 28 hours or so, with a massive overshoot, the CFU in the femur behaves differently. The initial growth rate

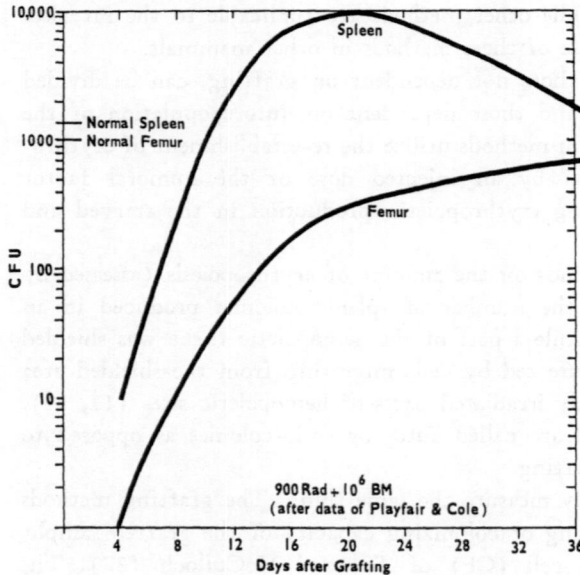

Fig. 1. Growth of CFU in spleen and femur after grafting into irradiated mice.

is fast, probably approaching that in the spleen, but it begins to slow down after 8 to 9 days. There is no overshoot above normal values in the femur, indeed the CFU values approach normal after 40 days (Fig. 1).

The growth rate, both in femur and in spleen, shows a different pattern if instead of a random repopulation only a moderate decrease in numbers is produced, *i.e.*, by 150 rad whole-body irradiation. This dose will reduce the CFU numbers only to about 15 to 20 percent of normal values. The recovery pattern will be characterized by a long post-irradiation lag and dip, lasting 4 to 6 days (23, 18), followed by a return to normal values by about the 14th to 16th day. Both splenic and femoral CFU behave similarly in this respect with no evidence of an overshoot (Fig. 2). A similar pattern of recovery was found in the repopulating capacity of rat femoral bone marrow cells (using ^{59}Fe incorporation into RBC as an end-point) after 200 rad by Blackett *et al.* (5). Clearly, from the kind of curve shown in Fig. 2, one cannot get a reliable estimate of the growth rate of CFU, but on the ascending slope a thirty-hour doubling time is a possible conjecture.

It is important to realize that while after 150 rad both femoral and splenic CFU recover to normal in a similar fashion, the pattern is different after a larger depopulation (*e.g.*, after 400 rad or grafting). In the latter case, the splenic CFU grow and overshoot with a doubling time of about 25 to 30 hours, but the femoral CFU appear to lag behind, not reaching normal values even after 30 days (Fig. 1). It should be remembered, however, that of the total CFU in the normal mouse the spleen contains only about 2000 (1:10^5 CFU and ~2 × 10^8 cells) while one femur alone contains about 2000 CFU (1:10^4 CFU and ~2 × 10^7 cells). One femur, however, is only about 5 percent of the total marrow cellularity. Hence if the proportion of CFU is the same in all bone marrow sites, the total CFU in the marrow of a mouse may be as much as 40,000, *i.e.*, 20 times as much as in the spleen.

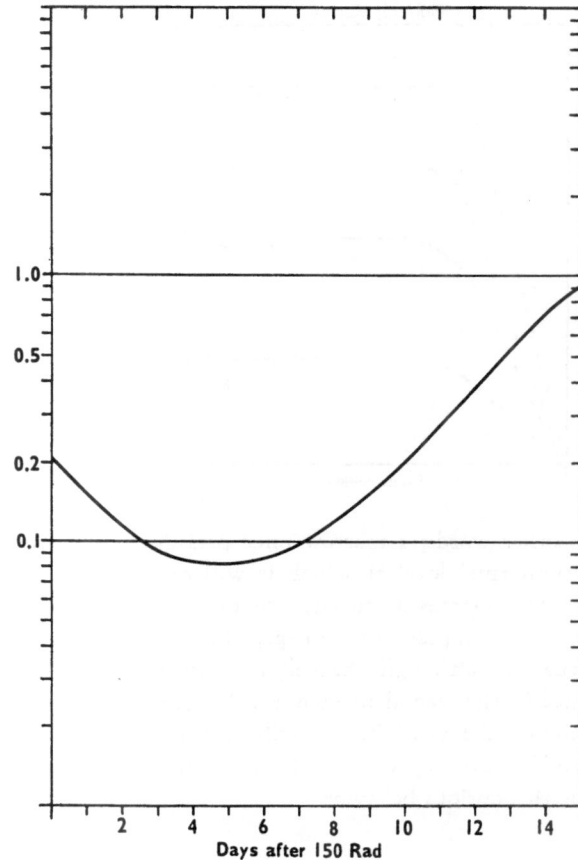

Fig. 2. Pattern of recovery of CFU in femur of mice receiving 150 rad wholebody irradiation, expressed as fraction of control.

Decline in Colonizing Capacity

The colonizing cells apparently do not possess unlimited proliferating capacity. It has been reported in the serial transplantation experiments of Ford, Micklem and Gray (10) that by the third transplant generation, the marrow had lost its restorative capacity. This work was extended by Siminovitch, McCulloch and Till (24) using the splenic colony assay. They have transplanted serially spleen cell suspensions at fourteen-day intervals (after an initial bone marrow grafting) and found practically no CFU content after the fourth passage. Pooling excised splenic colonies; they found an even faster decline of colonizing capacity: a drop from 22–27 to <2 CFU per colony in the first and second passage, respectively. Looking at individual (as opposed to pooled) colonies, the decline was even more marked. Of 21 samples from individual colonies, only 4 showed any colony forming capacity at the second passage. These observations were also confirmed by Cudkowicz, Upton, Shearer and Hughes (8) who noted the interesting fact that not only is the recolonizing capacity of the marrow gradually declining with serial passages, but that the subnormal repopulation found, *e.g.*, 30 days after the first or second graft persists for as long as 150 days.

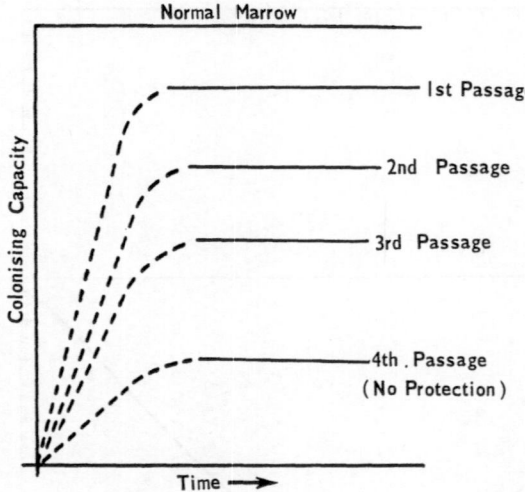

Fig. 3. Growth rate and plateau values for colonizing capacity of bone marrow grafts during repeated passages of grafting.

In other words, a marrow once passaged will restore the colonizing capacity only to a subnormal level at which it will remain.

This creates a curious situation, illustrated in Fig. 3. The curious aspect is that the graft appears to multiply, to a certain extent. It then maintains a subnormal situation, although the cell line has not lost its proliferative capacity completely, since in the second passage it will again start proliferating, although to an even more subnormal level. There it will remain, again, in spite of further (but more limited) proliferative capacity in the third passage. There is no good explanation at present for this curious behavior.

The CFU Growth Paradox

According to current concepts of the Toronto group of workers (28), after grafting bone marrow cells the individual colony forming cells settle in the spleen and begin proliferation and differentiation. This will result in a growth rate of CFU which is determined by the cell generation time of the CFU and by the loss of CFU for differentiation (Fig. 4a). The differentiating cells, however, have only a very limited proliferative capacity (5–10 cell cycles), hence, although initially they may "start off" with a cell cycle time as fast as that of the CFU, their number will only increase sharply at the beginning and then their rate of increase in number will have to parallel that of the CFU increase in the colony (Fig. 4b). With the increasing rate of differentiation, the CFU may even decrease in numbers in a colony. This would, of course, eventually halt growth of the colony and cause its disappearance. In any case, the proportion of CFU per 100 colony cells should decrease initially, then it should remain relatively constant while the colony grows in size (Fig. 4b).

The experimental observations, however, indicate that something is wrong with this concept. Playfair and Cole (21) found that the proportion of CFU in the colonies (CFU per 10^6 spleen nodule cells) *increases* between the seventh to tenth day after grafting, *i.e.*, at a time when these colonies grow in size. The same observation was made in our laboratories, and it was found that the rate of increase of proportion

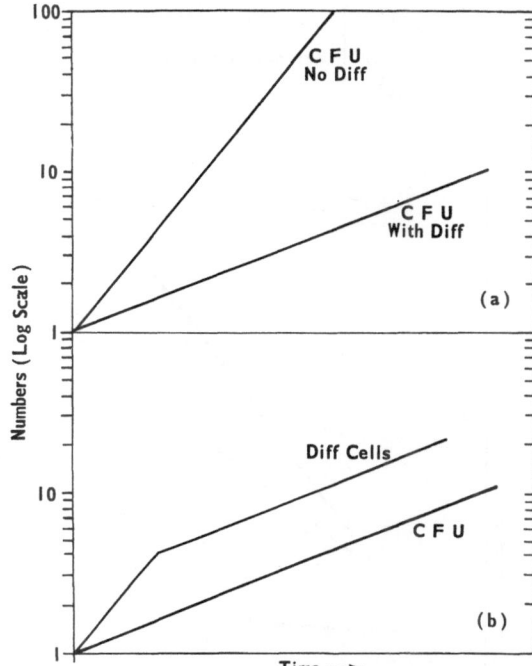

Fig. 4a. Theoretical growth of CFU with or without loss of cells for differentiation.
Fig. 4b. Theoretical growth of CFU and differentiated cells originating from it.

of CFU per 10^6 colony cells depends on the size of the initial graft (Fig. 5). With a small narrow graft the colonies grow and the proportion of CFU in them does not change between days 8 to 12, as would be theoretically expected. With larger initial grafts, the colonies growing at the same rate as the smaller grafts, the proportion of CFU in them increases with time, the rate of increase depending on graft size. Again, there is no good explanation at present to explain this apparently paradoxical phenomenon.

CFU Kinetics during Chronic Irradiation

In a kinetic model for a bone marrow stem cell population, it was proposed (17) that a major part of the stem cells will not be in a state of cell cycle, but will "rest" in a G_0 period (16, 11). This was experimentally confirmed by Becker, McCulloch, Siminovitch and Till (2) who found that in normal mouse marrow the proportion of CFUs which can be killed by ^{3}H-thymidine "suicide" is negligibly small.

In such a cell population the existence of a G_0 subpopulation acts as a "reservoir" for demands of faster cellular turnover, assuming that the feedback control system for population size is sensitive enough to detect the demand for increased turnover in any particular situation. After grafting marrow into an irradiated recipient the feedback mechanism clearly operates. This is indicated by a) the absolute growth of CFU in the grafted animal, and also by b) the high proportion of CFU in cell cycle: about 60 percent of the CFU on the sixth day after grafting can be destroyed by ^{3}H-thymidine suicide (2).

It could be expected, therefore, that a cell population with a large G_0 reservoir

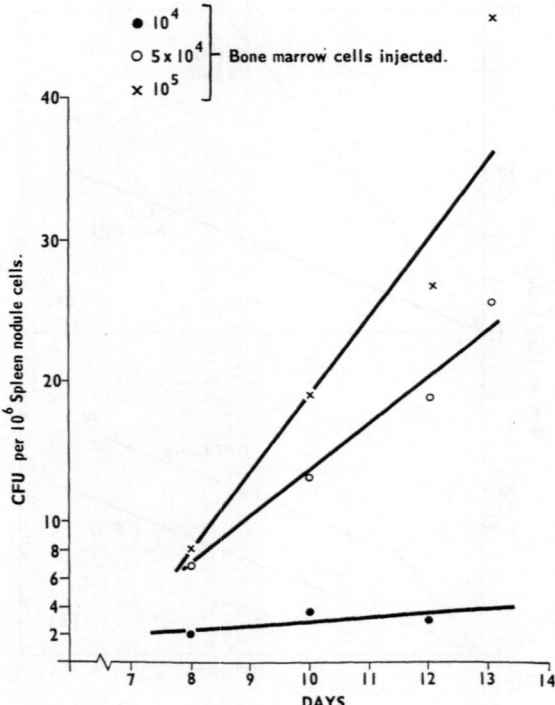

Fig. 5. Dependence of the proportion of CFU in splenic colonies on graft size.

in steady state (>90 percent in G_0) and capable of fast proliferation on grafting (>60 percent in S period) should be able to respond in an elastic fashion during a state of increased cell removal from the population, such as that produced by continuous irradiation.

Apparently this is not the case. A regime of 45–50 rad continuous irradiation depresses the repopulating capacity of the marrow to about 10 percent of the control in rats by the fifth week (5, 4) and a regime of daily 50 rad acute dose will result in eventual undetectability of repopulating capacity (after 30 days) in mice (23). Curiously enough, although the repopulating capacity in rats is maintained at 10 percent of the control level for 20 weeks of continuous irradiation, the damage is not irreversible (at least not after 10 weeks of irradiation) because on terminating the irradiation regime, the repopulating capacity returns towards normal with a doubling time of about 5 days (4).

It is understandable that even a regime of 50 rad per day can produce an initial depopulation of CFU. After all, most of the population is "sitting" in G_0 and there is little cell turnover to replace the sterilized cells. The unresolved question, however, is: why the long low plateau at 10 percent of the control value (or less)? Why cannot the CFU population cope with this low rate of radiation (which cannot kill 50 percent of the cells per cell cycle)? Apparently, it cannot, although it had "noticed" the depleted numbers, for on completion of radiation it begins to increase its numbers towards normal. Some further ^{3}H suicide experiments, in progress in our laboratory, will elucidate when the CFU population "notices" its depopulation.

Kinetics of Autorepopulation

The autorepopulation or autocolonizing test measures, in principle, the rate of release of colonizing cells from the shielded part of the hemopoietic tissue (*e.g.*, femur), and the rate of migration from an 8 mm shielded femur has been reported to be about 1.8 CFU per hour for the first 7 hours after irradiation and shielding (13). The immediate effect of a whole-body dose of 150 rad is to decrease the number of colony forming cells capable of seeding, but, with time this seeding capacity recovers and in normal mice overshoots to control values by a factor of 2–3 (23). The pattern of recovery of autocolonizing capacity is shown in Fig. 6, and it is clear that it is greatly different from the recovery curve after 150 rad found with the exocolonizing assay (Fig. 2). The two basic differences are: a) no postirradiation dip and lag with autocolonization (18) while it is marked with the exocolony assay, and b) a marked overshoot with autorecolonization. Since earlier experiments indicated a splenic enlargement in the autocolonization test 14 days after 150 rad (23), the experiments were repeated with splenectomized mice, using ^{59}Fe incorporation into RBC as an end-point. As can be seen in Fig. 6, splenectomy abolished the overshoot

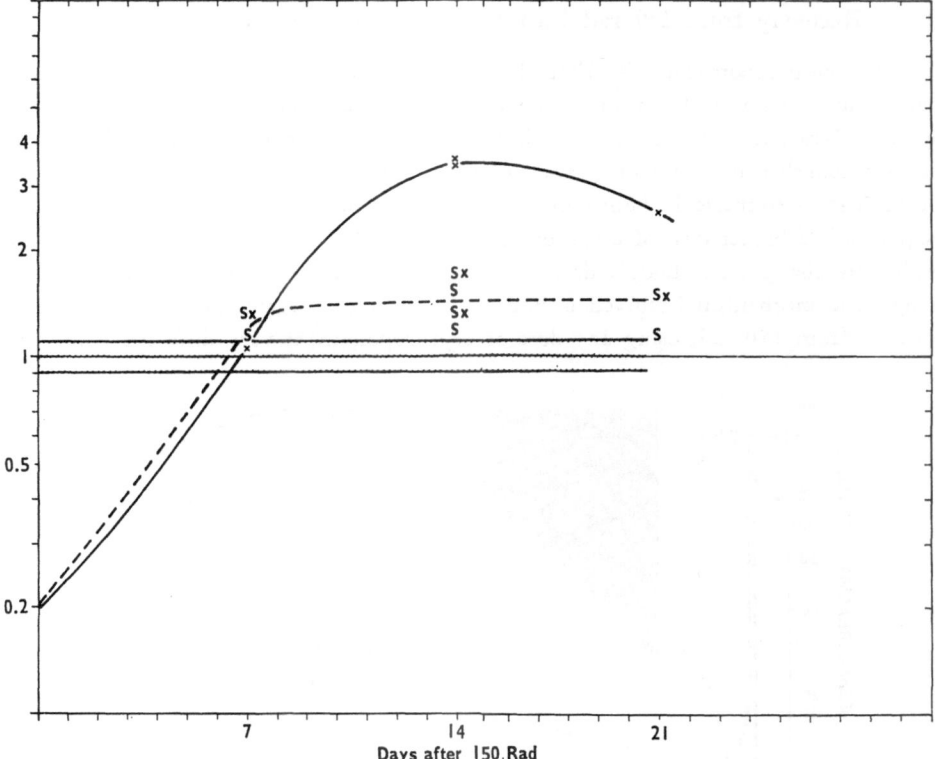

Fig. 6. Recovery of autorepopulating capacity in mice receiving 150 rad radiation:
Solid line—normal mice receiving 150 rad.
Interrupted line—splenectomized mice receiving 150 rad:
expressed as fraction of control.

but did not affect the pattern of early recovery. The number of cells capable of release and repopulation does not show the long postirradiation dip which is seen with grafting marrow or spleen after 150 rad. This may be only an apparent contradiction since the two techniques do not measure exactly the same thing. The exocolony assay measures the absolute number of CFU in the sample, while the autorepopulation assay measures a combination of changes in numbers and rates of release from the marrow. Although the number of cells available for seeding from the femur may be limited, as indicated by Hellman (14), variation of these two factors may complicate the interpretation of results in terms of pure numerical changes.

The role of the spleen in the overshoot seen with the autorepopulation assay is somewhat surprising. Apparently, the 150 rad whole body dose results in a spleen which 14 days later, in spite of 760 to 800 rad, will be more "receptive" to seeding cells from the shielded femur. However, the fact that splenectomy (performed 10 to 14 days before the priming 150 rad dose) abolishes the overshoot, indicates that the cells which would have seeded into the spleen, had it been there, cannot seed elsewhere in the hemopoietic system. If they could, there would be an overshoot even in splenectomized mice, with radioiron incorporation as the end-point.

Recovery from 150 rad Measured with the Erythropoietin Test

It has been reported earlier that the stem cells responding to erythropoietin recover quickly from 150 rad and respond with an overshoot by a factor of about 2 fourteen days later (1, 16, 23). Unlike the case of autorepopulation, splenectomy does not abolish this overshoot (23). However, the overshoot in this test clearly does not indicate a numerical change in stem cells responding to erythropoietin since it disappears if a higher dose of erythropoietin is used (Fig. 7). It appears that previous irradiation changes the body's dose response relationship to erythropoietin (7) although the mechanism involved is not yet understood. Again, however, the initial recovery from 150 rad, using any dose of erythropoietin, is very different from that

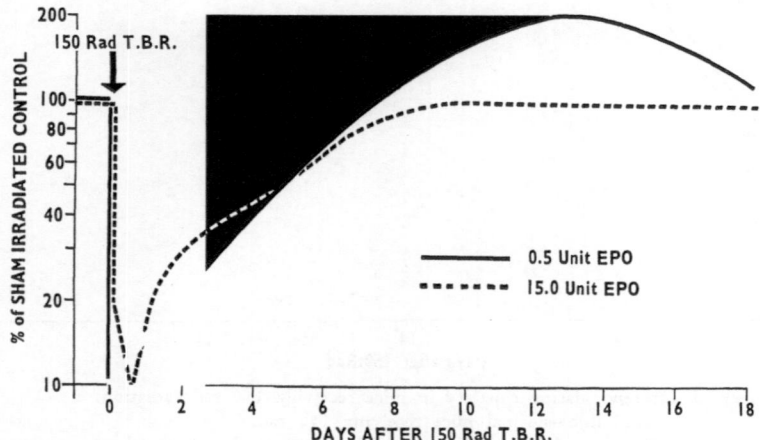

Fig. 7. Recovery of the response to erythropoietin following 150 whole-body radiation.

found with the exocolonizing assay, and it is very similar to that found with auto-repopulation.

Since there is mounting evidence that the erythropoietin-sensitive "stem" cell may not be identical with the recolonizing "stem" cell (6), a different pattern of recovery from 150 rad may not be surprising, even though the erythropoietin-sensitive cell originates from the colonizing cell.

Conclusions

The data presented above indicate that although a great deal of information has been gathered with new techniques on the proliferation kinetics of hemopoietic stem cells, the picture is far from clear. We understand, or believe we understand, a great deal about the colony forming cell, primarily due to the beautiful work of McCulloch and Till, and their colleagues. As has been shown here, however, there are still unresolved problems, even paradoxes to whet the appetite for further research. With the growing realization that the hemopoietic stem cell population may not be homogeneous but likely to consist of a "primitive pluripotential stem cell" (CF) and less primitive but still undifferentiated "committed precursor cells" (such as the erythropoietin-responsive cell: ECR), there is a great deal more work ahead before a reviewer may be bold enough to write a definitive and conclusive paper on the proliferative capacity of hemopoietic stem cells.

References

1. ALEXNIAN, R., PORTEOUS, D. D. and LAJTHA, L. G.: Stem cell kinetics after irradiation. Int. J. Radiat. Biol. 7, 87 (1963).
2. BECKER, A. J., McCULLOCH, E. A., SIMINOVITCH, L. and TILL, J. E.: The effect of differing demands for blood cell production on DNA synthesis by hemopoietic colony forming cells of mice. Blood 26, 296 (1965).
3. BECKER, A. J., McCULLOCH, E. A. and TILL, J. E.: Cytological demonstration of the clonal nature of spleen colonies derived from transplanted mouse marrow cells. Nature 197, 425 (1963).
4. BLACKETT, N. M.: Erythropoiesis in the rat under continuous γ-irradiation at 45 rads/day. Brit. J. Haemat. 13, 915 (1967).
5. BLACKETT, N. M., ROYLANCE, P. J. and ADAMS, K.: Studies of the capacity of bone marrow cells to restore erythropoiesis in heavily irradiated rats. Brit. J. Haemat. 10, 453 (1964).
6. BRUCE, W. R. and McCULLOCH, E. A.: The effect of erythropoietic stimulation on the hemopoietic colony-forming cells of mice. Blood 23, 216 (1964).
7. BYRON, J. W. and LAJTHA, L. G.: Estimation of hemopoietic stem cells with erythropoietin: A consideration of response curves. Brit. J. Haemat. 15, 47 (1968).
8. CUDKOWICZ, G., UPTON, A. C., SHEARER, G. M. and HUGHES, W. L.: Lymphocyte content and proliferation based on the growth of spleen colony forming cell. Proc. Nat. Acad. Sci., Wash. 51, 29 (1962).
9. CUDKOWICZ, G., UPTON, A. C., SMITH, L. H., GOSSLEE, D. G. and HUGHES, W. L.: An approach to the characterization of stem cells in mouse bone marrow. Ann. N.Y. Acad. Sci. 114, 571 (1964).

10. Ford, C. E., Micklem, H. S. and Gray, S. M.: Evidence of selective proliferation of reticular cell clones in heavily irradiated mice. Brit. J. Radiol. **32**, 280 (1959).

11. Gilbert, C. W. and Lajtha, L. G.: The importance of cell population kinetics in determining response to irradiation of normal and malignant tissue. *In:* Cellular Radiation Biology, VIII Annual Symposium on Fundamental Cancer Research. *For:* University of Texas M. D. Anderson Hospital and Tumor Institute, Houston, Texas. Williams and Wilkins Co., Baltimore, 474 (1965).

12. Gurney, C. W., Lajtha, L. G. and Oliver, R.: A method for investigation of stem cell kinetics. Brit. J. Haemat. **8**, 461 (1962).

13. Hanks, G. E.: *In vivo* migration of colony forming units from shielded bone marrow in the irradiated mouse. Nature **203**, 1393 (1964).

14. Hellman, S.: Circulating stem cells: Variation with duration of partial body X-irradiation. Nature **205**, 100 (1965).

15. Hodgson, G. S.: Radiosensitivity of marrow cells responsible for reestablishing erythropoiesis in lethally irradiated mice. Acta Physiol. Lat. Amer. **12**, 365 (1962).

16. Lajtha, L. G.: On the concept of the cell cycle. J. Cell. Comp. Physiol. **62**, 143 (1963).

17. Lajtha, L. G., Oliver, R. and Gurney, C. W.: Kinetic model of a bone marrow stem cell population. Brit. J. Haemat. **8**, 442 (1962).

18. Lajtha, L. G., Pozzi, L. V. and Schofield, R.: Comparison of methods of study of stem cell kinetics. *In:* Twenty-first Symposium on Fundamental Cancer Research, Houston, Texas. (In press.) 1968.

19. McCulloch, E. A. and Till, J. E.: Proliferation of hemopoietic colony-forming cells transplanted into irradiated mice. Radiat. Res. **22**, 383 (1964).

20. McCulloch, E. A. and Till, J. E.: The radiation sensitivity of normal mouse marrow cells determined by quantitative transplantation into irradiated mice. Radiat. Res. **13**, 115 (1960).

21. Playfair, J. H. L. and Cole, L. J.: Quantitative studies on colony forming units in isogenic radiation chimeras. J. Cell. Comp. Physiol. **65**, 7 (1965).

22. Porteous, D. D., Alexanian, R. and Lajtha, L. G.: The fasted mouse in the study of bone marrow stem cell kinetics. Int. J. Rad. Biol. **7**, 95 (1963).

23. Porteous, D. D. and Lajtha, L. G.: On stem cell recovery after irradiation. Brit. J. Haemat. **12**, 177 (1966).

24. Siminovitch, L., McCulloch, E. A. and Till, J. E.: The distribution of colony forming cells among spleen colonies. J. Cell. Comp. Physiol. **62**, 327 (1963).

25. Smith, L. H. and Vos, O.: Sensitivity and protection of bone marrow cells x-irradiated *in vitro*. Int. J. Rad. Biol. **5**, 461 (1962).

26. Till, J. E.: Quantitative aspects of radiation lethality at the cellular level. Amer. J. Roentgen. **90**, 917 (1963).

27. Till, J. E. and McCulloch, E. A.: A direct measurement of the radiation sensitivity of normal mouse bone marrow cells. Radiat. Res. **14**, 213 (1961).

28. Till, J. E., McCulloch, E. A. and Siminovitch, L.: A stochastic model of stem cell proliferation based on the growth of spleen colony-forming cells. Proc. Nat. Acad. Sci., Wash. **51**, 29 (1964).

Discussion

Colony Forming Units in the Bone Marrow of Partial Body Irradiated Mice *

A. L. Carsten and Victor P. Bond

Medical Department
Brookhaven National Laboratory
Upton, New York

An extensive series of experiments is under way at the Brookhaven National Laboratory, Medical Department, designed to investigate the relationship of cell survival, particularly of "stem cells," to the survival of the irradiated animal. In the short time available, two experiments from the series that bear on some of the material presented by Dr. Lajtha will be discussed. The first experiment was designed to study the effects of partial body shielding on the colony forming unit (CFU) or "stem cell" content of the right hind leg of the mouse subjected to whole body and partial body exposure. Evaluations are made over the first several days after exposure. The second experiment was similar in that the CFU content of the right hind leg was measured after whole body and partial body radiation, but in this case over a period of weeks and months after irradiation.

Materials and Methods

For both experiments, eight-week-old male mice of the Hale-Stoner BNL strain were used. All irradiations were done using a General Electric 250 kvp Maxitron x-ray machine operating at 250 kvp, 30 ma, and at a dose rate of approximately 120 rads per minute. Depth dosimetry to establish the efficiency of the various shielding geometries was verified using lithium fluoride, thermoluminescent dosimeters implanted into tissue equivalent phantoms. For the first irradiations (donor mice for later spleen colony determinations) animals were anesthetized using sodium pentobarbital at a dosage of 70 mg/kg. In the first experiment the exposure patterns were as follows:

GROUP 1. 100 rads whole body exposure in order to standardize the effect of this exposure on the whole marrow, when no migration or abscopal effect is present.

GROUP 2. 100 rads to the lower body to determine if seeding, recovery or local stimulation of the production of cells takes place in the irradiated tissue.

* Research supported by U.S. Atomic Energy Commission.

GROUP 3. 100 rads to the upper body to determine if there is an increased production of cells in the shielded area, *i.e.*, abscopal effect.

GROUP 4. 100 rads to the lower body and immediately 1000 rads to the upper body. This would eliminate any possible seeding from the upper body, with the result that any changes in stem cell population of the leg would be due to local effects, *i.e.*, recovery, stimulation or migratory loss to the more seriously injured upper body.

GROUP 5. 1000 rads to the right leg. This dose should reduce the local stem cell population to a point where if seeding from the outside takes place, it should be measurable.

In the second experiment one group of animals received 1400 rads to the upper body (xiphoid process—cephalad), a second group 1400 rads to the lower body and the third group 750 rads whole body. The 1400 rads partial body exposures are in the low lethal range whereas the 750 rads whole body is in the high lethal range. Following irradiation and at the time intervals indicated, donor mice were sacrificed by ether anesthesia, their right hind legs amputated, the femur and tibia removed and the marrow cells prepared for injection as previously described (7). Sixty thousand bone marrow cells thus obtained were then injected via the tail vein into donor mice which had just received a whole body x-ray exposure of 750 rads. After seven days, the recipient animals were sacrificed, their spleens removed, fixed in Bouin's solution and subsequently examined for the presence of spleen colonies. With some minor modifications, this is basically the method of Till and McCulloch (8).

Results

The results of the first experiment are shown in Figs. 1 and 2. It is emphasized that in each case it is the number of CFU's in the right hind leg of the mouse that was determined. In Fig. 1, the number of CFU's *per 60,000 nucleated cells* of the right hind leg are shown at various times postirradiation. The reproducibility of the methods involved is evident from the curve for the control animals. A dose of 100 rads to the upper body resulted in a significant decrease in CFU's as early as 30 minutes, with an apparent over-shoot beginning at 4 hours and lasting for the duration of the experiment. The initial drop is consistent with an early and significant influx of nucleated cells mobilized from the irradiated areas. Following this the "efficiency" of the marrow in terms of CFU per unit number of nucleated cells becomes greater than normal. The second change may be related to a relative increase in the number of nucleated nonstem cells flowing from the unirradiated right hind leg to the remaining irradiated portion of the body presumably in response to the overall reduction in total number of surviving nucleated cells.

The lower four curves in the figure represent exposure of the right leg, with and without irradiation of the remainder of the body. In each case in which the right leg received 100 rads, an initial and sharp decrease in the numbers of CFU's occurred. The three curves are not markedly dissimilar throughout the observation period, indicating that the stem cell content of the irradiated right lower leg was not in-

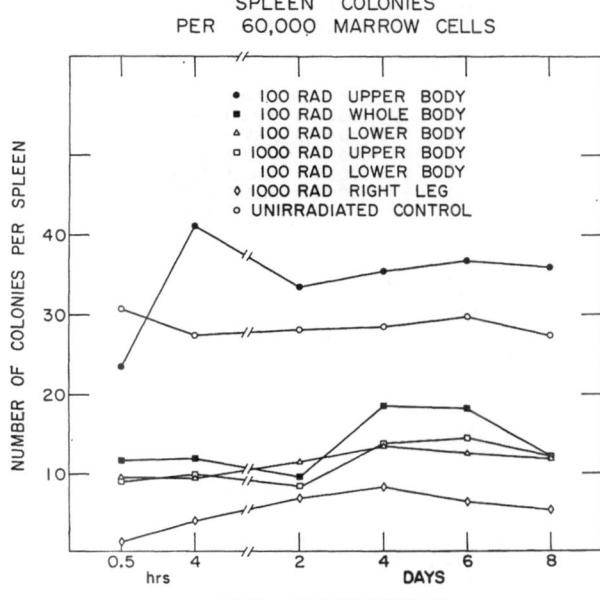

Fig. 1. Curves for number of spleen colonies per 60,000 injected marrow cells for each treatment group.

fluenced appreciably by the amount of radiation delivered to the remainder of the body. The number of stem cells per unit of total nucleated cells was reduced for a sustained period. The lower curve, representing the effect of 1000 rads to the right hind leg, showed an apparent increase in CFU's per unit of nucleated cells, reaching a maximum on day 4.

However, results shown in Fig. 1 can be misleading, since they are only an expression of the ratio of CFU's to nucleated cells. Since the total number of cells per leg is changing during this time, one cannot determine from these data alone the changes in the asbolute number of CFU's which is most probably the more interesting parameter. On this basis, the plot of the *absolute* number of CFU's per leg shown in Fig. 2 is more informative. From the upper two curves, there appears to have been an early drop in absolute number of CFU's in the right hind leg, within the first half hour, when the lower body is shielded and the upper body is irradiated. There then appears to be an over-shoot by four hours which is transient, with no evidence of a continuing over-shoot of CFU's in the nonexposed right hind leg, as might be deduced from the data presented in Fig. 1. Thus there seems to be no sustained measurable loss of CFU's to the irradiated upper body. Or alternatively, if a sustained loss is occurring, it may be just compensated by proliferation within the shielded leg.

From the group of three similar curves near the bottom of Fig. 2, all of which represent irradiation of both the examined leg and at least some of the remainder of the body, there was evidence of an early and severe depletion of CFU's within the irradiated leg. (The degree of fall was about what would be expected from the dose effect curve determined in this laboratory, representing numbers of CFU's in the bone marrow versus dose of radiation to the entire body.) There was no marked change in the number of CFU's over the time of observation, indicating no large or sustained

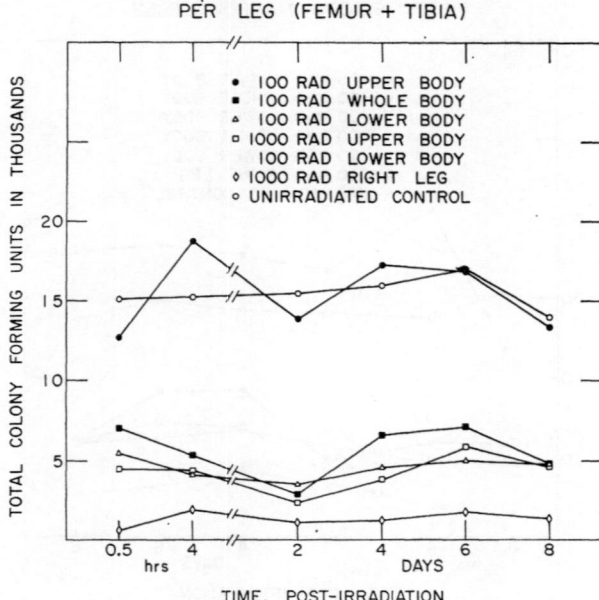

TOTAL COLONY FORMING UNITS
PER LEG (FEMUR + TIBIA)

- • 100 RAD UPPER BODY
- ■ 100 RAD WHOLE BODY
- ▲ 100 RAD LOWER BODY
- □ 1000 RAD UPPER BODY
-   100 RAD LOWER BODY
- ◇ 1000 RAD RIGHT LEG
- ○ UNIRRADIATED CONTROL

TOTAL COLONY FORMING UNITS IN THOUSANDS

TIME, POST-IRRADIATION

Fig. 2. Curves for absolute numbers of CFU per leg in each treatment group following x-irradiation. Early changes.

entrance of CFU's from the unirradiated marrow to the irradiated marrow. There appears to be a rise in the absolute number of CFU's from day 4 to 6, at the time that an increase in the absolute number of nucleated cells per leg is increasing. In the groups in which the right leg received 100 rads, the total number of nucleated cells was approaching normal limits by day 6 or 8 when the absolute number of CFU's per leg remained at about a third their normal value. This would indicate that a larger than normal number of stem cells was going the route of committed maturation, rather than that of reproducing stem cells.

From the work of Bruce (2), it would appear that normally not all stem cells are actively in the division cycle, but that some are either dividing with a markedly long generation time or are in the "G_0" phase. The results of this experiment are consistent with all of the stem cells being in the division cycle, presumably due to demands placed upon the pool.

The bottom curve represents that of animals receiving 1000 rads to the right leg only. If the entire body had received 1000 rads, the number of CFU's in the leg would have been reduced below the levels indicated at one half hour. However, in the animals receiving 1000 rads to the right hind leg only, approximately 600 CFU's were found to be present at this time. This is consistent with a rapid influx of cells from unirradiated marrow into the heavily irradiated marrow, as has been indicated also by the work of Hellman (3), and Robinson (5). A rapid exodus of stem cells from non-exposed marrow is seen in the fall in the absolute number of CFU's shown for animals that received no irradiation to the lower body, but 100 rads to the upper body. The results are consistent with the degree of stimulus for release of CFU's from unirradiated marrow being dependent on the dose received by the irradiated marrow. The influx was obvious to marrow that had received 1000 rads; it was minimal in marrow that had received 100 rads.

Experiment II

In this experiment designed to determine the absolute number of CFU's in partial body irradiated animals weeks and months after exposure, one group of animals was given 1400 rads to the upper body only, a second group 1400 rads to the lower body only and the third group 750 rads to the entire body. Assays were done in each case on the CFU content of right hind leg, and the results were expressed in absolute numbers of CFU's per leg.

The results are shown in Fig. 3, in which the absolute numbers of CFU versus time after exposure are plotted. The upper curve shows the absolute number of CFU's in the right leg of animals receiving 1400 rads to the upper body. There appears to have been a significant decrease at approximately 15 days with an increase above normal on day 30. There was then a secondary fall at day 60 followed by an increase from approximately 100 to 120 days. Beyond this time the numbers were in the normal range.

The curve for animals receiving 1400 rads to the lower body to some degree mirrored that for 1400 rads to the upper body. There was a sharp rise around day 15, followed by a sharp fall beginning around day 60. The absolute number of CFU's then remained well below normal until about day 160, when a sharp rise into the normal range occurred. Results are consistent with an increased content of stem cells in unirradiated marrow, when the CFU content of irradiated marrow is severely reduced and additional CFU's are needed.

The curve representing 750 rads to the entire body showed a delay in repopulation of CFU's over that seen with partial body radiation. The absolute numbers remain well below the normal range, and there appears to be a secondary fall beginning

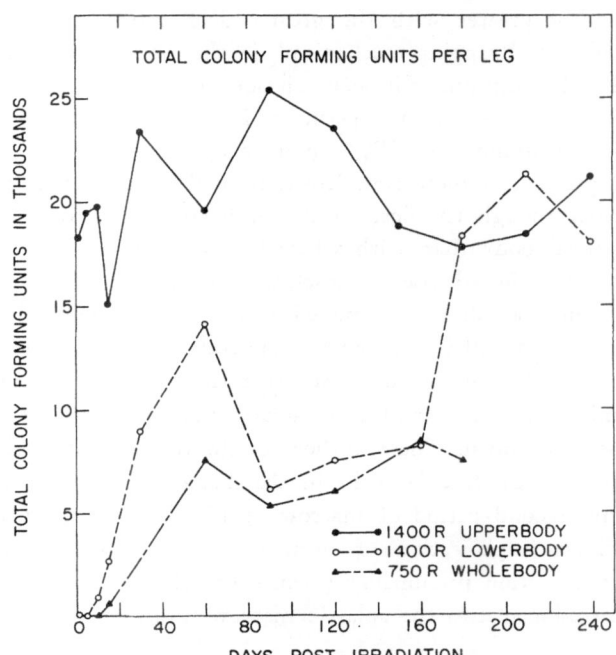

Fig. 3. Curves for absolute numbers of CFU per leg in each treatment group following x-irradiation. Late changes.

TOTAL COLONY FORMING UNITS PER LEG

TOTAL COLONY FORMING UNITS IN THOUSANDS

•——• 1400 R UPPERBODY
o---o 1400 R LOWERBODY
▲---▲ 750 R WHOLEBODY

DAYS POST IRRADIATION

around day 60. Partial recovery occurred around day 120; however, the total number of CFU's remained well below normal throughout the period of observation. In all groups, the absolute number of nucleated cells was normal or near normal from day 50 on. The fact that absolute number of CFU's remained well below normal throughout a large portion of this time is consistent with all available stem cells cycling, and the lack of a non-cycling "G_0" fraction of stem cells.

Discussions and Conclusions

Results of Experiment I indicate that data expressed as CFU's per unit of nucleated cells and that expressed as absolute number of CFU's per leg may lead to different conclusions. In relative terms, one might conclude that there is a marked and sustained increase in CFU's in shielded unirradiated marrow. Results expressed in absolute numbers of CFU's per leg indicate that no such sustained over-shoot occurs. If the leg is irradiated, the number of CFU's is reduced drastically, and does not show appreciable recovery even by day 8. The fact that total cellularity has approached the normal range by day 8 would indicate that fewer absolute number of stem cells are producing close to normal numbers of nucleated cells per unit time. Either the generation time is decreased, or alternatively one might postulate that more stem cells than normal are committed to maturation, and that there may be few or no stem cells in the "G_0" or non-cycling phase as appears to be the case normally (2).

The results of Experiment I are also consistent with a very rapid (within minutes) exodus of significant numbers of stem cells from shielded marrow into the unshielded marrow at the pressure of a rapid circulating pool. The numbers of stem cells appear to be somewhat dependent on the dose to the unshielded marrow, and is greater with the greater dose. Alternatively, one might postulate a more efficient "trapping mechanism" in the marrow receiving the higher dose. The reason for this stimulus, if it occurs, is not known.

With respect to Experiment II, the results are consistent with an initial increase in the number of CFU's in irradiated marrow. The increase occurs sooner, is more rapid, and is more complete if normal unshielded marrow is available in the animal, even though the dose to the unshielded irradiated marrow was much higher with partial body than with whole body exposure.

The initial rise in absolute numbers of CFU's is followed, however, with a secondary fall that occurred as late as approximately day 60. The reason for this secondary fall is not known; however, it may well be related to the work of Knospe et al. (4) who demonstrated that the leg of the rat given 4000 R recovered rapidly initially, but showed a secondary marrow aplasia at approximately 60 days which was sustained. These authors attributed the late aplasia to a slow turnover time perhaps of vascular cells in the marrow. Injection of normal marrow cells during this second period of marrow aplasia did not result in regeneration. However, the direct implantation of normal marrow into the aplastic marrow did result in regeneration presumably because vascular structures, perhaps relatively intact, were introduced into the aplastic marrow under these conditions.

The total marrow cellularity during the second period of marrow aplasia was close to normal, indicating that the remaining stem cells, even though few in number, were capable of dividing and differentiation. Alternatively, the marrow may have been populated at least in part by differentiated cells flowing into the right leg from other portions of the body.

The absolute number of CFU's in the right leg did not return to normal throughout the period of observation in the whole body irradiated group. In contrast, the group receiving 1400 rads to the lower body showed a dramatic increase in the number of CFU's into the normal range, but only as late as approximately 180 days. The reasons for this greatly delayed regeneration are not at all apparent.

The results of Experiment II, combined with the work of Knospe *et al.* (4), indicate that the microenvironment in which "stem cells" find themselves may strongly influence the degree to which these cells can proliferate. Data are also available indicating that the microenvironment may also influence type of maturating cells that stem cells will produce, *i.e.*, whether granulocytic, erythrocytic or megakaryocytic colonies are formed (9, 10, 6, 1).

References

1. BRECHER, G., SMITH, W. W., WILSON, S. and FRED, S.: Kinetics of colchicine-induced hemopoietic recovery in irradiated mice. Rad. Res. **30**, 600 (1967).

2. BRUCE, W. R. and MEEKER, B. E.: Comparison of the sensitivity of normal hematopoietic and transplanted lymphoma colony forming cells to tritiated thymidine. J. Natl. Cancer Inst. **34**(6), 849 (1965).

3. HELLMAN, S.: Circulating stem cells: Variation with duration of partial body x-irradiation. Nature **205**, 100 (1965).

4. KNOSPE, W. H., BLOM, J. and CROSBY, W. H.: Aplastic anemia. Dependence of function on structure in the bone marrow. Amer. Soc. of Haemat., Toronto, Ontario, Dec. 3–5, 1967. Abstract #6, 29.

5. ROBINSON, C. V., COMMERFORD, S. L. and BATEMAN, J. L.: Evidence for the presence of stem cells in the tail of the mouse. Proc. Soc. Exptl. Biol. & Med. **119**, 222 (1965).

6. SILINI, G., PONS, S. and POZZI, L. V.: Quantitative histology of spleen colonies in irradiated mice. Brit. J. Haemat. **14**, 489 (1968).

7. STONER, R. D. and BOND, V. P.: Antibody formation by transplanted bone marrow, spleen, lymph node and thymus cells in irradiated recipients. J. Immunology **91**, 185 (1963).

8. TILL, J. E. and McCULLOCH, E. A.: A direct measurement of the radiation sensitivity of normal mouse bone marrow cells. Rad. Res. **14**, 213 (1961).

9. WOLF, N. S., TRENTIN, J. J. and CHENG, V.: Effect of marrow donor irradiation and erythropoietic stimulation of the recipient on spleen colony and number and type. Exptl. Hematol. **15**, 88 (1968).

10. WOLF, N. S. and TRENTIN, J. J.: Hemopoietic colony studies. V. Effect of hemopoietic organ stroma on differentiation of pluripotent stem cells. J. Exptl. Med. **127**, 205 (1968).

Cellular Proliferation in the Liver *

J. W. GRISHAM †

Department of Pathology
Washington University
St. Louis, Missouri

This report discusses cellular proliferation in the liver of the rat during postnatal growth and during induced growth following partial hepatectomy. Space limitations preclude a comprehensive survey of the literature. The reader is referred to recent reviews (6, 7, 26, 40).

The Replicative Cycle in Hepatocytes

The proportion of hepatocytic nuclei that incorporates tritiated thymidine after pulse labeling or that is in mitosis falls rapidly after birth (Fig. 1). After a short lag, cellular proliferation then increases to a peak at about 3 weeks of age (12, 19, 30), following which a second rapid decline to the adult level occurs. The peak of cellular proliferation at 3 weeks is correlated with the period of maximal postnatal hepatic growth (12). Some authors have described a steady fall in cellular proliferation from a maximal level at birth (35, 38). This has probably resulted from too infrequent sampling to detect the biphasic changes. Both hepatocytic labeling and mitosis are subject to diurnal variation with maxima occurring in the early morning and minima in the late evening (32).

The hepatocytic replicative cycle lengthens as rats age (19, 38, 39, 47) (Table 1). One-day-old rats complete 3 replicative cycles in the same time that it takes 3 to 8 week old rats to complete 2 cycles (39). Although the data are conflicting, the replication time may be further lengthened in very old rats (32, 39). However, evaluation of mitotic labeling is unreliable in old rats because of the low rate of hepatocytic proliferation. The fraction of hepatocytes participating in the replicative cycle (the growth fraction) decreases as rats age (19, 38) (Table 2). Slowing of postnatal growth is correlated with a decrease in the hepatocytic growth fraction and with an increase in the replication time of these proliferating cells. Once formed, hepatocytes exist for virtually the entire life of the rat, the life span of hepatocyte and organism being similar (28). Since its cellular population progressively, but slowly increases, the liver has been termed an expanding tissue (32).

* Supported by U.S.P.H.S. Grant No. AM-07568 and by a grant from the John A. Hartford Foundation.

† John and Mary R. Markle Scholar in Academic Medicine.

28

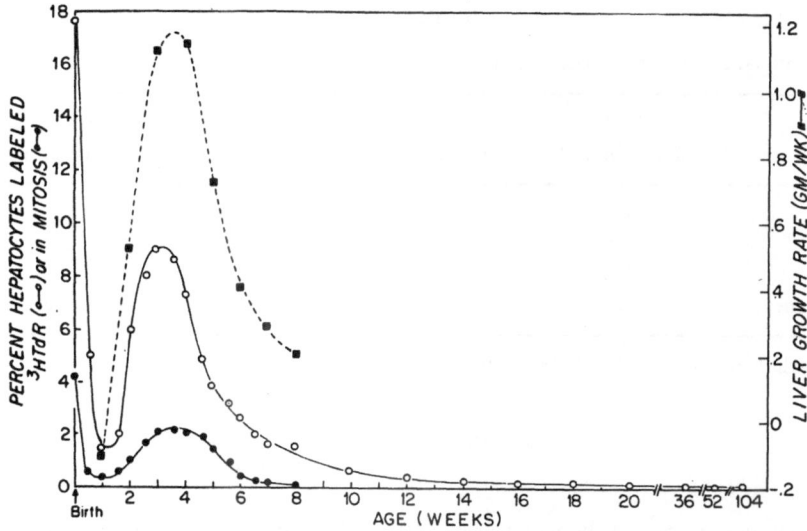

Fig. 1. Proliferation of hepatocytes and postnatal growth rate in male Wistar rats. Each point is the mean value from 3 to 5 rats.

After partial hepatectomy of 8 to 10 week old rats (young adults), significantly increased numbers of labeled hepatocytes are first seen between 15 and 18 hours after surgery (13, 20, 36) (Fig. 2). At this time there is a sudden increase in the number of labeled nuclei, reaching a peak at 20 to 25 hours and gradually declining over the next 24 hours. A slightly elevated rate of labeling continues for several days. Appearance and peak occurrence of mitosis follows that of labeled cells by 6 to 8 hours and both curves are similar in shape though different in magnitude. The augmented rate of proliferation is correlated with the most rapid rate of hepatic

TABLE 1

LENGTH OF THE REPLICATIVE CYCLE AND ITS PHASES IN
RAT HEPATOCYTES DURING POSTNATAL GROWTH

Age (or weight) and strain	Cycle time (hours)	Phase times (hours)				Reference
		G_1	S	G_2	M	
1 day, Wistar	13.75	4.95	7.0	1.5	0.3	38
3 week, Wistar	21.5	9.0	9.0	1.3	1.7	38
5 to 6 week, Wistar	21.0	8.5	9.0	$(G_2 + P)$ 2.5	1.0	19
8 week (and older), Wistar	21.5	9.0	9.0	1.8	1.7	39
8 week, Long-Evans	—	—	8.2	>2.0	0.77	13
260 gm., Sprague-Dawley or B-D II	—	—	15–18	2.5	5.5	47

TABLE 2

SIZES OF GROWTH FRACTIONS OF RAT HEPATOCYTES DURING POSTNATAL GROWTH

Age	Cycle time (hours)	Synthesis time (hours)	Percent of nuclei labeled	Growth fraction * (percent)
1 day	13.75	7.0	16–18	32–36
3 weeks	21.5	9.0	4–9	10–20
8 weeks	21.5	9.0	1.5–2.5	4–6
4–6 months	21.5	9.0	0.2	0.5

* Growth fraction calculated from the formula:

$$\text{Growth fraction} = \frac{\text{Percent nuclei labeled} \times \text{Cycle time}}{\text{Synthesis time}}$$

growth following partial hepatectomy (19). Cellular proliferation is maximal at its onset and is steadily retarded, remaining proportional to the number of cells to be formed; between 75 and 100 percent of removed hepatocytes are replaced after partial hepatectomy (4, 43). Diurnal variation in rate of hepatocytic proliferation following partial hepatectomy is similar to that occurring in intact liver during post-natal growth (25).

Enumeration of labeled mitotic figures after tagging a group of cells with tritiated thymidine demonstrates that the replication time of hepatocytes proliferating after 68 percent hepatic resection is shorter than that in intact livers of similarly

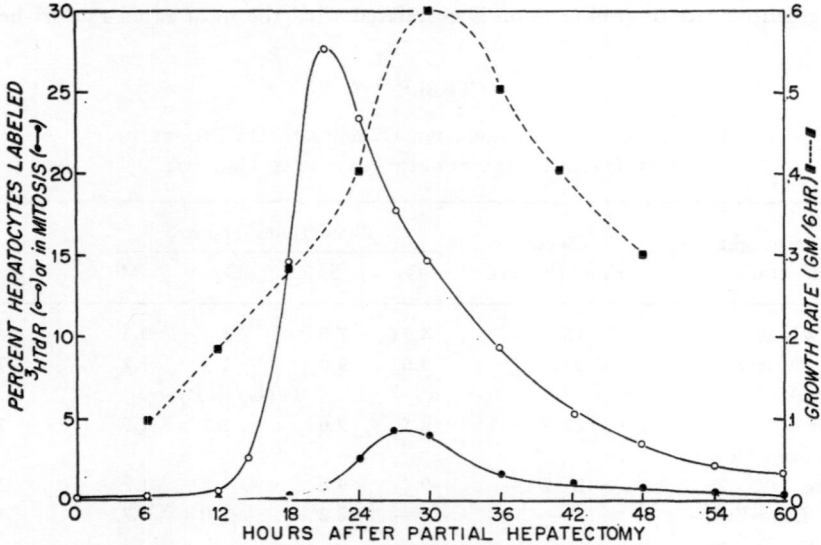

Fig. 2. Proliferation of hepatocytes and hepatic growth rate in young adult (as defined in text) male Wistar rats. Each point is the mean value from 5 to 10 rats.

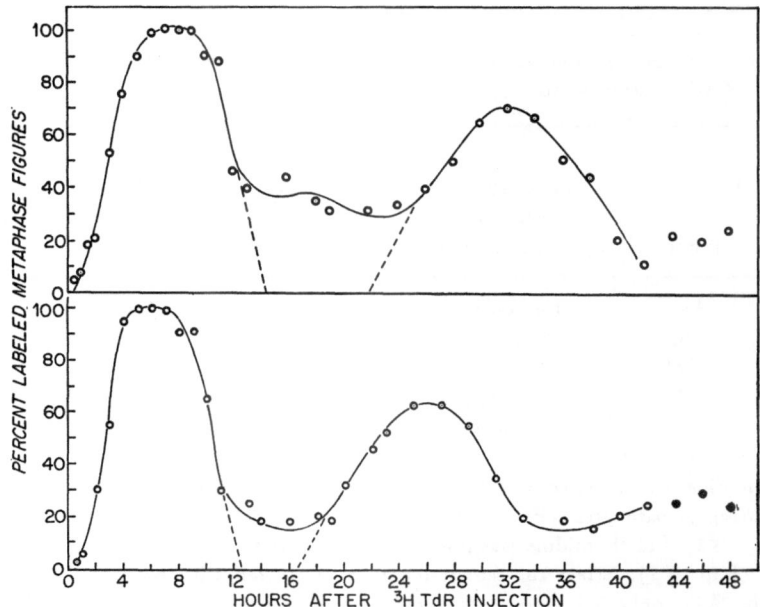

Fig. 3. Appearance of labeled metaphase figures after tagging hepatocytes with ³HTdR in 60 gm. male Wistar rats before (top) and at 18 hours after (bottom) 68 percent resection of liver.

aged animals (16, 19, 46) (Fig. 3). Reduction of the cycle time in regenerating hepatocytes is accomplished predominantly by shortening the G_1 phase, although the S phase is also somewhat shorter than in hepatocytes of intact livers (Table 3).

Labeling begins a few hours earlier in 3 to 4 week old (weanling) rats than in young adults, reaching a peak at 18 to 20 hours; this peak is followed by a second, lower, peak at about 36 hours (9). Rats more than 1 year old (old rats)

TABLE 3

LENGTH OF THE REPLICATIVE CYCLE AND ITS PHASES IN
RAT HEPATOCYTES FOLLOWING PARTIAL HEPATECTOMY

Age (or weight) and strain	Cycle time (hours)	Phase time (hours)				M	Reference
		G_1	S	G_2			
6 to 8 week, Wistar	16.5	5.5	8.0	$(G_2 + P)$ 2.5		1.0	19
6 to 8 week, Wistar	—	—	8.0		$(G_2 + M/2)$ 3.0		16
2 month, Long-Evans	—	—	8.5	>2.0		0.9	13
330 gm., strain unknown	—	—	7.2	2.0		4.0	46

TABLE 4

LABELING OF HEPATOCYTES PROLIFERATING AFTER PARTIAL HEPATECTOMY WITH ^{14}C- AND
^{3}H-THYMIDINE DURING TWO SEPARATE REPLICATIVE CYCLES *

Experiment number	Isotope	Time after surgery when thymidine injected	Time after surgery when animal killed	^{14}C or ^{14}C + ^{3}H labeled nuclei (percent)	^{3}H labeled nuclei (percent)
#1	^{14}C	18 hours	19 hours	25.6 †	—
#2	^{14}C	18 hours	39 hours	48.2	—
#3	^{3}H	38 hours	39 hours	—	11.9
#4	^{14}C	18 hours			
	^{3}H	38 hours	39 hours	52.4	3.8

* ^{14}C-thymidine was injected at 18 hours after partial hepatectomy to tag a group of early replicating hepatocytes (Exp. #1). Nineteen hours later most of these cells had divided (Exp. #2). ^{3}H-thymidine was injected at 38 hours to tag a group of late replicating hepatocytes (Exp. #3). When the same animals were treated with both ^{14}C- and ^{3}H-thymidine (Exp. #4), only 3.8 percent of the late replicating hepatocytes were tagged with ^{3}H alone. The remainder of the cells proliferating at this time were derived from the first replicative cycle and, thus, also tagged with ^{14}C.

† Each value in the table represents the mean from 3 animals. Radioactive nuclei were detected by autoradiography with two layers of emulsion.

respond more slowly, as regards both initiation of labeling and occurrence of the peak level, the latter occurring between 28 and 32 hours (9). Labeling of hepatic DNA or of hepatocytic nuclei following removal of various fractions of liver (from 9 to 68 percent) is directly related to the amount removed in weanling and old rats, but in young adult rats labeling is only slightly increased, as compared to that in intact livers, until about 40 percent of the liver is removed (8, 19, 29). After this point is passed the response is linear. The reason for this atypical proliferative response to partial hepatectomy in young adult rats is obscure; it may occur because rats of this age have an unusually large hepatocytic growth fraction relative to hepatic growth rate (19). It may be possible to considerably increase hepatic growth in rats of this age merely by speeding the replicative cycle.

Depending on the age of the animal, labeled hepatocytes in livers of growing rats pass consecutively through 1 to 3 replicative cycles during 48 hours. Consecutive replication of individual hepatocytes in regenerating livers also varies with age. The pattern of DNA labeling at different times after partial hepatectomy in weanling rats indicates that two cycles of hepatocytic proliferation occur (9). Two cycles of labeled mitotic figures were noted during a 48 hour period in 60 gm. partially hepatectomized rats whose hepatocytes were initially tagged with thymidine at 18 hours after surgery (19) (Fig. 3). In older rats only one cycle of labeled mitotic figures was detected (16, 46). However, results of a double-labeling experiment, in which proliferating cells were labeled with different isotopes during two separate replicative cycles provide direct evidence that some hepatocytes labeled early after partial hepatectomy in adult rats replicate at least one more time (19) (Table 4). Of the hepatocytes proliferating at 38 hours after partial hepatectomy, about 70 percent were the progeny of cells originally tagged during the earlier cycle of proliferation. The rate of hepatocytic proliferation is low by 38 hours, however, and hepatocytes resulting from a second division of originally tagged cells represent only a small fraction of the total number of parenchymal cells formed after partial hepatectomy of adult rats.

Binuclearity and Polyploidy

At birth the murine hepatocytic population is composed almost entirely of diploid (2n = 42 chromosomes) mononuclear cells (1, 34, 35). Hepatic parenchyma of adult rats contains a heterogenous population of hepatocytes as regards the number and the ploidy of the nuclei they contain (1, 34, 35) (Table 5). Evolution of binuclearity and polyploidy is initiated during the most rapid phase of postnatal growth (1, 34, 35). Polyploidization of hepatocytic nuclei predominantly results from fusion of the two mitotic plates in binuclear cells passing through a replicative cycle (34). Formation of binuclear cells of one ploidy class always precedes development of the next higher class, the appearance of which correlates with cellular proliferation and with a corresponding decline in binuclear cells (1, 34). Other postulated mechanisms for development of polyploid cells have not been conclusively demonstrated (35). DNA synthesis without subsequent mitosis would lead to formation of hepatocytes with doubled amounts of DNA arrested in G_2 (these nuclei would not be polyploid since chromosomes are not separated, but would be indistinguishable from polyploid cells during interphase). There is no evidence of a G_2 population of hepatocytes in normal liver. Neither endomitosis following DNA synthesis nor nuclear fusion in binuclear cells without occurrence of DNA synthesis has been clearly demonstrated.

The effect of partial hepatectomy on binuclearity and polyploidy depends on the number and type of binuclear cells in the liver at the time of operation (18, 34).

TABLE 5

PROPORTIONS OF POLYPLOID AND BINUCLEAR HEPATOCYTES IN
LIVERS OF DIFFERENT AGED RATS

Age	Diploid		Tetraploid		Octoploid	
	Mononuclear	Binuclear	Mononuclear	Binuclear	Mononuclear	Binuclear
1 week	90–98	1–10	0–2	0	0	0
3 weeks	80–90	8–15	2–5	0	0	0
4 weeks	35–40	40–50	10–15	0–4	0	0
4 months and older	4–10	5–10	60–80	5–15	4–10	0

Partial hepatectomy apparently does not cause formation of binuclear cells but, by stimulating pre-existing binuclear cells to replicate, results in production of nuclei of higher ploidy and a concomitant decrease in binuclear cells (34). In rats less than 3 weeks old (hepatocytes uniformly mononuclear diploid) partial hepatectomy does not alter the cytologic composition of the liver (34). Between 3 weeks and 4 months of age (when the adult level of binuclear and polyploid cells is established), partial hepatectomy speeds the development of the adult status by causing the large number of binuclear cells present during this interval to proliferate (34). Partial hepatectomy in adult rats produces further modest increases in polyploid nuclei (18, 34). Decrease in binuclear cells and increase in mononuclear cells of higher ploidy is precisely correlated with the occurrence of cell division after partial hepatectomy (34).

Cellular proliferation occurs from hepatocytes with diploid nuclei (either mononuclear or binuclear) during early postnatal growth (39). During postnatal growth in older rats (10) and after partial hepatectomy (18, 31, 34) both diploid and tetraploid hepatocytes proliferate although diploid cells may compose the major fraction.

Proliferation of Nonparenchymal Hepatic Cells

Of the nonparenchymal cells, littoral cells (cells lining sinusoids whether actively phagocytic or not) form the largest fraction (11). In intact livers of adult rats, tritiated thymidine labels from 2 to 5 times as many littoral cells (0.8 to 2.3 percent) as it does hepatocytes (13, 20, 32, 36). Other nonparenchymal cells (bile duct cells, endothelial cells, fibroblasts, etc.) have been largely ignored in studies of cell proliferation in liver during postnatal growth. These cells seem to be labeled at a rate somewhat higher than hepatocytes (13, 19). Studies of replicative cycles of nonparenchymal cells have not been reported.

After partial hepatectomy nonparenchymal cells undergo proliferation in total magnitude similar to that of hepatocytes. Areas under labeling curves for hepatocytes and for littoral and bile duct cells are nearly identical (13, 20) (Fig. 4). However, proliferation of nonparenchymal cells occurs later than proliferation of hepatocytes, initiation of increased labeling and attainment of the peak rate of labeling occurring about 15 to 20 hours later (13, 20, 36, 41).

All nonparenchymal cells are mononuclear diploids (11) and this situation is not altered by partial hepatectomy. Bile duct cells do not differentiate into hepatocytes after partial hepatectomy (23).

Lobular Localization of Proliferating Hepatic Cells

The localization within the lobule or acinus of proliferating littoral cells is random during growth both postnatally and after partial hepatectomy (13, 20). The majority of the remaining nonparenchymal cells are confined to Glisson's capsule (including portal tracts) in normal liver and their proliferation, of course, takes place in this location.

Proliferating hepatocytes are concentrated in the periportal half of the paren-

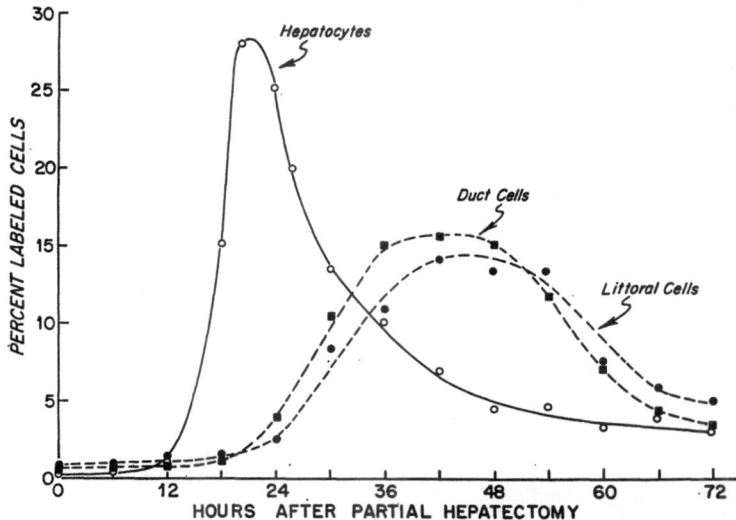

Fig. 4. Labeling of hepatocytes, duct cells, and littoral cells with ^{3}HTdR at different times after 68 percent hepatic resection.

chyma during the most active phases of proliferation during postnatal growth (19, 30) and following partial hepatectomy (8, 13, 15, 20, 24, 36, 41). When the rate of proliferation is low, dividing cells appear to be randomly distributed within the lobule or acinus (8, 13, 20). This is clearly demonstrable after partial hepatectomy; at the time of peak proliferation labeled hepatocytes are confined to the one-third to one-half of the parenchyma nearest to terminal portal venules (8, 13, 15, 20, 36, 41). As parenchymal proliferation wanes, some hepatocytes near terminal hepatic veins are labeled and the location of labeled cells becomes diffuse by 48 hours after surgery (15, 20, 36). Mitotic figures are similarly located (24).

Results of studies utilizing heterotopically placed partial hepatic autografts indicate that the localization of proliferating hepatocytes is determined by the site at which afferent blood enters the parenchyma. Partial autografts of canine liver can be placed in the neck, connected to the carotid artery and jugular vein, in such a fashion that they are perfused through the portal vein in the normal manner (forward flow) or through the hepatic vein (reverse flow) (44). Resection of part of the liver remaining within the abdomen elicits a burst of hepatocytic proliferation in grafts comparable to that occurring in residual liver (27, 45, 48) (see below). In grafts with forward flow of blood, proliferating hepatocytes are concentrated about terminal portal venules, as in residual liver (44). However, in grafts in which the flow of blood is reversed, proliferating hepatocytes are concentrated around terminal hepatic veins and not, as in residual liver, around terminal portal venules (44). These findings demonstrate that all hepatocytes are capable of proliferating after partial hepatectomy and that the stimulus to proliferate affects most intensively those cells that first contact perfusing blood.

Following the initiation of cellular proliferation in periportal parenchyma, a wave-like front of steadily diminishing hepatocytic proliferation progresses along

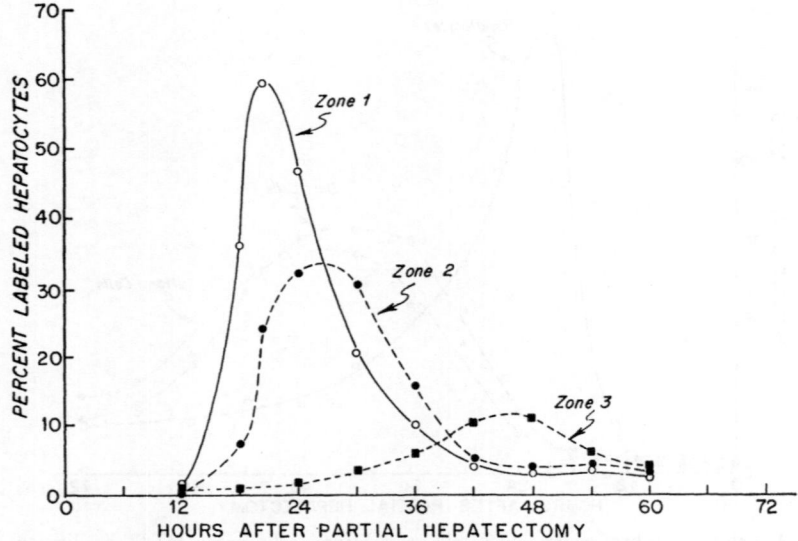

Fig. 5. Proportions of hepatocytes in different areas of the lobule or acinus that are labeled with ^{3}HTdR at different times after 68 percent resection in 60 gm. male Wistar rats. Zone 1 is the third of the lobule nearest terminal portal venules and Zone 3 is the third nearest terminal hepatic veins; Zone 2 is intermediate in location. See Reference 20 for similar data from somewhat older rats.

hepatic plates toward terminal hepatic veins. This view is supported by the observation that the time of peak labeling of interphase nuclei (20) or of mitotic figures (15) occurs progressively later in hepatocytes located in each third of the hepatic plate distant from terminal portal venules (Fig. 5). The overall peak rate of labeling has already passed before those hepatocytes in the inner third of the lobule are maximally labeled (20). Consequently, the earliest labeled hepatocytes (periportal) produce the majority of the total number of new hepatocytes formed after partial hepatectomy (20).

The sharp periportal localization of nuclei labeled at the time of maximal proliferation becomes somewhat more diffuse when examined at successively longer intervals after initial labeling (15, 20, 36, 42). This spreading results from mitotic division of labeled cells and is correlated in time with a progressive decrease in average grain count over individual nuclei (15, 20, 42). Some labeled cells are apparently forced from periportal areas by population pressure resulting from localized formation of new cells. Most of this apparent migration, however, may be erroneous. It is possible that the lightly labeled cells seen in centrolobular areas at late intervals after partial hepatectomy and initial labeling result from reutilization of label by these late replicating hepatocytes (5).

Regulation of Hepatocytic Proliferation

The precision of regulation of hepatocytic proliferation is evident from the foregoing discussion. Regulation of cellular proliferation in the organism is complex with many facets operating simultaneously and coordinately at the levels of cell, tissue, and organism. Control of hepatocytic proliferation is ultimately regulated through the events occurring at the beginning of or early during G_1. Intrinsically regulated reactions in hepatocytes during G_1 (see references 6 and 7 for details of reactions occurring in hepatocytes between the time of partial hepatectomy and the beginning of DNA synthesis) are similar to those that occur in any proliferating cells and, thus, confer no specificity to control of hepatocytic proliferation. Although organismic control is exerted on these subcellular events, alone they do not provide for the coordination between organism and hepatocyte demanded, for instance, by the close relationship between body size and hepatic mass. Since the entire structure and function of the liver are intimately related to hepatic blood flow (3), it seems likely that the blood has a function in the feedback mechanism relating liver size and body size.

Since all hepatocytes are capable of proliferating, the localization of proliferating cells to the site at which afferent blood enters the parenchyma further suggests a role for the blood in initiating proliferation. The rate of blood flow per gram liver increases after partial hepatectomy since total hepatic blood flow is determined by extrahepatic factors and tissue mass is reduced by the operation (2, 3). The nearly reciprocal relationship between hepatic mass and hepatic tissue perfusion has led many investigators to implicate the latter in triggering hepatocytic proliferation (3, 6). Perhaps the most incisive evidence that increased portal flow or pressure alone is not responsible for initiating hepatocytic proliferation after partial hepatectomy has come from experiments utilizing heterotopic partial autografts of liver. Partial hepatectomy of an animal bearing an autograft of liver located in any of several sites in the body produces an hepatocytic proliferative response in the graft similar to that in the residual liver (27, 45, 48) (Fig. 6). This occurs even though the graft is located outside the portal bed and, therefore, does not receive portal

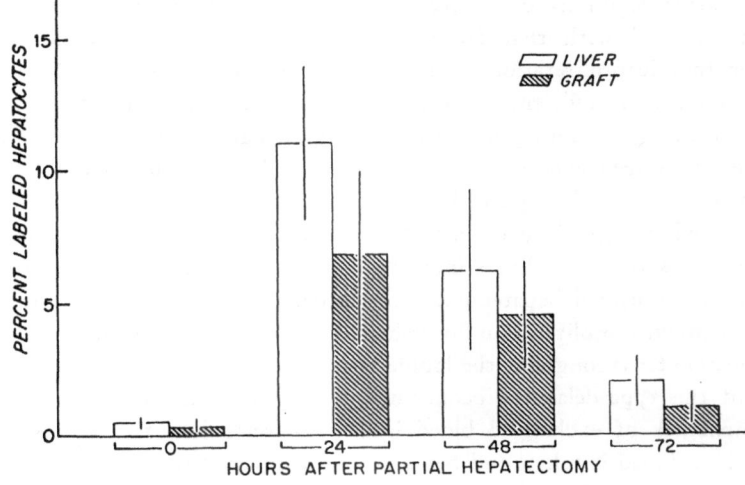

Fig. 6. Labeling of hepatocytes with ³HTdR in livers and subcutaneous partial hepatic autografts at intervals after partial hepatectomy. See Reference 27 for details.

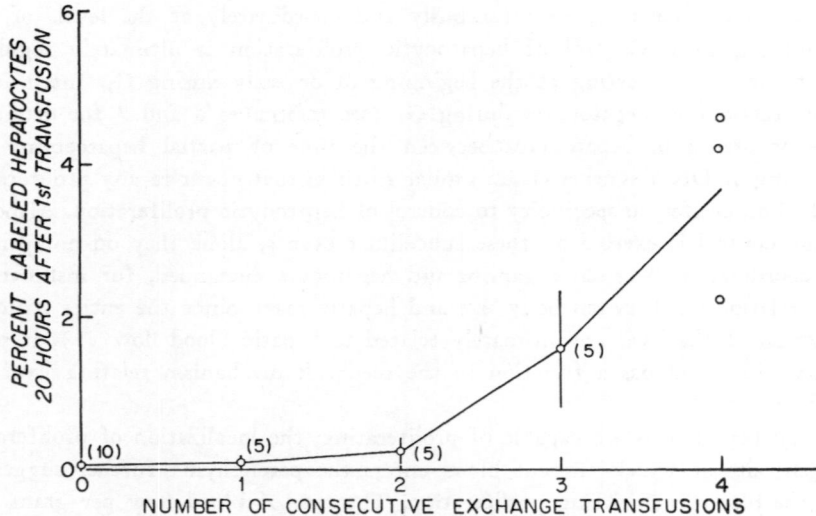

Fig. 7. Labeling of hepatocytes with ³HTdR in intact livers of rats subjected to exchange transfusion with blood from animals partially hepatectomized 24 hours before.

blood and is not subjected to the perturbations of blood flow and pressure to which the residual liver is exposed. These results suggest that following partial hepatectomy there is a change in the composition of the blood and that this change affects hepatocytic proliferation.

Direct, though not conclusive, support for this hypothesis comes from studies utilizing exchange transfusion (19, 22, 49) or direct cross circulation via carotid artery—jugular vein connection (33). Continuous cross circulation for at least 12 hours between an animal with an intact liver and a partner that has been partially hepatectomized results in significantly enhanced labeling of DNA in the intact liver at 20 hours after beginning cross circulation (33). Similarly, replacement of blood of an intact animal with that from a partially hepatectomized donor results in elevated hepatocytic proliferation in the recipient of the transfusion (19) (Fig. 7). One transfusion is insufficient to increase proliferation and 3 or 4 consecutive exchanges are necessary before increased labeling occurs. These results indicate the necessity for prolonged exposure of intact liver to blood from partially hepatectomized animals before DNA synthesis is induced.

Studies in which the blood of partially hepatectomized rats was exchanged with blood from rats with intact livers indicate that the proliferative response that normally occurs after partial hepatectomy can be delayed (22, 49). After the delay is overcome hepatocytic proliferation "overshoots" the peak rate seen in control rats and involves hepatocytes throughout the lobule at its initiation (Fig. 8). Two consecutive exchanges of this type delay the occurrence of peak proliferation even further. The delaying capability of exchanged blood is directly related to the liver mass of the rat from which blood is taken and has a rapid turnover, with a half-life of activity of about 1 hour (22). DNA labeling is maximally delayed when blood is exchanged

4 to 6 hours after surgery (14 to 18 hours prior to maximal DNA labeling in non-transfused, partially hepatectomized rats) and transfusion is partially effective in delaying DNA labeling when made as late as 10 to 12 hours after partial hepatectomy (22). This implies that critical G_1 events occur at this interval. The reproducibility of exchange transfusion experiments has been questioned (33) and recent studies suggest that more consistent results can be achieved if test animals are subjected to 30 percent, rather than 68 percent, resection of the liver (49).

Both of these properties of blood can be demonstrated by the effect of serum on proliferation of cultured hepatic cells (21). A significant increase in nuclear labeling occurs in static cultures of liver exposed to serum from partially hepatectomized rats (Fig. 9). In actively proliferating cultures a slight inhibition of proliferation is effected by serum from rats with intact livers (19). Preliminary evidence indicates that the stimulatory activity is associated with a molecular species small enough to pass through a dialysis membrane (19). Although these results seem superficially analogous to those demonstrated *in vivo*, this remains to be demonstrated.

The data reviewed are consistent with the viewpoint that there is a critical relationship between the ratio of hepatic mass to body size and the hepatocytic growth fraction. All hepatocytes are apparently capable of proliferating "on demand"; organismic control of hepatocytic proliferation is probably effected by a humoral mechanism that is almost instantaneously responsive to changes in the liver weight to body weight ratio. The evidence suggests that the mechanism of

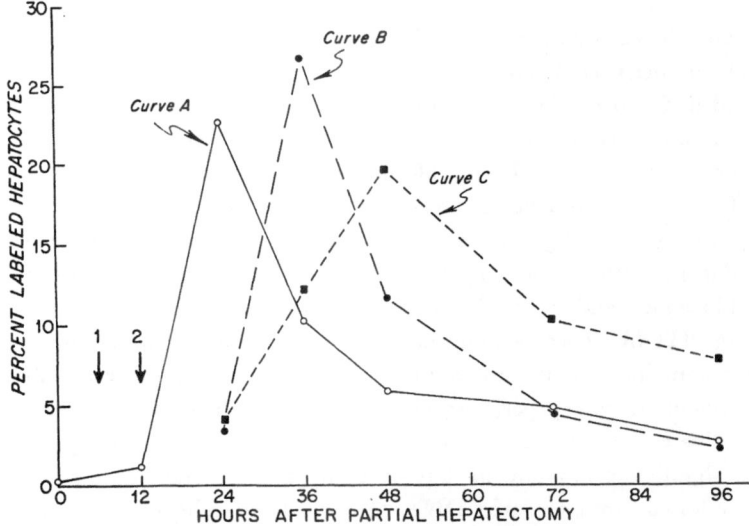

Fig. 8. Labeling of hepatocytes with ^{3}HTdR after 68 percent hepatic resection in rats subjected to one (Curve B) or two (Curve C) exchange transfusions with blood from animals with intact livers. Transfusions were performed at the times indicated by the arrows. Curve A represents labeling in control animals not transfused. See Reference 22 for details.

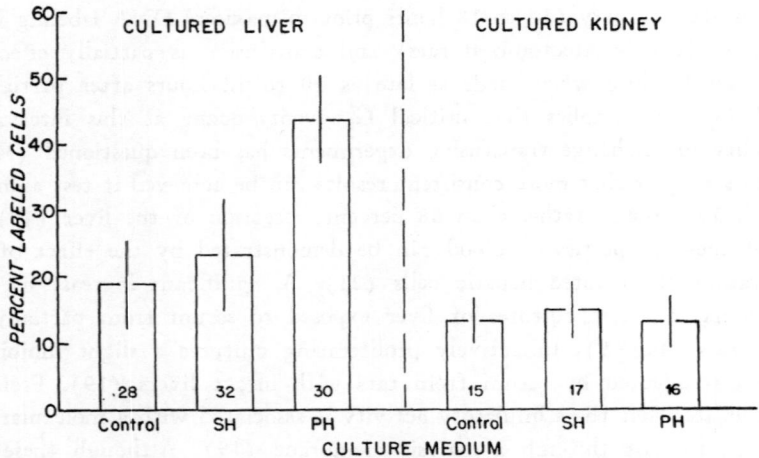

Fig. 9. Response of cells in explants of liver and kidney to serum from animals sham-operated or partially hepatectomized 24 hours earlier. See Reference 21 for details.

organismic control is mediated by interaction between interphase hepatocytes (G_0 or slowed G_1) and some property of the blood perfusing them. This interaction possibly involves clearance by hepatocytes of some decisive substance which then affects the molecular events in the cell and leads to DNA synthesis. Better understanding of the hepatocytic replicative cycle will allow more rational experimental examination of this hypothesis.

Addendum: Since submission of this paper for publication two reports have appeared which merit comment. Evidence for a population of hepatocytes slowed in an extended G_2 period in normal mouse liver has been presented (37). This interpretation results from the finding that not as many colchicine-arrested, labeled mitotic figures accumulated during 60 hours after initial labeling of hepatocytes with [3]HTdR as there were labeled interphase nuclei. Arrest of mitoses was attempted with colchicine (1 mg/kg) given every 12 hours. The authors assumed that colchicine did not affect the length of the S or G_2, that no cells escaped the colchicine blockade, and that all labeled hepatocytes were tagged shortly after administering [3]HTdR. These assumptions are open to serious question. The hepatotoxicity of colchicine is well known (14); the decreasing number of labeled nuclei with time, noted in this paper, suggests that tagged hepatocytes were killed and disappeared. The assumption that all cells were labeled shortly after injecting [3]HTdR ignores the significant amount of late labeling that results from reutilization of metabolites released from tritiated DNA of short-lived cells (5). Considering these limitations, a normal G_2 population of hepatocytes cannot be considered as being conclusively demonstrated.

The kinetics of proliferating cells in regenerating liver have been reconsidered and extended (17). The conclusions of this study essentially agree with those presented here and reported earlier by various authors (13, 15, 20, 36, 41).

References

1. ALFERT, M. and GESCHWIND, I. I.: The development of polysomaty in rat liver. Exp. Cell Res. **15**, 230 (1958).

2. BENACERRAF, B., BILBEY, D., BIOZZI, G., HALPERN, B. N. and STIFFEL, C.: The measurement of liver blood flow in partially hepatectomized rats. J. Physiol. (London) **136**, 287 (1957).

3. BRAUER, R. W.: Liver circulation and function. Physiol. Reviews **43**, 115 (1963).

4. BRUES, A. and MARBLE, B. B.: An analysis of mitosis in liver restoration. J. Exp. Med. **65**, 15 (1937).

5. BRYANT, B. J.: Reutilization of lymphocyte DNA by the cells of intestinal crypts and regenerating liver. J. Cell. Biol. **18**, 515 (1963).

6. BUCHER, N. L. R.: Regeneration of mammalian liver. Intern. Rev. Cytol. **15**, 245 (1963).

7. BUCHER, N. L. R.: Experimental aspects of hepatic regeneration. New England J. Med. **277**, 686 and 738 (1967).

8. BUCHER, N. L. R. and SWAFFIELD, M. N.: The rate of incorporation of labeled thymidine into the deoxyribonucleic acid of regenerating rat liver in relation to the amount of liver excised. Cancer Res. **24**, 1611 (1964).

9. BUCHER, N. L. R., SWAFFIELD, M. N. and DiTROIA, J. F.: The influence of age upon incorporation of thymidine-2-C^{14} into the DNA of regenerating rat liver. Cancer Res. **24**, 509 (1964).

10. CARRIERE, R.: Polyploid cell production in normal adult rat liver. Exp. Cell Res. **46**, 533 (1967).

11. DAOST, R.: The cell population of liver tissue and the cytological reference bases. *In:* Liver Function. R. W. Brauer (ed.). American Institute of Biological Sciences. Washington, 3 (1958).

12. DOLJANSKI, F.: The growth of the liver with special reference to mammals. Intern. Rev. Cytol. **10**, 217 (1958).

13. EDWARDS, J. L. and KOCH, A.: Parenchymal and littoral cell proliferation during liver regeneration. Lab. Invest. **13**, 32 (1964).

14. EIGSTI, O. J. and DUSTIN, P.: Colchicine in Agriculture, Medicine, Biology and Chemistry. Iowa State College Press, Ames (1955).

15. FABRIKANT, J. I.: The spatial distribution of parenchymal cell proliferation during regeneration of the liver. Johns Hopkins Med. Bull. **120**, 137 (1967).

16. FABRIKANT, J. I.: The effect of prior continuous irradiation on the G_2, M and S phases of proliferating parenchymal cells in regenerating liver. Radiat. Res. **31**, 304 (1967).

17. FABRIKANT, J. I.: The kinetics of cellular proliferation in regenerating liver. J. Cell. Biol. **36**, 551 (1968).

18. GESCHWIND, I. I., ALFERT, M. and SCHOOLEY, C.: Liver regeneration and hepatic polyploidy in the hypophysectomized rat. Exp. Cell Res. **15**, 232 (1958).

19. GRISHAM, J. W.: Unpublished observations.

20. GRISHAM, J. W.: A morphologic study of deoxyribonucleic acid synthesis and cell proliferation in regenerating rat liver. Autoradiography with thymidine-H^3. Cancer Res. **22**, 842 (1962).

21. GRISHAM, J. W., KAUFMAN, D. L. and ALEXANDER, R. W.: ^{3}H thymidine labeling of rat liver cells cultured in plasma from sham- or partially hepatectomized rats. Fed. Proc. **26**, 624 (1967).

22. GRISHAM, J. W., LEONG, G. F., ALBRIGHT, M. F. and EMERSON, J. D.: Effect of

exchange transfusion on labeling of nuclei with thymidine-^{3}H and on mitosis in hepatocytes of normal and regenerating rat liver. Cancer Res. 26, 1476 (1966).

23. Grisham, J. W. and Porta, E. A.: Origin and fate of proliferated hepatic ductal cells in the rat: Electron microscopic and autoradiographic studies. Exp. Molec. Path. 3, 242 (1964).

24. Harkness, R. D.: The spatial distribution of dividing cells in the liver of the rat after partial hepatectomy. J. Physiol. (London) 116, 373 (1952).

25. Jaffe, J.: Diural mitotic periodicity in regenerating rat liver. Anat. Rec. 120, 935 (1954).

26. Leduc, E. H.: Regeneration of the liver. In: The Liver: Morphology, Biochemistry, Physiology. C. Rouiller (ed.). Academic Press, Vol. 2, New York, 63 (1964).

27. Leong, G. F., Grisham, J. W., Hole, B. V. and Albright, M. F.: Effect of partial hepatectomy on DNA synthesis and mitosis in heterotopic partial autografts of rat liver. Cancer Res. 24, 1496 (1964).

28. MacDonald, R. A.: "Lifespan" of liver cells. Arch. Int. Med. 107, 335 (1961).

29. MacDonald, R. A., Rodgers, A. E. and Pechet, G.: Regeneration of the liver. Relation of the regenerative response to size of partial hepatectomy. Lab. Invest. 11, 544 (1962).

30. McKellar, M.: The postnatal growth and mitotic activity of the liver of the albino rat. Am. J. Anat. 85, 263 (1949).

31. Makino, S. and Tanaka, T.: Chromosome features in regenerating rat liver following partial extirpation. Texas Reports Biol. Med. 11, 588 (1953).

32. Messier, B. and Leblond, C. P.: Cell proliferation and migration as revealed by radioautography after injection of thymidine-H^3 into male rats and mice. Am. J. Anat. 106, 247 (1960).

33. Moolten, F. L. and Bucher, N. L. R.: Regeneration of rat liver: Transfer of a humoral agent by cross circulation. Science 158, 272 (1967).

34. Nadel, C. and Zajdela, F.: Polyploidie somatique dans le foie de rat. I. Le role des cellules binucléées dans la genese des cellules polyploides. Exp. Cell Res. 42, 99 (1966).

35. Naora, H.: Microspectrophotometry of cell nuclei stained with the Feulgen reaction. IV. Formation of tetraploid nuclei in rat liver during postnatal growth. J. Biophys. Biochem. Cytol. 3, 949 (1957).

36. Oehlert, W., Hämmerling, W. and Büchner, F.: Der zeitliche Ablauf und das Ausmass der desoxyribonukleinsäure—Synthese in der regenerierenden Leber nach Teil-hepatektomie. Beitr. Path. Anat. 126, 91 (1962).

37. Perry, L. D. and Schwartz, F. J.: Evidence for a subpopulation of cells with an extended G_2 period in normal adult mouse liver. Exp. Cell Res. 48, 155 (1967).

38. Post, J. and Hoffman, J.: Changes in the replication times and patterns of the liver cell during the life of the rat. Exp. Cell Res. 36, 111 (1964).

39. Post, J. and Hoffman, J.: Further studies on the replication of rat liver cells in vivo. Exp. Cell Res. 40, 333 (1965).

40. Post, J. and Hoffman, J.: Hepatic cell replication during growth and regeneration. In: Progress in Liver Diseases. H. Popper and F. Schaffner (eds.). Grune and Stratton, Vol. 2, New York, 154 (1965).

41. de Recondo, A. M. and Frayssinet, C.: Étude auto-historadiographique après injection de thymidine tritée des cellules synthétisant de l'ADN dans le foie de rat in hypertrophie compensatrice. J. Physiol. (Paris) 55, 242 (1963).

42. de Recondo, A. M. and Frayssinet, C.: Mise en évidence de lignées cellulaires dans le foie au cours de l'hypertrophie compensatrice apres hépatectomie partielle. J. Physiol. (Paris) 57, 685 (1965).

43. SHEA, S. M.: Kinetics of hepatocytic proliferation in the early stages of liver regeneration. Exp. Cell Res. **36**, 325 (1964).

44. SIGEL, B., BALDIA, L. B., BRIGHTMAN, S. A., DUNN, M. R. and PRICE, R. I. M.: The effect of blood flow reversal on liver cell formation. Gastroenterology **52**, 1142 (1967).

45. SIGEL, B., BALDIA, L. B., DUNN, M. R. and MENDUKE, H.: Humoral control of liver regeneration. Surg. Gynec. Obst. **124**, 1023 (1967).

46. STÖCKER, E. and BACH, G.: Zur Proliferationsmodus des Leberparenchyms nach Teilhepatektomie. Naturwiss. **52**, 663 (1965).

47. STÖCKER, E. and HEINE, W. D.: Über die Proliferation von Nieren- und Leberepithel unter normalen und pathologischen Bedingungen. Beitr. Path. Anat. **131**, 410 (1965).

48. VIROLAINEN, M.: Mitotic response in liver autograft after partial hepatectomy in rat. Exp. Cell Res. **33**, 588 (1964).

49. WEINBREN, K.: Problems in restoration of the liver. *In:* Wound Healing, A Symposium based upon the Lister Centenary Scientific Meeting. C. Illingworth (ed.). Little, Brown and Company, Boston, 69 (1965).

Discussion

Cellular Proliferation in the Liver *

NANCY L. R. BUCHER, FREDERICK L. MOOLTEN, THEODORE R. SCHROCK

John Collins Warren Laboratories
Huntington Memorial Hospital
Harvard University
Boston, Massachusetts

Dr. Grisham has presented a fine compilation of data pertaining to various aspects of hepatic growth. At the end he dwelt upon the crux of the matter—the quest for the mechanisms that control the growth process.

In the adult rat the hepatocytes comprise a population of essentially non-growing cells, but a burst of intense proliferative activity can be easily induced by partial hepatectomy. This "turning on" of the replicative machinery—or in more technical terms, this derepression of the part of the genome that controls cellular reproduction—has parallels in many other biological systems in which non-growing cells are led to divide in response to specific stimuli. In such systems there is generally an initial "lag" period during which changes are thought to occur in the quantity and/or quality of the RNA being synthesized, as well as alterations in the character of the proteins formed, including activation and probably *de novo* synthesis of a

---

* This is publication No. 1318 of the Cancer Commission of Harvard University.

number of enzymes on the pathway serving DNA replication. About the time the latter enzymes are augmented, DNA synthesis begins and mitosis ensues. Knowledge of the particular mechanisms that set the growth process in motion is almost totally lacking. In the case of hepatocyte proliferation, the obvious tailoring of liver size to the metabolic demands of the organism has long suggested that the regulatory influences must arise from extra hepatic sources. Firm evidence for humoral control is relatively recent and rests upon the elegant autograft studies that Dr. Grisham has described.

A brief digression in order to review certain quantitative aspects of liver growth stimuli may be helpful in the further discussion of humoral control. In 1936 Dr. Brues made an important observation, recorded in a classical study, that the several lobes of the liver bear a constant relation to the total hepatic mass (1). By resecting lobes singly or in combination, quite precise degrees of hepatic deficiency can be achieved (2). When the response is determined by incorporation of labeled thymidine into DNA, small stimuli (9 percent or 34 percent deficiencies) are found to result in slow, prolonged responses, whereas larger ones (43 percent or 68 percent deficiencies) cause a high initial burst of activity followed by a slower phase after part of the deficit has been restored. Radioautographs show that the size of the response reflects the number of hepatocytes undergoing DNA replication. The timing of the response is not affected by the size of the hepatectomy up to 68 percent (2), but excision of 82 percent of the liver tends to result in a considerable delay (4). Weinbren and his co-workers found the maximum rate of DNA labeling in these subtotally (82 percent) hepatectomized animals to be retarded by about 14 hours (4). The cause of this delay is not known, but there are greater hemodynamic changes, additional surgical trauma and other debilitating aspects attendant upon subtotal hepatectomy that may temporarily overwhelm the repair mechanisms. The requirement for seeking a humoral factor might therefore be expected to include a relatively large stimulus, perhaps acting over an extended period of time, to produce a significantly large response; but if the stimulus were of overwhelming magnitude, inhibitory or delaying influences might be encountered.

With this information as background, we attempted to demonstrate transmission of a humoral factor for regulation of hepatocyte proliferation from one rat to another by means of cross circulation of blood. Approximately 6 week old female rats weighing about 150 gm were connected to partners via polyethylene cannulas running from carotid arteries to external jugular veins. The animals were kept in individual restraining cages. The rate of blood flow was determined by placing the cages on opposite pans of a balance, clamping one of the cannulas and timing the resulting change in weight. The flow was 2–2.5 ml/minute quite consistently. Since the total blood volume of such animals is around 7.5 ml, the exchange rate approximated 30 percent of the blood volume/minute. Partially hepatectomized partners were connected to normal partners within 1½–2 hours after the hepatic resection and cross circulation was maintained for 19 hours. The partners were then separated, given 0.8 μc of C^{14}-thymidine intravenously and sacrificed after a 1 hour incorporation period. The results in Table 1 show that DNA labeling in normal-to-normal

TABLE 1

Rats	dpm/mg DNA	
	Normal partners	Partially hepatectomized partners
Single	489 ± 47 (3)	15,000 ± 3,783 (4)
Normal–normal pairs	331 ± 27 (8)	
68%–68% hepatectomized pairs		6,580 ± 841 (4)
Normal–34% hepatectomized pairs	309 ± 44 (3)	991 ± 245 (3)
Normal–68% hepatectomized pairs	1,056 ± 413 (5)	11,860 ± 1,720 (5)
Normal–85% hepatectomized pairs	2,591 ± 568 (6)	4,566 ± 1,710 (6)

Specific activity of hepatic DNA determined in rats that were cross circulated for approximately 19 hours, then separated and sacrificed 1 hour after injection of 0.8 μc of thymidine-2-C^{14} (specific activity 30 μc/μmole). Results expressed as mean specific activities ± standard errors of means; numbers of rats in parentheses; dpm, disintegrations per minute. Normal partners of 68% or 85% hepatectomized rats both differ significantly from normal rats cross circulated with each other (p < 0.01, rank test) (3).

partners was a little less than in normal single rats. In 68-percent-hepatectomized-to-68-percent-hepatectomized partners, the values were much lower than in single 68 percent hepatectomized animals. It appears that the experimental procedure is in itself suppressive. In spite of this inhibitory influence, it is possible to demonstrate a stimulation of DNA labeling in the livers of normal rats following cross circulation with partially hepatectomized partners, and the response appears to be dose-related, i.e., maximal when the partners were 85 percent hepatectomized, less but still significant when partners were 68 percent hepatectomized and nil when 34 percent hepatectomized. The hepatectomized partners seemed to benefit from exchange with normal animals, as shown by the higher response in 68 percent hepatectomized partners of normal rats compared to 68 percent hepatectomized partners of 68 percent hepatectomized rats (3).

The average values for hepatectomized partners tended to be higher than for corresponding normal partners. Thus, even at the high rate of blood exchange present in these experiments, the factor failed to equilibrate; it must therefore be biologically unstable and rapidly renewed.

It is important to note that cross circulation experiments cannot distinguish the rise of a growth stimulating agent as a result of partial hepatectomy from the fall of a circulating inhibitor below levels normally present when livers are intact. Such experiments merely confirm the effectiveness of a change in the composition of the blood in initiating hepatocyte proliferation. For simplicity we refer to a humoral agent or factor, but there may be a single or a combination of factors, inhibitory or stimulatory.

In this connection, Dr. Grisham has presented evidence that might suggest both stimulatory and inhibitory factors in experiments involving single or multiple exchange blood transfusions. Because of the debilitating conditions already noted, we are at present unable to determine whether the normal partners exert any inhibitory influence upon the partially hepatectomized rats. For reasons that are frustratingly obscure to Dr. Grisham and ourselves, we have been completely unable, in spite of repeated attempts, to confirm his observation that exchange blood transfusions from normal donors into partially hepatectomized recipients exerts an inhibitory effect. We have not attempted to repeat the experiments that he has just reported, using partially hepatectomized donors in transfusions which stimulated normal recipients.

As stated above, the experimental conditions for cross circulation are debilitating and tend to depress the level of response. I have purposely chosen the vague term "debilitation" because we do not know precisely what it entails. We know that among suppressive conditions are: inappropriate age of animals (those younger than the specified age are too fragile, those older do not tolerate restraint as well), the degree of restraint, dehydration, and sedation. Use of barbiturate sedation may account for the failure of Alston and Thomson to demonstrate a humoral influence in experiments otherwise similar to those we have reported. Results of further efforts to define debilitating aspects of the experimental procedure are shown in Table 2. The data are of a preliminary nature but clearly indicate that sham-neck operations and prolonged restraint tend to suppress the response in animals already subjected to a partial hepatectomy. Added insults seem to be more or less cumulative and probably for this reason the 85 percent hepatectomized animals are especially susceptible to suppressive influences.

For growth initiation, not only must the stimulatory factor be present in the blood but the hepatocytes must be capable of responding to it. It may be that debilitating conditions affect especially the competence of the hepatocytes to proliferate, because in several isolated instances (not shown in Table 1) the livers of normal rats were found to synthesize DNA more rapidly than those of their partially hepatectomized partners.

The proliferative response achieved in the normal partners of cross-circulated pairs exhibits characteristics of regenerating liver described by Dr. Grisham; by

TABLE 2

Single rats	dpm/mg DNA
Sham	462 ± 32 (3)
Sham + restraint	356 ± 34 (4)
68% Hepatectomy	14,200 ± 1,720 (5)
68% Hepatectomy + sham	9,150 ± 1,670 (6)
68% Hepatectomy + sham + restraint	3,530 ± 2,260 (4)
85% Hepatectomy	3,700 ± 1,810 (6)
85% Hepatectomy + restraint	62 ± 62 (2)

Effects of sham-neck cannulation (including saline and heparin injections) and 18 hours in restraining cage on normal, 68% and 85% hepatectomized rats.

Fig. 1. Specific activity of hepatic DNA in normal members of cross circulated pairs as a function of the duration of continuous cross circulation. Partners were connected approximately one hour after 85% hepatectomy and cross circulated for the times shown. They were then separated, and at 20 hours after the start of the cross circulation injected with 0.8 μc of thymidine-2-C14 (specific activity 52.4), and killed one hour later. Vertical bars show standard errors of the means: numbers of rats in parentheses. ■———■ normal numbers of 85%-hepatectomized-to-normal pairs; ●———● normal members of normal-to-normal pairs.

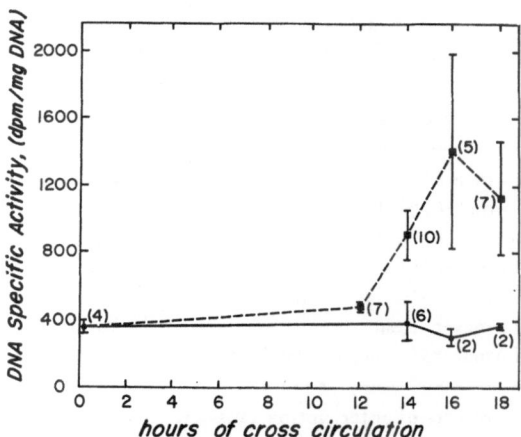

radioautography the distribution of hepatocyte labeling following incorporation of H³-thymidine into DNA exhibits the typical periportal pattern. Mitotic activity is found almost exclusively in the parenchymal cells.

For transmission of the regenerative impetus, prolonged cross circulation seems to be necessary. Under the conditions of our experiments it must endure for more than 12 hours (Fig. 1). Preliminary trials suggest that this interval does not include time needed for the factor to reach a critical level in the partially hepatectomized partners, but further studies are needed.

We wondered whether interrupting the cross circulation for a 2–4 hour interval during the required 12–14 hour period would permit the growth initiating process to regress towards the time zero level or to remain stationary or even to progress onwards from the previous level. Preliminary results, marred by distressing variability, are shown in Tables 3 and 4. Continuous exchange for 12 hours seemed insufficient to establish DNA synthesis irreversibly. However, in several instances when the total exchange time was 12 hours with a hiatus of 2 hours, we did

TABLE 3

Rat pairs	Cross circulation schedule (12 hrs total elapsed time)		Normal partners dpm/mg DNA
Normal–85% hepatectomized	Continuous	12 hrs	466 ± 22 (7)
Normal–85% hepatectomized	Interrupted *	6–2–4 hrs	823 (1)
Normal–85% hepatectomized	Interrupted	6–4–2 hrs	352 (1)
Normal–85% hepatectomized	Interrupted	8–2–2 hrs	843 ± 121 (2)
Normal–normal	Interrupted	8–2–2 hrs	341 ± 18 (2)

Effects of interrupting cross circulation during a 12 hour period.

* Interrupted 6–2–4 hrs means rats were cross circulated for 6 hours, disconnected from each other and self-shunted for 2 hours by connecting the free ends of the rats' own arterial and venous cannulas, then reconnected to the same partner for an additional 4 hours. Injected with 0.8 μc of thymidine-2-C14 at 20 hours after start of cross circulation and sacrificed one hour later.

TABLE 4

Rat pairs	Cross circulation schedule (14 hrs total elapsed time)		Normal partners dpm/mg DNA
Normal–85% hepatectomized	Continuous	14 hrs	900 ± 154 (10)
Normal–85% hepatectomized	Interrupted	6–2–6 hrs	369 (1)
Normal–85% hepatectomized	Interrupted	6–4–4 hrs	585 ± 38 (2)
Normal–normal	Interrupted	6–4–4 hrs	313 ± 31 (2)
Normal–85% hepatectomized	Interrupted	8–4–2 hrs	1,171 ± 575 (3)
Normal–normal	Interrupted	8–4–2 hrs	264 ± 48 (2)
Normal–85% hepatectomized	Interrupted	10–2–2 hrs	445 (1)

Effects of interrupting cross circulation during a 14 hour period. See footnote to Table 3.

observe activation of DNA synthesis (Table 3). Possibly the hiatus allowed some recovery from the trauma attendant upon maintaining a balanced circulation against a partner, and hence facilitated progression of the initiating factor. Similar trends were apparent when the total elapsed time of cross circulation was 14 hours with interruptions of 4 hours' duration. It seems from these very preliminary observations as if the process of initiating DNA synthesis progresses in stages; the partial "turning on" that occurs during 6–8 hours of cross circulation persists and does not regress during a 2–4 hour interruption so that an additional few hours of cross circulation makes final entry into the "S" phase irrevocable. Again more work is needed, but we have temporarily suspended further cross-circulation studies until we can find the cause of and reduce the large variability inherent in our present experimental set-up.

We conclude that the cross-circulation experiments support the concept of a humoral mechanism for initiation of regeneration. From preliminary attempts to characterize the mechanism we suggest that prolonged exposure to a large volume of stimulus-bearing blood is required. "Turning on" of the growth process may occur in stages. It is not rapidly reversible. The factor in the blood is probably subject to rapid renewal; its nature and mode of operation remain completely obscure.

References

1. BRUES, A. M., DRURY, D. R., and BRUES, M. C.: A quantitative study of cell growth in regenerating liver. Arch. Pathol. 22, 658 (1936).
2. BUCHER, N. L. R., and SWAFFIELD, M. N.: The rate of incorporation of labeled thymidine into the deoxyribonucleic acid of regenerating rat liver in relation to the amount of liver excised. Cancer Research 24, 1611 (1964).
3. MOOLTEN, F. L., and BUCHER, N. L. R.: Regeneration of rat liver: transfer of humoral agent by cross circulation. Science 158, 272 (1967).
4. WEINBREN, K., and WOODWARD, E.: Delayed incorporation of ^{32}P from orthophosphate into deoxyribonucleic acid of rat liver after subtotal hepatectomy. Brit. J. Exper. Path. 45, 442 (1964).

Cell Proliferation in the
Intestinal Epithelium *

SAMUEL W. LESHER and JANIE BAUMAN

Department of Radiology
Allegheny General Hospital
Pittsburgh, Pennsylvania

The intestinal epithelium which lines the inner surface of the mammalian small intestine is a continuous membrane that is formed by a layer of simple columnar epithelial cells. This epithelial membrane covers the villi that project out into the intestinal lumen and lines the crypts that invaginate into the lamina propria from the base of each villus (Fig. 1).

As early as 1892 Bizzozero noted that dividing cells were confined to the crypt, but their fate was not known until Leblond and Stevens (1948) using ^{32}P as a DNA label showed that cells produced in the crypts moved up the sides of the villus and were extruded when they reached the villus tip. Because of this carefully regulated balance between cell production and cell death, the intestinal epithelium is a good example of a steady-state cell renewal system.

Cell turnover is probably higher in the intestinal epithelium than in any other *in vivo* cell population. A number of investigators (4, 5, 7, 8, 12) have shown that the production of cells is sufficient to completely replace the entire mucosal membrane of the small intestine in $1\frac{1}{2}$ to 2 days. Although cell production is continuous and constant, the relationship between proliferative and non-proliferative cell populations is highly critical and any factor which affects this relationship leads to a change in proliferative rate.

Advancement in our understanding of cell population kinetics over the past decade has been rapid. This advancement stems from the biological utilization of radioactivity labeled metabolic precursors, the perfection of high resolution auto-radiography, and the development of new quantitative techniques to study the behavior of labeled and non-labeled cells in *in vivo* and *in vitro* cell populations. It is now possible using such compounds as ^{3}H- or ^{14}C-uridine, -cytidine, -thymidine or any one of several amino acids to determine which cells are involved in DNA, RNA and/or protein synthesis, the rate at which the synthesis takes place, the relationship and interdependence these processes have to each other, and how they are affected by intrinsic and extrinsic factors.

* Work supported by the U.S. Atomic Energy Commission.

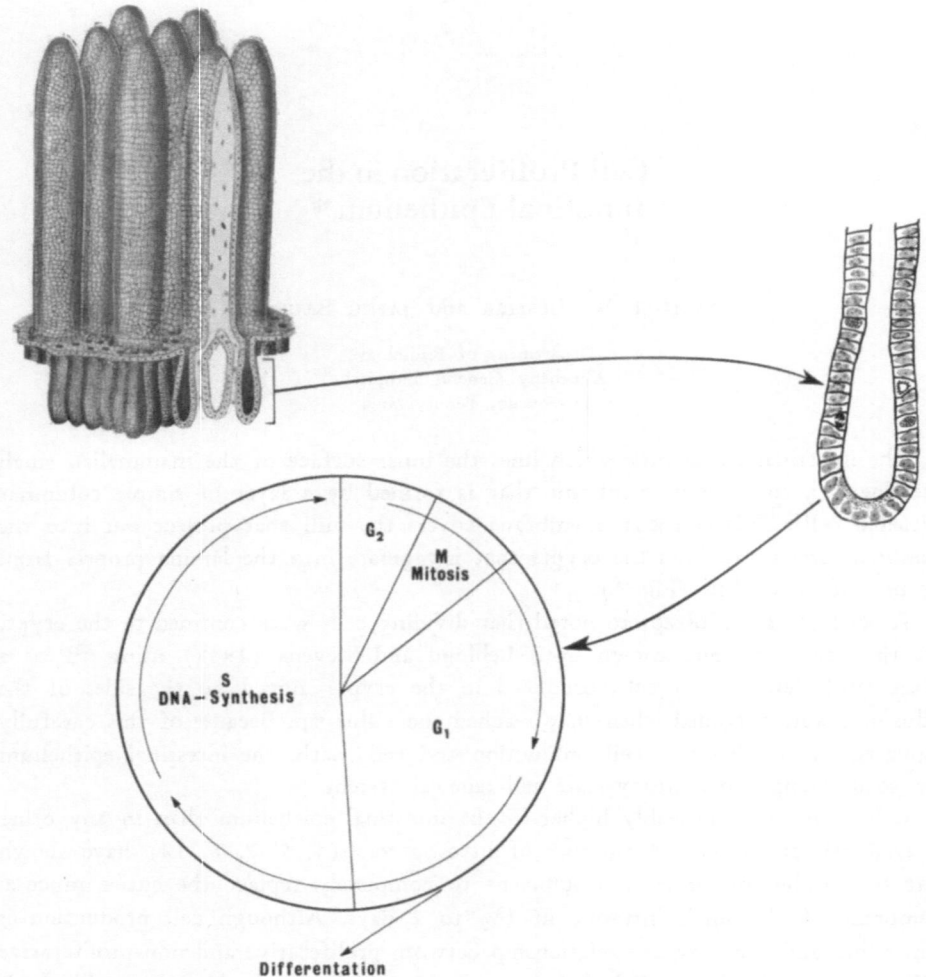

Fig. 1. Schematic drawing showing the relationship of crypts to villi in the mouse upper small intestine. As shown the epithelial membrane is a continuous sheet of columnar cells covering the villi and lining the crypts. Cell proliferation is confined to well defined compartments within the crypts, and in these compartments all cells are in one of the four phases of the generation cycle (G₁, S, G₂, M).

Functional Characterization of the Intestinal Epithelium

Although our knowledge of the functional characteristics of the non-proliferative epithelial cells within the crypt and on the villus is in a preliminary state, experiments in progress (2) using tritiated-uridine, -cytidine, -thymidine, and -leucine alone and in various combinations suggest that there is a well-defined and orderly metabolic sequence as the cells move from their place of origin in the crypts to the extrusion zone at the villus tip. Within the crypt the cells can be divided into three major compartments (Fig. 2): the **Paneth Cell Compartment** (F_p zone)

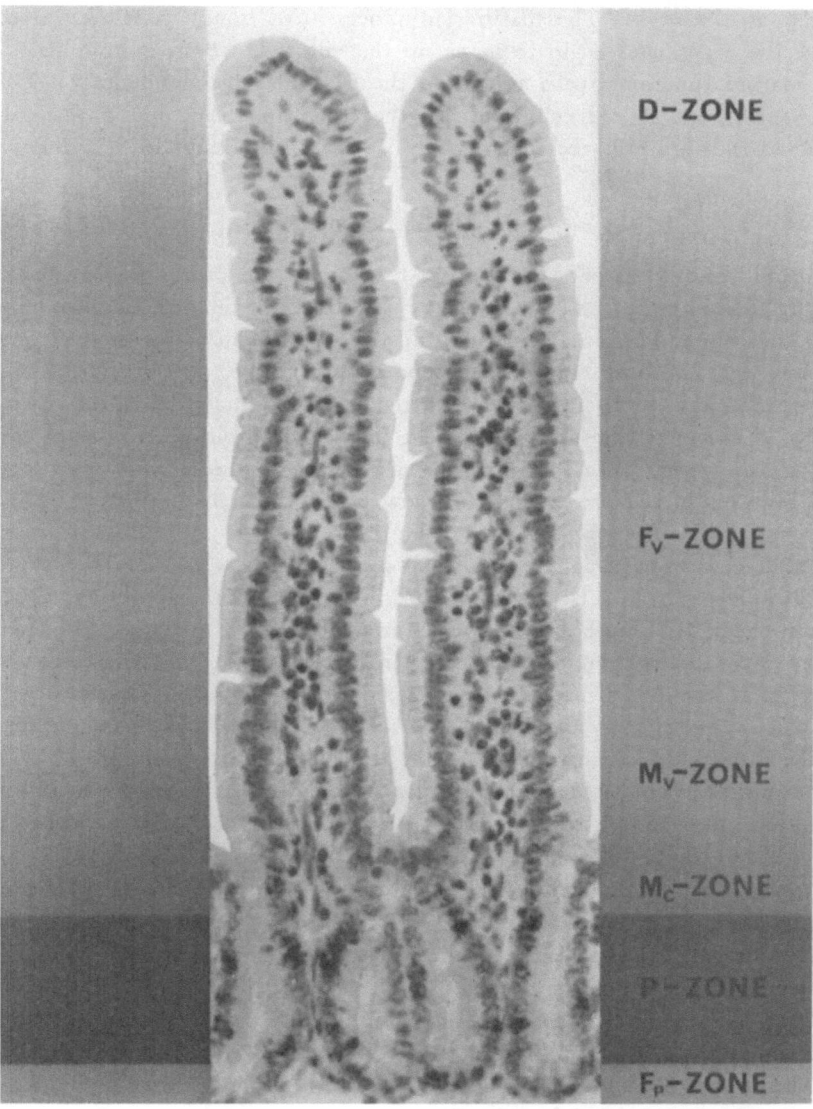

Fig. 2. A photomicrograph through a longitudinally cut section of the upper small intestine. The cells of the intestinal epithelium can be divided into five functional compartments; namely, (1) F_p-zone, which contains the secretory Paneth cells; (2) the P-zone, which contains the proliferative cells; (3) the M_c-zone and the M_v-zone, both in the crypt and villus, all cells are undergoing differentiation; (4) the F_v-zone, which contains the mature functional cells; and (5) the D-zone, which contains cells near the end of their life span.

includes less than 10% of the total crypt population; the **Proliferative Compartment** (P zone, 55 to 60%); and the **Maturation Compartment** (M_c zone, 30 to 35%) at the top of the crypt. The maturation process (M_v zone) continues after the cells leave the crypts and begin to move up the villus; however, most of the villus cells are mature functional cells and lie in the F_v zone which includes 75–85% of the villus epithelium. As the cells approach the villus tip, their functional capability decreases and they are near the end of their life span when extruded (D zone).

Cell Proliferation

For many years, research emphasis has been upon the proliferative capacity of the rapidly dividing cells within the crypts and their ability to maintain the intestinal epithelium in spite of various insults that disturb the balance between proliferative and non-proliferative cell populations. Hence, our knowledge of cell kinetics within the proliferative compartment is far more extensive than our knowledge of the metabolic activity of cells in the non-proliferative compartments. In this section we will deal with the nature of the proliferative population, the processes involved in cell production, and how production rate is affected by various factors.

Although cell proliferation in the small intestine is confined to the crypt, the proliferative cells can only be identified during mitosis (M) and during the DNA synthesis period (S). The S cells however are only identifiable in autoradiographs since they incorporate thymidine and appear labeled. The remaining proliferative cells will be in the DNA preparatory phase G_1 or the mitotic preparatory phase G_2 and will be morphologically identical to cells which are undergoing differentiation in the maturation compartments. After the G_0 stem cell pool for the erythropoietic system was postulated by Lajtha (8, 5), speculation began as to the possibility of such a system existing for the intestinal epithelium, however, recent work seems to indicate that it does not.

In theory, if all of the cells in the proliferative compartments are participating in cell production, and if tritiated thymidine (^{3}HTdR) is made available at closely spaced time intervals, then when cells which were in G_2 at time of the first injection have passed through the remainder of G_2, M, G_1, and into S all the cells within the compartment would be labeled. This interval of G_1, G_2, and M ranges from 6 to 8 hours in the 100 day old BCF_1 mouse.

A series of 100 day old BCF_1 mice were given 5 μCi, intraperitoneal injections of ^{3}HTdR (0.36 Ci/mM Schwartz Bioresearch, Inc.) every two hours. Thirty minutes after each injection 2 mice were sacrificed, tissue samples fixed, and both crypt squash and section autoradiographs prepared. Tissue sections' autoradiographs show that the proliferative compartment lies in the midsegment of the crypt (Fig. 3) and that all cells in this zone appear to be labeled after five injections (Fig. 4). Therefore, it can be assumed that the proliferative compartment does not contain a G_0 compartment. This experiment further suggests that all cells within the proliferative compartment are at all times in one of the four phases of the generation cycle; *i.e.*, G_1, S, G_2, or M.

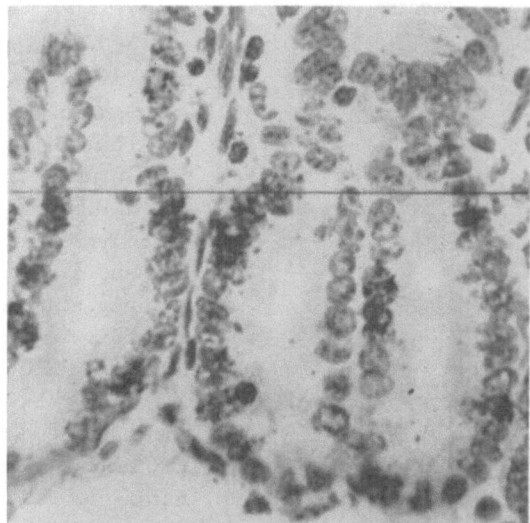

Fig. 3. Labeled nuclei in crypts after single injection of ^{3}HTdR. Proliferative compartment lies below the topmost labeled nuclei marked by horizontal line. Cells above the line lie in the maturation compartment.

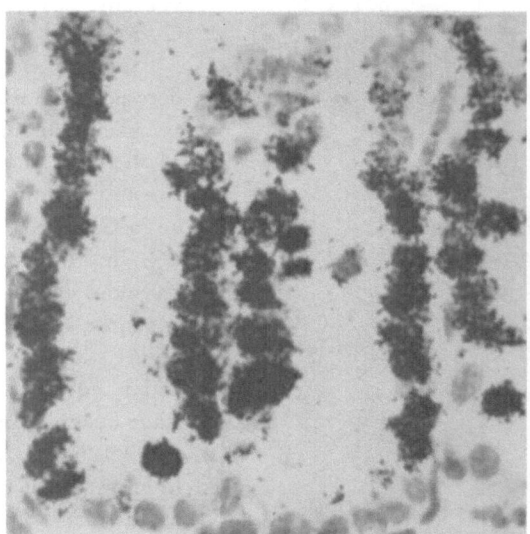

Fig. 4. Heavily labeled nuclei following 5 injections of ^{3}HTdR (5 μCi each) 2 hours apart. All cells in proliferative compartment labeled. Labeled cells have moved into the maturation zone. No Paneth cells labeled.

The labeled mitosis method (11) was used to obtain estimates of the generation cycle (GT) and the four phases of the cycle: G_1, S, G_2 and M. To use this method, a series of animals must be injected with ^{3}HTdR and sacrificed at ½ to 1 hour intervals after injection, autoradiographs prepared from fixed tissue samples, mitotic figures scored as to labeled or not labeled, and the percent of labeled mitotic figure data plotted against time after injection. The cyclic labeled mitosis curve obtained for a 100 day old BCF_1 mouse is shown in Fig. 5. The critical segments of the labeled mitosis curve are the first and second rising arms and the first descending

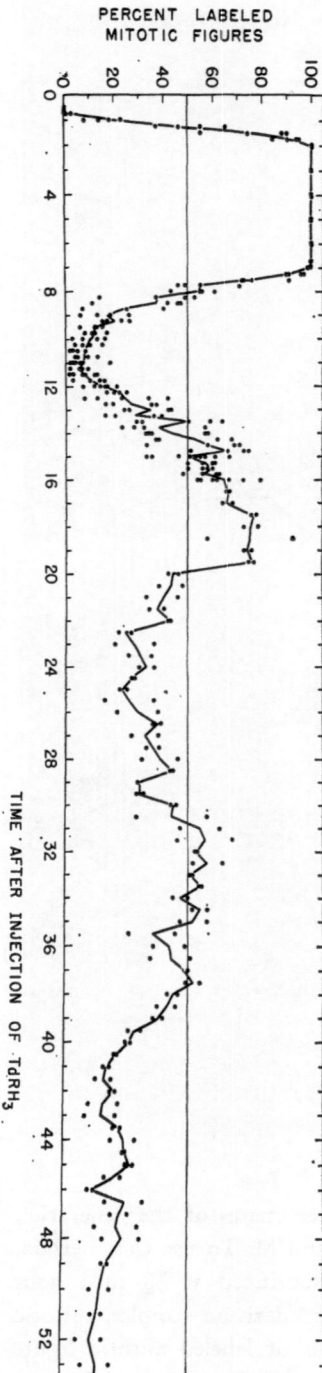

PERCENT LABELED
MITOTIC FIGURES

TIME AFTER INJECTION OF TdRH3

arm. To obtain accurate estimates of GT, G_1, S, G_2 and M, the interval between sacrifices must be decreased and the number of animals at each sacrifice increased during the time intervals covered by the three critical segments.

To further increase the accuracy of these estimates and to minimize the selection bias of the estimator, a linear regression line can be fitted to the first rising arm and a quadratic regression line to the first descending arm and the second rising arm. The point at which the regression line for the first rising arm intersects the 0% labeled time axis is t_0, while t_1, t_2, and t_3 are the points at which the regression lines for the first ascending arm, the first descending arm and the second ascending arm cross the 50% labeled mitosis levels. Using these values: $GT = t_3 - t_1$; $G_1 = t_3 - t_2 - 2t_1 + t_0$; $S = t_2 - t_1$; $G_2 = t_0$; and $M = 2(t_1 - t_0)$. This gives a value of 13.1 hours for GT, 4.6 hours for G_1, 6.9 hours for S, 1.0 hour for G_2 and 0.7 hour for M (9).

Since it seems highly probable that the P zone does not contain a G_0 complement of cells it can be assumed that all cells are in one of the four phases at all times. Using the above estimates of GT, G_1, S, G_2, and M approximately 30 to 35% of the cells will be in G_1, 50 to 55% in S, 8 to 12% in G_2, and 4 to 6% in M. If the proliferative population is asynchronous and GT is not affected by time of day then it can be assumed that the proportion of cells in different stages of the cell cycle is the same at any time and is equal to the proportion of time which that stage occupies in the whole cycle. Using the estimate of 13.1 hours for GT and 6.9 hours for S and the mean number of initially labeled nuclei per whole crypt squash a calculated estimate of 126 cells/crypt in the P zone is obtained.

Fig. 5. A labeled mitosis curve obtained (after injecting 100 day old BCF$_1$ mice with 10 μCi of ^{3}HTdR) by plotting percent labeled mitosis figures against time at closely spaced intervals.

Changes in Cell Production

Although cell proliferation is extremely high in the crypts of the intestinal epithelium, the rate is sensitive to various factors, such as environmental conditions, nutritional level, presence or absence of bacteria, metabolic inhibitors, partial resection, irradiation, etc. The proliferative cells appear to have threshold tolerances such that within certain levels there seems to be no effect. However, if the stress is beyond this threshold level and period of exposure is extended, the cell production rate changes.

This has been shown by Adelstein's (1) low temperature experiments in which he studied cell proliferation in the small intestinal crypts of the hibernating dormouse finding that there was a pronounced reduction in number of cells in S and M which suggests an increase in GT. Generation time is also longer in the duodenal crypts of germ free mice than in conventional animals of the same strain (10). On the other hand, there is an acceleration of the generation cycle and an increase in the size of the proliferative population in mice and rats after irradiation or following partial resection. An analysis of irradiation experiments shows that as the exposure level increases and more cells are killed, the greater the reduction in the generation cycle time and the larger the increase in the proliferation population.

In general, it would appear that a stress beyond the normal threshold tolerance level which affects metabolic rates or produces cell death leads to a reduction in GT and hence an increase in cell proliferation. Furthermore, this change in production rate appears to be directly related to the need for cells. If there is a need, production increases; but if the need decreases, cell production is reduced. Reduction in proliferative rate appears to be accomplished by a simple increase in the generation cycle time without a noticeable change in the proliferative compartment size. However, increased production by shortening the duration of the generation cycle is limited even if G_1 is eliminated and S is reduced. Maximum reduction observed at 72 hours after 1000R whole body x-ray was from 13.1 to 7.5 hours and this would not double production. Hence, the size of the proliferative compartment must increase and it does. The increase after 1000R is 6—8 times normal four days after exposure. Mechanisms which lead to this amazing compensatory cell behavior are unknown, but changes in cell mass and/or the ratio of nonproliferative to proliferative cell populations may trigger-off the feedback reactions.

References

1. ADELSTEIN, J., LYMAN, C. P. and O'BRIEN, R. C.: Variation in the incorporation of thymidine into the DNA of some rodent species. Comp. Biochem. Physiol. 12, 223 (1964).
2. BAUMAN, J. and LESHER, S.: (unpublished data).
3. BIZZOZERO, G.: Ueber die schlauchförmigen Drüsen des Magendarmkanals und die Beziehungen ihres Epithels zu der Oberflächenepithel der Schleimhaut. Arch. Mikr. Anat. 40, 325 (1892).

4. FRY, R. J. M., LESHER, S. and KOHN, H. I.: Influence of age on the transit time cells of the mouse intestinal epithelium. Lab. Invest. 11, 289 (1962).

5. FRY, R. J. M., LESHER, S. and KOHN, H. I.: Age effect on cell-transit time in mouse jejunal epithelium. Amer. J. Physiol. 201, 213 (1961b).

6. LAJTHA, L. G.: Bone marrow stem cell kinetics. Editions du Centre National de la Reserche Scientifique, VII, 411 (1963).

7. LEBLOND, C. P. and STEVENS, C. E.: The constant renewal of the intestinal epithelium in the albino rat. Anat. Rec. 100, 357 (1948).

8. LESHER, S., FRY, R. J. M. and KOHN, H. I.: Influence of age on transit time of mouse cells intestinal epithelium. Lab. Invest. 10, 291 (1961a).

9. LESHER, S. and SACHER, G. A.: Changes in cell proliferation produced by 12 Roentgens of ^{60}co. gamma irradiation per day in the intestinal crypt cells of 100-, 400-, and 825-day-old BCF$_1$ mice. Rad. Res. 30, 654 (1967).

10. LESHER, S., WALBURG, H. E. and SACHER, G. A.: Generation cycle in the duodenal crypt cells of germ-free and conventional mice. Nature 202, 884 (1964).

11. PAINTER, R. B. and DREW, R. M.: Studies on deoxyribonucleic acid metabolism in human cancer cell cultures (HeLa). The temporal relationship of deoxyribonucleic acid synthesis to mitosis and turnover time. Lab. Invest. 8, 278 (1959).

12. QUASTLER, H. and SHERMAN, F. G.: Cell population kinetics in the intestinal epithelium of the mouse. Exp. Cell Res. 17, 420 (1959).

Discussion

Proliferation of Gastrointestinal Cells

MARTIN LIPKIN

Department of Medicine
Cornell University
New York, New York

This discussion continues the description of cell proliferation kinetics in gastrointestinal mucosa, particularly as it applies to man.

Dr. Lesher has described characteristics of proliferation in rodents, including the duration of the generative cycle and its phases, the size of the proliferative pool and the location of proliferative and non-proliferative cells. I should like to point out some of the similarities and differences in these characteristics both in different parts of the gastrointestinal tract, and between man and rodents. I should also like to mention some alterations in cell proliferation during the development of mucosal disease, and the possible relationships to the development of malignancy.

In measuring the phases of the proliferative cell cycle after injecting tritiated thymidine and constructing labeled mitosis curves, we have found longer duration of the cell cycle in man than in rodents. Durations of the G$_2$ phase in proliferating gastrointestinal cells of man have extended from around 1–7 hours, S phase from 10–20 hours, G_1 phase in the order of 10 or 20 hours, and the entire cell cycle in the order of 1–2 days (13, 14). We have also seen a longer G_2 duration, extending to 15 hours in a villous papilloma. In another instance, the G_2 duration of a rectal carcinoma was within previously observed normal limits, while G_2 of the histologically normal adjacent tissue was prolonged. The S phase durations of both cell types were normal. The specific metabolic alterations occurring during G_2 that lead to delay in the onset of mitosis have not been defined. Important metabolic events occurring include synthesis of RNA and proteins needed for mitosis (11, 20). The probability that cells normally stop in G_1, and that G_2 arrest is usually abnormal, has been referred to during this symposium.

Additional insight into the nature of proliferating populations of cells may be gained by constructing theoretical labeled mitosis curves having known population elements and comparing them to experimental curves. We have studied the proliferative cycle in different areas of the gastrointestinal tract in this manner. Our data derived from newborn hamsters and man are compatible with approximately 2:1 spreads of cycle durations among the cells that comprise the proliferating population. In hamsters, the proliferative rates were fastest in the small intestines and slowest in the sigmoid colon. In different regions of the same column of proliferating cells, marked changes in cell cycle duration did not develop as cells migrated toward the lumen (14, 15). The possibility that levels of nucleic acid enzymes differ in different areas of the gastrointestinal tract is also being examined (6).

Proliferative rates therefore vary in different areas of the gastrointestinal tract. Fewer cells re-entered the proliferative cycle shortly after cell division in the sigmoid colon and stomach than in small intestine (15). This finding is of interest in view of the fact that carcinomas in man are more common in the sigmoid colon and stomach while rare in the small intestine. A more rapid re-entry into the proliferative cycle, less decay of synchronization of the repetitive cycles, and more efficient removal of cells from the mucosa appear to be associated with a lower incidence of carcinomas.

Earlier in this symposium, Dr. Lamerton emphasized the importance of considering regulatory factors affecting the organization of cells in tissues, in addition to those concerned with metabolic events within cells. Our studies of disease in man have revealed instances of alterations in both, contributing to the development of abnormalities in gastrointestinal mucosa. The alterations may be transient or permanent. For example, in the large intestine and stomach, cell proliferation takes place in the deep portion of the crypts and gastric pits. From there, maturing cells migrate to the luminal surface of the mucosa to be extruded. These cells undergo maturation and cease to make new DNA or undergo mitosis. In a number of diseases that have been considered precancerous, i.e., familial polyposis, gastric atrophy of pernicious anemia, and villous papilloma, this is not so. Epithelial cells continue to synthesize DNA when present on the surface of the mucosa where they have characteristics of mature cells. In some instances, histologically normal mucosa adjacent to mucosal excrescences also contains maturing cells that continue to synthesize DNA. This is also true of tissues undergoing early hyperplasia, and continued DNA synthesis in these cells appears to be an early sign of this change (2).

In the opposite direction, decreased DNA synthesis and mitosis have been observed before and during the development of experimental stress erosions of gastric mucosa (10). Here, the application of a whole body restraining procedure induces a sequence of events within the cells that leads to a decrease in DNA synthesis throughout most of the gastrointestinal tract. In gastric cells RNA is also lost shortly after the external stress is applied. The rates of synthesis of RNA and mucoprotein decline, and cellular necrosis and erosions develop in the mucosa (7). The action of stress on the cells of the mucosa may be mediated in part by events within the central nervous system, for lesions in the central nervous system also depress cell proliferation (16).

Analysis of the critical pathways through which proliferating cells and elements in their environment interact to influence the cell cycle, should provide interesting areas for future research. Events occurring within proliferating cells critical to initiation of DNA synthesis and mitosis will be the subject of additional discussions at this symposium. Within recent years a number of important events have been clarified, although all steps necessary for initiation of DNA synthesis have not been elucidated. It is known, however, that enzymes leading to DNA synthesis are elaborated in G_1 phase in a number of cell systems. Specific RNA's and proteins are also produced before DNA synthesis begins (4, 17, 12, 18, 9), and it has been suggested that protein synthesis as well as a specific protein are necessary for the initiation of replication (3, 8, 19). At the present time the sequence of alterations leading to synthesis of DNA in certain maturing gastrointestinal cells has not been clarified. Normally, the factors mentioned above and others unknown influence the initiation of DNA synthesis, with asynchronous replication of chromosomes at multiple sites and activation of genetic units of transcription to yield messenger RNA (1, 5, 21). As noted above, physiological changes within the organism may bring about a decrease as well as an increase in some of these activities, demonstrating transient or permanent alterations together with the expressions of different forms of disease.

References

1. BEERMAN, W.: Structure and function of interphase chromosomes. Proc. Intl. Cong. Genetics 2, 375 (1963).
2. DESCHNER, E., LIPKIN, M. and SOLOMON, C.: Study of human rectal epithelial cells in vitro. II. H³ thymidine incorporation into polyps and adjacent mucosa. J. Natl. Cancer Institute 36, 849 (1966).
3. HANAWALT, P. C., MAALOE, O., CUMMINGS, D. J. and SCHAECHTER, M.: The normal DNA replication cycle. II. J. Molec. Biol. 3, 156 (1961).
4. HOTTA, Y.: Molecular facets of mitotic regulation. I. Synthesis of thymidine kinase. Proc. Natl. Acad. Sci. 49, 648 (1963).
5. HSU, T. C.: Mammalian chromosomes in vitro. XVIII. DNA replication in the Chinese hamster. J. Cell. Biol. 23, 53 (1964).
6. IMONDI, A. R., LIPKIN, M. and BALIS, M. E.: Distribution of enzymes involved in nucleic acid metabolism in the gastrointestinal tract (abstract). Federation Proc. 27, No. 2, 787 (1968).

7. IMONDI, A. R., BALIS, M. E. and LIPKIN, M.: Nucleic acid metabolism in the gastro-intestinal tract of mice during restraint stress (abstract). J. Clin. Invest. 47, 50a (1968).

8. KILLANDER, D. and ZETTERBERG, A.: A quantitative cytochemical investigation of the relationship between cell mass and initiation of DNA synthesis in mouse fibroblasts *in vitro*. Exp. Cell. Res. 40, 12 (1965).

9. KILLANDER, D. and ZETTERBERG, A.: Quantitative cytochemical studies on interphase growth. I. Exp. Cell Res. 38, 272 (1965).

10. KIM, Y. S., KERR, R. and LIPKIN, M.: Cell proliferation during the development of stress erosions in mouse stomach. Nature 215, 1180 (1967).

11. KISHIMOTO, S. and LIEBERMAN, I.: Synthesis of RNA and protein required for the mitosis of mammalian cells. Exp. Cell. Res. 36, 92 (1964).

12. LIEBERMAN, I. and OVE, P.: Deoxyribonucleic acid synthesis and its inhibition in mammalian cells cultured from the animals. J. Biol. Chem. 237, 1634 (1962).

13. LIPKIN, M.: Cell replication in the gastrointestinal tract of man. Gastroenterology 48, 616 (1965).

14. LIPKIN, M. and BELL, B. Cell proliferation. *In:* Handbook of Physiology, Section 6, The Alimentary Canal. W. Heidel and C. F. Code (ed.). American Physiological Society, Washington, D.C. Vol. 5, Chapter 138, 2861 (1968).

15. LIPKIN, M. and DESCHNER, E.: Comparative analysis of cell proliferation in the gastrointestinal tract of newborn hamster. Exp. Cell Res. 49, 1, 1968.

16. LIPKIN, M.: (unpublished data).

17. MAZIA, D.: Synthetic activities leading to mitosis. J. Cellular Comp. Physiol. 62 (Suppl. 1), 123 (1963).

18. STONE, G. E. and PRESCOTT, D. M.: Cell division and DNA synthesis in tetrahymena pyriformis deprived of essential amino acids. J. Cell Biol. 21, 275 (1964).

19. TAYLOR, E. W.: Control of DNA synthesis in mammalian cells in culture. Exp. Cell. Res. 40, 316 (1965).

20. TAYLOR, E. W.: Relation of protein synthesis to the division cycle in mammalian cell cultures. J. Cell Biol. 19, 1 (1963).

21. TAYLOR, J. H.: Asynchronous duplication of chromosomes in cultured cells of Chinese hamster. J. Biophys. and Bioch. Cytol. 7, 455 (1960).

General Discussion

Symposium on Normal and Malignant Cell Growth

DR. FRY: All of the papers which we've heard this morning are open for general discussion.

DR. BASERGA: I have a question for Professor Lamerton. You have shown some nice symmetrical labeled mitoses curves. Recently we have seen more of these curves that are very asymmetrical or curves that never reach 100 percent labeled. For instance, curves for the shope papilloma stimulated epithelial culture or some of the minimal deviation hepatomas that grow slowly, never reach the 100 percent labeled level. Would you like to comment on what causes this?

PROFESSOR LAMERTON: One of the reasons is that you can get a very considerable spread in G_2 in the cell cycle. Even temporary arrest may occur between the end of synthesis and the beginning of mitosis. I think there are some very odd labeled mitoses curves in the literature, particularly for the ascites tumors. You yourself have obtained a curve in which the fraction of mitoses labeled increases and then stays up for a very long time. These curves are rather difficult to understand. Under certain conditions it may be due to a greatly prolonged DNA synthesis.

DR. BOND: I would like to ask Dr. Lesher a question. You have shown, very beautifully, after irradiation the absolute number of labeled cells, presumably stem cells, increases in the crypt. To draw an analogy in the bone marrow, the absolute number of labeled cells could increase either by an increase in the stem cells or by an increase in cells that are committed but can only become mature cells. Do you have any information to indicate that in the crypt this increase in labeled cells is in fact stem cells or an increase in the number of perhaps some intermediate pool destined to become mature cells?

DR. LESHER: I feel that this tremendous increase in the proliferative population is due primarily to the fact that they do not differentiate; they retain their capability of dividing and they divide 6–8 times before going out onto the villus and therefore the crpyt becomes enormous in size.

DR. HALEY: *Loyola Medical School.* I would like to ask a question of either Dr. Bucher or Dr. Grisham. At what stage are we in the identification and isolation of humoral factors that may appear after hepatectomy?

DR. GRISHAM: We are still in the dark ages.

DR. MARUYAMA: *University of Minnesota.* Is every hepatocyte potentially capable of division or is there a stem cell compartment which is responsible for the regeneration of liver following subtotal hepatectomy?

DR. GRISHAM: Well, I guess it depends on how you define stem cells and therefore it becomes a semantic problem which I am not qualified to judge. I think, however, in the way I understand the definition of stem cells, I would say "no" that there is not a stem cell population. I think any hepatocyte is capable of proliferating, but yet only a certain number of them are triggered to divide. The ones that are triggered appear to go through several proliferative cycles.

DR. BERTALANFFY: Dr. Grisham, what sort of rates of cell formation did you obtain in the liver at the time of maximum proliferation after partial hepatectomy?

DR. GRISHAM: Twenty-five to 30 percent labeled cells, after flash labeling, is the maximum.

DR. BASERGA: Dr. Grisham, the evidence you and Nancy Bucher presented is very interesting, but the concentrations of albumin in the blood is completely controlled by the liver and as soon as partial hepatectomy is performed, the cells of the liver are pouring albumin into the blood. If you have a heterograft, you may be doing the same. It has been shown that albumin does appear in the blood after partial hepatectomy and does come from the cells of the liver. It has also been shown that after plasmaphoresis cells of the liver go into DNA synthesis. So all of your results could be compatible simply with the loss of proteins, albumin and maybe other proteins from liver cells.

DR. GRISHAM: I think the possibilities are wide open. I try to retain an open mind, but I think the kinetics change in albumin synthesis after partial hepatectomy. The fall in albumin concentration in the peripheral blood is too slow to really explain the results. With plasmaphoresis you take many things out of the blood besides albumin, and I doubt seriously that it is the explanation. I seem to recall, that in rats hypertransfused with albumin, albumin doesn't feedback on its own synthesis. If the level of albumin in the blood doesn't control its own synthesis, it seems unlikely that it controls proliferation. I think that it is all speculation at the present time.

DR. SCHWEPPE: *Chicago.* I would like to ask if there is any change in lysine or arginine histone in regenerating liver and if there is any evidence of change in the turnover of these substances.

DR. BUCHER: I don't know of any specific studies.

DR. SCHWEPPE: I think there is a change in total DNA histone ratio, but I think there is also some work on the relationship of arginine and lysine histones to cell proliferation. I wonder if there is any evidence from studies on regenerating liver.

DR. BUCHER: I don't know of any data on that specific point.

DR. SCHREK: Dr. Lajtha, in measuring the number of cells that can form colonies, you seem to be measuring two capacities of the cells: First, the capacity to multiply and second, the capacity to, you might say, transplant and it seems that the second capacity is more easily destroyed by insults than the first. This might explain some of the peculiarities of the number of cells that produce colonies.

DR. LAJTHA: I think that is a very real possibility. One of the main problems really is, as Dr. Bond has pointed out, that after radiation where the limb has been shielded you get a tremendous loss of colony forming cells in that limb. The number of these cells goes down to about a third or so of the control value, which is about a 1000 colony formers per femur. As far as the seeding rate is concerned, in Hanks' original experiments (Hellman confirmed the results) it is about 2–3 per hour into the spleen. Though not detectable, there is a loss of cells which go somewhere where they don't take. So we are dealing with an extremely difficult situation where the cells can go to the spleen and take there with a certain efficiency which may not be the same as the F factor with exografting. It could be that the mode doesn't change after radiation. We are trying to measure a combination of things; the actual proliferation where the cells take, and where the cells go when they don't take, and why they don't take.

DR. FRY: What is a colony forming unit cell when it is at home?

DR. LAJTHA: It does exactly the same thing in the spleen or in the bone marrow. It proliferates when there is some chance for it to proliferate, and it can give rise to a differentiated line of cells.

DR. FRY: You said that it didn't proliferate when in the marrow?

DR. LAJTHA: Under normal steady state conditions most of them do not proliferate. Most of them do not proliferate anywhere. The growth fraction is probably between 10 and 20 percent in normal steady state in the mouse.

DR. DeGOWIN: *Univ. of Chicago.* Dr. Lajtha, would you comment on the relationship of the capacity of stem cells to form colonies and their capacity to respond to erythropoietin and differentiate.

DR. LAJTHA: Once upon a time in the good old days, I believed that these two could be correlated. I have come to the very regrettable conclusion that they cannot be correlated at the moment. The reason for this is that we are probably dealing with two different kinds of cells. There is an increasing amount of evidence that the colony forming stem cell is a pluripotent primary stem cell. In the mouse, we have evidence that the colony forming cell certainly can form erythroid cells, myeloid cells, platelets and probably even immunocytes. In man, we know that it can form platelets, granulocytes, erythrocytes, but certainly not lymphocytes. The Philadelphia chromosome made it possible to show this. Now these stem cells apparently give rise to a secondary stem cell population which is essentially a transient population which has between 10 and 20 divisions. These cells are committed cells, but not completely differentiated. This is the cell which can respond to erythropoietin which Cliff Gurney termed the ERC—erythropoietin responsive cell. There is very good evidence from Professor Lamerton's department that the proliferative state of these two populations is very different. A large fraction of the colony forming cells are in G_0 perhaps 80–90 percent. While practically none of the secondary stem cells, ERCs, are in G_0. Now the question is do these secondary stem cells just proliferate madly for 20 divisions and then die or are they proliferating and their proliferation is counteracted by the normal erythropoietin level pulling them out for erythropoiesis. I think the evidence which Frank Trobaugh and his group have shown is that they are proliferating and die because in the grafted polycythemic mouse you can reinstate the large erythropoietic colonies straight away with erythropoietin so these secondary stem cells are there in large numbers. What has to be done now is some very careful, patient histology by heroic Ph.D. students to look at these small colonies and identify morphologically those committed but not yet differentiated secondary stem cell populations. There are two different cell lines, one of course originating from the other.

DR. J. F. BOHORQUEZ: *Michael Reese Hospital.* I would like to ask Dr. Lesher whether there was any relationship between the increase in labeled cells with the dose of radiation and if there was any difference between giving total body irradiation and localized irradiation to a small segment of the intestine?

DR. LESHER: In answer to the first question: yes; to the second question: we don't know. There is a very intimate relationship between the dose and the response. The higher the dose, the longer the length of inhibition of mitosis. The higher the dose, the greater the overshoot.

DR. GRISHAM: Dr. Lajtha, how do you distinguish G_0 cells from G_1 cells?

DR. LAJTHA: Conceptually, it is very easy; experimentally, it is very difficult. However there is experimental proof for it now from a paper which is going to be published very soon by Dr. Brown from Oxford. If you plot against time the proportion of labeled cells in a population which has been continuously labeled and if you have a true G_0 population in which cell can be pulled out of or put into the cell cycle, you should get an increasing line which approaches 100 percent but never reaches it. If you are dealing with a long G_1, which varies in length, but nevertheless has a finite length, then the curve should initially be very similar; it might start a little bit steeper but it will certainly reach 100 percent. In the hamster cheek pouch epithelium Dr. Brown found that this is the case. There was quite a bit of argument whether there is a G_0 or a long G_1 and from the experimental data Brown has indicated that it is probably a long G_1.

DR. LAMERTON: Dr. Grisham, in one of the tables you showed the growth fraction and cell cycle for rats of different ages; the rat of 8–12 weeks had a cell cycle of something like 21 hours and a very small growth fraction. How did you measure the cell cycle? You have a very, very low mitotic index, and I don't see how you did it.

DR. GRISHAM: These are the data reported in the literature. They are not my own. I think the report with the lowest rate of proliferation is by E. Stöcker.[*] He didn't measure the cycle from the labeled mitoses curve but he computed it from the duration of DNA synthesis of 15–18 hours in the very old rats. I think it has to be taken with a grain of salt.

DR. LAMERTON: I have not been convinced by determinations of cell cycles by that method.

DR. GRISHAM: Well, I certainly agree with that.

DR. BASERGA: Dr. Lipkin, the DNA polymerase activity that you reported is higher in the liver than in the small intestine. This is strange unless it is a regenerating liver. Could you please explain this?

DR. LIPKIN: We have a small amount of data for a number of enzymes, but the data that we do have is, I think, compatible with that in the literature on enzymes of this type. The level of the enzyme is not necessarily correlated with the proliferative activity. Of course in the case of DNA polymerase, its exact role and whether it is a regulatory enzyme or not is the question. But, in general, the levels of enzymes concerned with DNA synthesis do not always reflect the rate of proliferative activity in liver and various parts of the gastrointestinal tract. This appears to be a peculiar finding, but I believe that in the case of the measurements made on tumor tissue reported in the literature it also appears to be so.

DR. WISSLER: I can't restrain myself from asking Nancy Bucher what the restraint does. It seems to me that the most remarkable effects that you showed were those due to restraint, and this certainly is a very large effect and might work for malignant tissues or other kinds of cells.

DR. BUCHER: Well, restraint has more of an effect, if you remember, in animals that have already been insulted. It is sort of the straw that breaks the camel's back. I don't know what restraint does; we are trying to find out because it would help us a great deal.

DR. WISSLER: Can you do the same thing with corticoids?

---

* Stöcker, E.: Der Proliferationsmodus in Niere und Leber. Verhandl. Deutsch. Gesellsch. f. Path. **50**, 53–74 (1966).

DR. BUCHER: We haven't yet tried. We have really just begun work on this. At the moment, we are looking at endotoxins to find out if they get to the liver and whether that has something to do with it. I haven't any data to give you yet.

DR. LIPKIN: May I add that restraint also appears to have a very profound effect on the incorporation of thymidine into the gastrointestinal mucosa and restraint in the small animals appears to depress the incorporation of thymidine into DNA in all areas of the gastrointestinal tract.

DR. FRY: Presumably due to vasoconstriction.

DR. PHILIPS: I have heard, although I have never seen it myself, that if you restrain a rat without anesthesia overnight or for 24 hours by the next day it may have a stomach ulcer and be near death.

DR. BUCHER: That has been reported a number of times and I think it is true. That is supposed to be related to the endotoxins and is why we are looking at them.

DR. WISSLER: I would also like to ask either Dr. Bucher or Dr. Grisham whether any work has been done so far on the hepatomas that Morris has produced in terms of their response to a humoral factor.

DR. BUCHER: I don't know.

Proliferation of Antibody-Forming Cells

DAVID W. TALMAGE

Departments of Microbiology and Medicine
University of Colorado
Denver, Colorado

I want to stress two things in my brief comments. First, it is clear that cell division is essential to the process of antibody formation, just as it is to the maturation of most cells. Second, I want to stress that we know very little else about the cellular dynamics of antibody formation. However, there are a few interesting things about what we don't know, and these I would like to mention.

What is the evidence for the necessity of cell division in the process of antibody formation? Burnet and Fenner (1) were the first to point out many years ago that the serum antibody titer expressed on a log scale rose in a straight line with a doubling time of 6–8 hours. At that time the doubling time of mammalian cells was not known, but Burnet and Fenner made the suggestion that a replicating unit was essential to the process of antibody formation. It has also been known for many years that the process of antibody formation is very sensitive to x-rays and to radiomimetic drugs. Perhaps Dr. Rowley will comment on his experiments with colchicine. The extreme sensitivity of antibody formation to x-ray and related agents certainly is consistent with the idea that antibody formation requires cell division. Another indirect piece of evidence is the appearance of antibody forming cells in clusters in the lymph nodes and spleen. This was pointed out many years ago by Albert Coons with the fluorescent antibody technique (3). More recently it has been possible to demonstrate this clumping with two interesting techniques, one by Playfair, Papermaster and Cole (9) and the other by Kennedy, Till, Siminovitch and McCulloch (6).

The latter technique is illustrated in Fig. 1. This is an agar plate with sheep red cells in the agar. A mouse was subjected to whole body x-radiation, injected with a limited number of spleen cells from a normal animal and then immunized with the sheep red cell antigen. The spleen was taken out after a few days and sliced on a microtome and the serial sections of the mouse spleen overlayed on the agar plate. The spleen sections were floated off an hour later by a solution of complement. The colonies of antibody forming cells producing lysis in the antigen agar can be clearly seen extending through several sections of the spleen.

The incorporation of tritium labeled thymidine into precursors of antibody forming cells is further evidence of cell proliferation (8). One of the most impressive pieces of evidence that cell division is essential in the maturation of antibody forming cells is the recent work by Dutton and Mishell (5) using their *in vitro* technique of

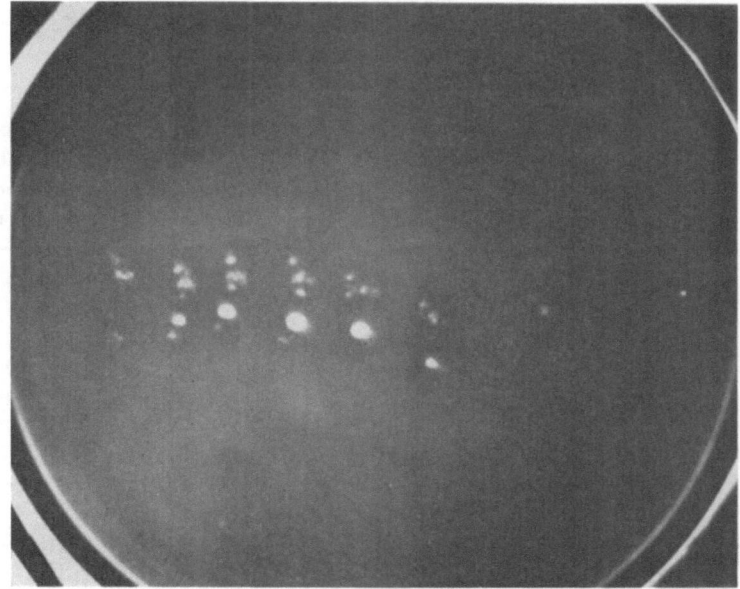

Fig. 1. Colonies of antibody forming cells demonstrable in serial frozen sections of a spleen by the technique of Kennedy, Till, Siminovitch and McCulloch.

antibody formation. With this technique these workers were able to show that very high specific activity tritium labeled thymidine could abolish the antibody response *in vitro*. I'll say more about this later because I think the timing of the action is very important.

Now I would like to review for you very briefly some data on the effects of x-ray on the antibody response that was collected by Dixon's (4) and Taliaferro's groups (12) simultaneously in 1951. This data was difficult to explain 17 years ago, and I still don't understand it today. Anything that is inexplicable for that long is worth looking at again.

Table 1 illustrates the extreme sensitivity of the antibody response to small doses of whole body radiation, both by the peak antibody titer, which is shown in the last column, and in the fraction of animals showing an immune elimination of the radioactively labeled antigen. All normal animals showed this immune elimination between day 5 and day 7. There was no significant effect from 25 r. The effects of 50 r and 75 r were questionable with a suggestion of some delay plus a drop in peak titer. With 125 r there was a very definite prolongation and a marked suppression of peak titer. With 200 r there was an extremely marked drop in the peak titer and a markedly prolonged response. With 300 r there was little if any response.

This sensitivity, I think, is important. If one assumes a 90 percent destruction of the precursor cells similar to that of mammalian cells in culture, then the remaining cells should reconstitute their number in 3 or 4 divisions. Since it appears that peak titer is determined by a feedback shut off by antibody, this value is a relatively poor reflection of the number of precursor cells at the start. With a 90 percent reduction

TABLE 1

Dose of X-Ray and Antibody Response

Experimental group	No. of animals	Fraction of rabbits showing immune antigen disappearance rate				Maximum antibody concentration
		4–7 Day	7–9 Day	9–11 Day	11–13 Day	
Control	16	16/16				16.4 ± 10
25 r	9	9/9				14.5 ± 7
50 r	8	7/8	7/8			15.8 ± 10
75 r	8	7/8	8/8			10.2 ± 5
125 r	8	4/8	7/8	7/8		5.2 ± 4
200 r	12	0/12	5/12	9/12	12/12	0.5 ± 1.4
300 r	22	0/22	3/22	12/22	16/22	0
400 r	8	0/8	0/8	0/8	2/7	0
600 r	11	0/11	0/11	2/10	2/10	0

From Dixon *et al.* (reference 4).

in precursor cells, there should be only a 1-day delay in the response and not necessarily any drop in peak titer. The marked reduction in peak titer and also the marked delay, much more than 1 day, in the rise of antibody, is difficult to explain.

The next point, illustrated in Table 2, is that the timing of the exposure x-rays with respect to the injection of antigen is important. If 400 r was given 6 hours after

TABLE 2

Time of X-Ray and Antibody Response

Experimental group	Fraction of rabbits showing immune antigen disappearance rate				Maximum antibody concentration
	4–7 Day	7–9 Day	9–11 Day	11–13 Day	
Controls	16/16				16.4 ± 10
400 r 6 hrs after antigen	9/9				14.2 ± 7
400 r simultaneously with antigen	12/18	17/18	18/18		12.7 ± 5
400 r 5 hours before antigen	4/9	8/9	9/9		7.7 ± 4
400 r 12 hours before antigen	0/9	3/9	6/9	9/9	2 ± 2
400 r 48 hours before antigen	0/8	0/8	0/8	2/7	0
800 r 3 days after antigen	0/29	27/29	29/29		16.1 ± 21
800 r 1 hour after antigen	0/8	2/8	6/8	8/8	6.4 ± 6

From Dixon *et al.* (reference 4).

the antigen, there was almost no significant delay or drop in peak titer. If x-ray and antigen were given almost simultaneously, there was a little delay but very little drop in titer. If the exposure to x-rays was 5 hours before the antigen, there was some effect; at 12 hours there was an extremely sharp effect. Something happens to the animal between 5 and 12 hours after exposure to x-rays to make it much less sensitive to the injection of antigen.

Table 3 summarizes the data from Taliaferro's group. The data are very similar to those in Table 2, although they used a different antigen. If the exposure to x-rays was 2 days to 8 hours after the antigen, there was no effect; at 6 hours, there was actually enhancement of the peak titer, although there was a delay. If the exposure to x-rays was 3–6 hours before the antigen, there was a very slight drop while at 12 hours before antigen the response was essentially abolished. In summary I think we can say that there is something unusually complicated about the sensitivity of the immunocompetent cell. It appears that something happens to this cell after exposure to x-radiation which requires some 6–12 hours and that during this time it becomes insensitive to antigen. One possible explanation for the extreme sensitivity of the antibody response to x-ray is that there are two interacting processes involved and that the irradiation is affecting both of them.

Figure 2 shows a model that attempts to explain some of the facts of the antibody response. There are three major kinds of lymphoid cells in a lymph node: small lymphocytes, large lymphocytes and plasma cells, or pyroninophilic antibody forming cells. The arrows here are hypothetical. This model would explain the sensitivity of the antibody to x-radiation if the multiplication of the large lymphocyte were sensitive to x-ray to the same degree as any other dividing cell, and if one also assumed that the transformation of the small lymphocyte to a large cell is also sensitive to x-ray. Thus, there would be two different sites at which the x-radiation would act and this would increase the sensitivity. The model also explains the observation that phytohemagglutinin and antigen produce transformation of small lymphocytes. It explains the fact that tritium labeled thymidine is incorporated into the antibody-forming cell at this stage before it becomes completely mature, and it also explains the timing of the killing or the abolishing of the antibody response in Mishell and Dutton's experiments that I referred to a few minutes ago.

TABLE 3

TIME OF X-RAY AND ANTIBODY RESPONSE

Time of X-ray	Peak titer $\times 10^{-3}$
Control-No X-ray	$3.43 \pm .37$
+2 days	3.65 ± 1.86
+1 day to 8 hr.	5.25 ± 1.68
+6 hr. to 10 min.	6.95 ± 1.17
−3 to 6 hours	2.96 ± 1.0
−12 hr. to 7 days	0.0

FROM Taliaferro et al. (reference 12).

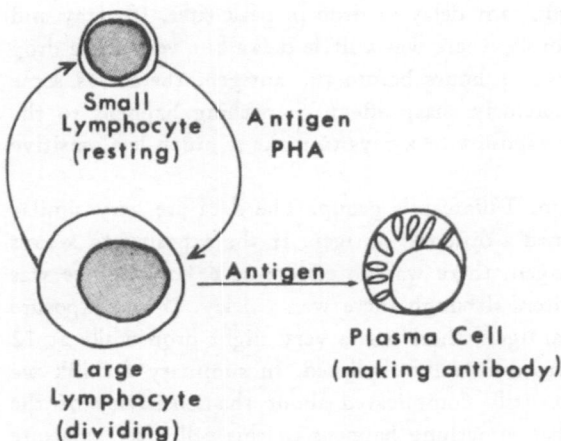

Fig. 2. A model of the cellular dynamics of antibody formation.

In these experiments, a very high specific activity tritium labeled thymidine was used which killed any cell which incorporated labeled thymidine. It was found that if the tritiated thymidine was added before the antigen, it had no effect at all on the antibody response. Presumably the precursor cells were not killed because they were not dividing. If the antigen was given 36 hours before the labeled thymidine, the antibody response was abolished completely.

The only trouble with the model illustrated in Fig. 2 is that it is too simple. For example, it says nothing about an interaction between cells. Claman, Chaperon and Triplett (2) reported two years ago that the immune competence of an irradiated animal could be reconstituted with a combination of thymus cells and bone marrow cells but not with either cell type alone. This work has recently been confirmed by Mitchell and Miller (7) and in addition these authors showed that it was not the thymus cell that was making the antibody but the bone marrow cell. This certainly suggests a complicated interaction between two cell types.

I want to introduce another question at this point; namely, the question of the specificity of the antigen responsive cell. The question is whether one cell responds to more than one antigen. This, of course, has been argued for many years. Nearly everyone would agree that at some stage the cell becomes specific for one antigen, but many think that at an earlier stage it is uncommitted. Figure 3 illustrates the controversy. According to the clonal selection hypothesis there is a precursor cell which has no competence to make antibodies. In the thymus, through the action of the thymic hormone, this cell becomes randomly committed to individual antigens so that there are many different cells, each responding to a different antigen. Most people in this field would agree with the two ends of this line but they think that there is an intermediate step. This intermediate cell is multipotential and capable of responding to many antigens. Following exposure to the antigen this cell becomes restricted in its capabilities.

There is not time to discuss this issue in any length. However, I thought the clonal selection theory was a good idea 10 years ago, and I still think it is a good idea. It is almost impossible to prove the theory because of the difficulty in proving

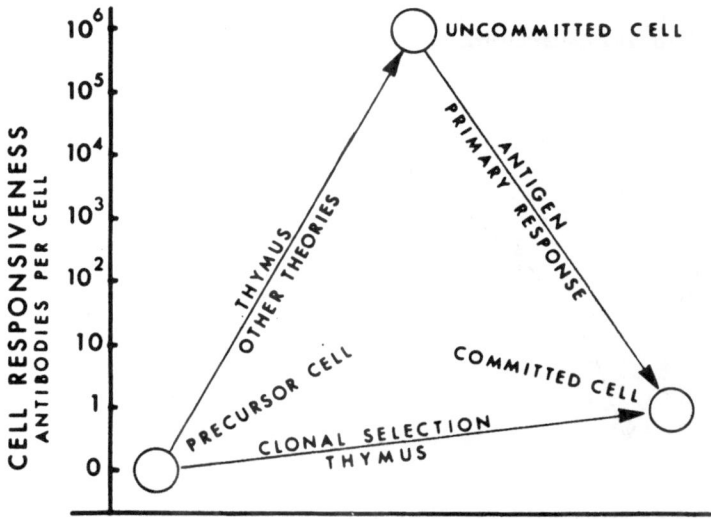

Fig. 3. A diagrammatic representation of the two major hypotheses of cell specificity.

the absence of the multipotential cell. For this reason it would be much easier to disprove the clonal selection theory than to prove it, assuming it were wrong. There have been many efforts to demonstrate the existence of a multipotential cell and one of the claims is based on the fact that if two different antigens are given simultaneously there is some tendency of competition and if one gives the two antigens at different times, there is sometimes a very pronounced suppression of the response to the second antigen.

Figure 4 shows some of our own experiments on antigenic competition (11). We gave two different antigens, sheep and horse red blood cells to LAF_1 mice and varied the interval between the two injections. Four days after the second injection we measured the number of plaque forming cells to the second antigen in the spleen. Compared to the control where only one antigen was given, there was little, if any, competition if the two antigens were given simultaneously, but there was a marked competition if there was a 4 day interval between the two antigens.

Although it is possible to explain the suppression as a competition for a multipotential cell, it also could be a competition for some humoral factor. There are other possible explanations such as a feedback by some humoral factor made in response to the first antigen which suppresses the cell responding to the second antigen. We attempted to get some idea of the mechanism with the experiment described in Table 4 by transferring the competition to an irradiated animal. We transferred two doses of normal spleen cells (10 million) which is about a tenth of a spleen and 50 million cells, about a half of a normal spleen. As indicated in Table 4, in one group sheep red cells only were given on day 0, in another sheep red cells on day 4, and in a third group the two antigens were given, one on day 0 and the other on day 4. There was a much greater depression of the response to the second antigen when 50 million cells were injected than when 10 million cells were injected. Since dilution should in-

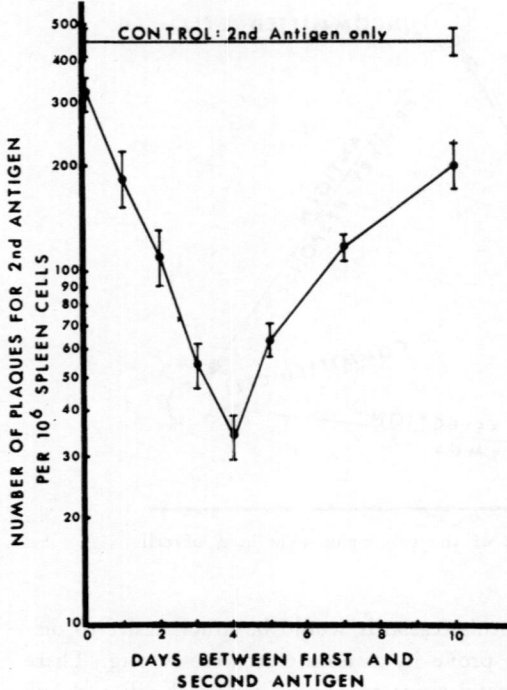

Fig. 4. The response of mice to sheep red blood cells (S-RBC) at various time intervals after the injection of horse red blood cells (H-RBC). Vertical bars indicate standard error.

crease competition for a limited number of cells, but decrease competition for a humoral factor, we concluded that the results were in favor of the latter.

Aside from negating the evidence for a multipotential cell, the experiment above gave additional evidence for cellular interaction. The unit response with 50 million cells transferred was higher than with 10 million. This looked like some kind of synergistic effect, and we decided to investigate this phenomenon a little more (10).

TABLE 4

Response to S-RBC of CO^{60} Irradiated Recipients Receiving Spleen Cells and H-RBC and S-RBC at Various Time Intervals after Cell Transfer

Group	10 × 10⁶ Cells transferred		50 × 10⁶ Cells transferred	
	No. of mice	PFC *	No. of animals	PFC *
I S-RBC Day 0	8	66 ± 14	7	218 ± 25
II S-RBC Day 4	7	181 ± 49	8	102 ± 17
H-RBC Day 0	11	58 ± 7	12	12 ± 5

* Mean PFC for S-RBC per million cells transferred in spleen of recipients 6 days after injection of S-RBC ± S.E. Five irradiated recipients given S-RBC on day 4 but no spleen cells averaged 8 PFC per spleen.

From Radovich et al. (reference 10).

TABLE 5

SIX DAYS ANTIBODY RESPONSE OF CO⁶⁰ IRRADIATED LAF₁ MICE INJECTED I.V. WITH NORMAL SPLEEN CELLS AND S-RBC

Number of animals	Spleen cells transferred $\times 10^{-6}$	Nucleated cells per spleen $\times 10^{-6}$	No. of PFC per 10^6 spleen cells transferred
10	1	15 ± 0.90	4 ± 6
5	7	31 ± 4	57 ± 11
5	50	136 ± 10	204 ± 39

FROM Radovich *et al.* (reference 10).

As indicated in Table 5 we transferred 1 million, 7 million or 50 million normal spleen cells to irradiated mice and the number of plaques per million spleen cells transferred was definitely not constant. There were hardly any plaques with one million cells transferred and more than 200 per million transferred at the highest dose. This type of effect suggests that there are at least two cell populations within the spleen involved in the antibody response. The next experiment, illustrated in Table 6, showed that one of the cell types is present in the bone marrow. If bone marrow cells are injected alone, there is very little response, that is these cells do not reconstitute the immune competence of the irradiated animal. However, if bone marrow cells are added to varying numbers of spleen cells, the unit response per million spleen cells is constant. The same thing was true when experiments were done with spleen cells from immunized animals (Table 7) except that fewer spleen cells were needed and the unit response was about ten times higher.

TABLE 6

ENHANCEMENT OF SIX DAY ANTIBODY RESPONSE BY BONE MARROW CELLS INJECTED I.V. INTO CO⁶⁰ IRRADIATED LAF₁ MICE WITH NORMAL SPLEEN CELLS AND S-RBC

Number of animals	Spleen cells transferred $\times 10^{-6}$	Bone marrow cells transferred $\times 10^{-6}$	Nucleated cells per spleen $\times 10^{-6}$	No. of PFC per 10^6 spleen cells transferred
10	1	0	15 ± 0.95	4 ± 6
5	1	5	118 ± 11	311 ± 259
5	7	0	42 ± 2	181 ± 50
5	7	5	174 ± 11	294 ± 55
5	50	0	181 ± 37	348 ± 172
5	50	5	229 ± 30	287 ± 60

FROM Radovich *et al.* (reference 10).

TABLE 7

ENHANCEMENT OF SIX DAY ANTIBODY RESPONSE BY BONE MARROW CELLS INJECTED I.V.
INTO CO^{60} IRRADIATED LAF_1 MICE WITH IMMUNE SPLEEN CELLS AND S-RBC

Number of animals	Spleen cells transferred $\times 10^{-6}$	Bone marrow cells transferred $\times 10^{-6}$	Nucleated cells per spleen $\times 10^{-6}$	No. of PFC per 10^6 spleen cells transferred
5	.1	0	12 ± 0.65	190 ± 187
5	.1	5	124 ± 12	2,480 ± 1,180
5	.3	0	16 ± 0.98	103 ± 39
5	.3	5	107 ± 12	3,120 ± 562
5	.7	0	18 ± 0.82	1,104 ± 159
5	.7	5	170 ± 9	3,470 ± 1,031
5	5	0	49 ± 4	472 ± 71
5	5	5	260 ± 10	1,702 ± 236

FROM Radovich *et al.* (reference 10).

In summary, the antibody response involves cell division, cell maturation and commitment and cellular interaction. Beyond that very little is known about its cellular dynamics.

References

1. BURNET, F. M. and FENNER, F.: *The Production of Antibodies*. MacMillan and Co., London (1941).
2. CLAMAN, H. N., CHAPERON, E. A. and TRIPLETT, R. F.: Thymus marrow cell combinations. Synergism in antibody production. Proc. Soc. Exp. Biol. Med. **122**, 1167 (1966).
3. COONS, A. F.: The cytology of antibody formation. J. Cell. Comp. Physiol. **52**, 55 (suppl. 1) (1958).
4. DIXON, F. J., TALMADGE, D. W. and MAURER, P. H.: Radiosensitive and radiophases in the antibody response. J. Immunol. **68**, 693 (1952).
5. DUTTON, R. W. and MISHELL, R. I.: Cell populations and cell proliferations in the *in vitro* response of normal mouse spleen to heterologous erythrocytes. Analysis by the hot pulse techniques. J. Exper. Med. **126**, 443 (1967).
6. KENNEDY, J. C., TILL, J. E., SIMINOVITCH, L. and McCULLOCH, E. A.: The proliferative capacity of antigen-sensitive precursors of hemolytic plaque forming cells. J. Immunol. **96**, 973 (1966).
7. MITCHELL, G. F. and MILLER, J. F. A. P.: Immunologic activity of thymus and thoracic duct lymphocytes. Proc. Nat. Acad. Sci. **59**, 296 (1968).
8. NOSSAL, G. J. and MÄKELÄ, O.: Autoradiographic studies on the immune response. I. The kinetics of plasma cell formations. J. Exper. Med. **115**, 209 (1962).
9. PLAYFAIR, J. H. L., PAPERMASTER, B. W. and COLE, L. J.: Local antibody production by transferred spleen cells in irradiated mice. Science **149**, 998 (1965).

10. RADOVICH, J., HEMINGSEN, H. and TALMADGE, D. W. J.: J. Immunol. 100, 756 (1968). (In press.)
11. RADOVICH, J. and TALMADGE, D. W.: Antigenic competition: cellular or humoral. Science 158, 512 (1967).
12. TALIAFERRO, W. H., TALIAFERRO, L. G. and JANSSEN, E. F.: The localization of x-ray injury to the initial phases of antibody response. J. Infect. Dis. 91, 105 (1952).

Discussion

The Proliferation of Antibody-Forming Cells

DONALD A. ROWLEY, FRANK W. FITCH and DONALD E. MOSIER

Department of Pathology
University of Chicago
Chicago, Illinois

These points will be made: 1) the increase in numbers of antibody-forming cells following immunization is due to cell division, 2) the magnitude of an antibody response is determined primarily by the rate of division of responding cells and their progeny, and 3) the rate of division of antibody-forming cells may be determined by the rate of interaction of 2 or more cell types required for the antibody synthesis.

Antibody-forming cells increase exponentially during the early primary immune response. Numerous investigations have confirmed this observation first made by Jerne and Nordin who developed a simple, elegant technique for enumerating cells releasing specific antibody (5). Rats or mice are immunized with sheep erythrocytes. Dispersed spleen cells from the immunized animals are mixed in a sheep erythrocyte-agar culture medium and poured in a thin layer. After brief incubation, the addition of a complement causes lysis of sheep erythrocytes immediately surrounding individual cells which have released anti-sheep erythrocyte hemolysin. The foci or "plaques" of lysis can be readily identified and enumerated. The sensitivity of the method is remarkable. For example, 500 plaque-forming cells mixed with 10^8 or 10^9 other lymphoid cells can be rapidly and accurately enumerated.

One day after intravenous injection of sheep erythrocytes, rat or mouse spleens contain about 10^2 plaque-forming cells; between 1 and 4 days, the numbers increase exponentially with doubling times ranging from about 5.5 to 12 hours. By the 4th day spleens contain 10^4 to 10^6 plaque-forming cells. Titers of circulating antibody, first detectable on the 3rd or 4th day depending on the magnitude of the response, correlate well with numbers of spleen plaque-forming cells.*

---

* The kinetics of the response after the 4th day and during the secondary response are much more complex and to our knowledge not fully worked out; therefore, only the early primary response is considered here.

Models accounting for the increase in antibody-forming cells must conform to the exponential growth law. The simplest models assume either exponential recruitment of cells, or exponential division of cells. Many immunologists suggest that recruitment of cells must occur because cell cycle times of 5 to 6 hours are too short for mammalian cells (2–7). This argument is supported by the experimental work of Sterzl (13) and Tannenberg (15, 6) who prepared autoradiographs of plaque-forming cells obtained from immunized animals injected with radioactive nucleotides. On the basis of analysis of the autoradiograph of spleen cells, they conclude that plaque-forming cells arise in large part from cells which have not undergone recent mitosis. These contentions are challengeable. First, the general argument based solely on an assumed maximum rate of division of mammalian cells is invalidated by recent observations that one population of lymphocytes in calf thoracic duct lymph has cycle times of 5.5 to 6.0 hours (16, 12). Second, Szenberg and Cunningham, using the same general experimental approach as Sterzl and Tannenberg, conclude that most plaque-forming cells have undergone recent mitosis (14). Third, Dutton and Mishell (4), using a high specific activity label technique which caused death of dividing cells, conclude that essentially all plaque-forming cells appearing in *in vitro* immunized cultures of mouse spleen cells could arise by cell division (4, 8).

We have devised a different method using mitotic blocking agents for estimating cell cycle times of plaque-forming cells (13). Two, three or four days after immunization, rats are injected intravenously with colchicine or Velban. The animals are sacrificed 2.5 to 7 hours after drug injection. The numbers of plaque-forming cells in the spleens of these animals are compared with the number in similarly immunized but non-drug-treated controls. Drug treatment causes a reduction in the number of spleen plaque-forming cells, the extent of reduction being directly proportional to the duration of drug treatment. The drug effects are consistent with assumptions that: 1. plaque-forming cells arrested in mitosis do not release sufficient antibody to be detected, 2. mitotic blocking agents by arresting plaque-forming cells in metaphase prevent not only detection of these cells but also the increase in numbers of cells which would have resulted from cell division, and 3. mitotic blocking agents do not affect release of antibody by cells in interphase. Cell cycle times based on the extent of reduction of plaque-forming cells per unit time of drug treatment are estimated using a mathematical model appropriate for exponentially increasing populations of cells.

Cell cycle times estimated 2, 3 or 4 days after immunization with various doses of antigen or antigen and an adjuvant agree well with cell doubling times calculated from the increase in plaque-forming cells. With low doses of antigen, cell cycle and cell doubling times were 10 to 11 hours while with high doses of antigen and an adjuvant the times were 5.5 to 6.0 hours. Similar results were obtained using mitotic blocking agents to estimate cell cycle times of *in vitro* immunized mouse spleen cell cultures; furthermore, it was possible to determine with reasonable certainty that reduced recovery of plaque-forming cells from cultures was caused by the drugs blocking these cells in mitosis (11). We conclude that: 1. the increase in antibody-forming cells is due to exponential division of cells and 2. the magnitude of the antibody response is determined almost entirely by the rate of division of responding cells and their progeny; *i.e.*, higher antigen doses or treatment of animals with an adjuvant increases the antibody response by increasing the rate of division of cells rather than by causing recruitment of additional cells or by increasing the rate of synthesis of antibody by individual cells.

The mechanism whereby antigen dose or an adjuvant regulates the rate of division of responding cells is not known. However, many immunologists assume that the interaction of two different cell types is required for antibody synthesis; one type phagocytizes and "processes" antigen to provide the stimulus for a second type, the lymphoid cells which synthesize specific antibody. These 2 cell types are indeed required for the *in vitro* immunization of dispersed spleen cells (10). It seems likely that the problem is more complicated than this. Miller and Mitchell present compelling evidence for 2 classes of lymphoid cells, each required for antibody synthesis (7, 9). One cell type, the "antigen reactive cell," is thymus derived or dependent, has a long generation time, and is highly sensitive to x-irradiation. "Antigen reactive cells" are considered to be recognition cells; the number of such cells which specifically recognize any one antigen is relatively small. These cells do not produce antibody, but interact with a second cell type which is derived from bone marrow, has a short generation time, and is relatively insensitive to x-irradiation. These cells, the antibody-forming cells, under the direction of the "antigen reactive cells," proliferate and synthesize specific antibody. Thus, the interaction of at least 2 and possibly 3 cell types may be required for antibody synthesis. Conceivably, antigen dose or an adjuvant may affect the magnitude of an antibody response by regulating the nature or rate of interaction between different cell types required for antibody synthesis.

References

1. BAKER, J. P. and LANDY, M.: Brevity of the inductive phase in the immune response of mice to capsular polysaccharide antigens. J. Immunol. **99**, 687 (1967).

2. BERENBAUM, M. C.: Role of mitosis and mitotic inhibition in the immunosuppressive action of thioguanine. Nature 210, 41 (1966).

3. CLAFLIN, A. J. and SMITHIES, O.: Antibody-producing cells in division. Science 157, 1561 (1967).

4. DUTTON, R. W. and MISHELL, R. I.: Cell populations and cell proliferation in the *in vitro* response of normal mouse spleen to heterologous erythrocytes. J. Exptl. Med. **126**, 443 (1967).

5. JERNE, N. K. and NORDIN, A. A.: Plaque-formation in agar by single anti-body producing cells. Science 140, 405 (1963).

6. MALAVIYA, A. and TANNENBERG, W. J. K.: The proliferation rate of 19 S antibody-forming cells during the primary and secondary response. Fed. Proc. 26, 751 (1967).

7. MILLER, J. F. A. P.: The thymus—yesterday, today and tomorrow. The Lancet **II**, 1299 (1967).

8. MISHELL, R. I. and DUTTON, R. W.: Immunization of normal mouse spleen cell suspensions *in vitro*. Science **153**, 1004 (1966).

9. MITCHELL, G. F. and MILLER, J. F. A. P.: Immunological activity of thymus and thoracic duct lymphocytes. Proc. Nat. Acad. Sci. **59**, 296 (1968).

10. MOSIER, D. E.: A requirement for two cell types for antibody formation *in vitro*. Science **158**, 1573 (1967).
11. ROWLEY, D. A., FITCH, F. W., MOSIER, D. E., SOLLIDAY, S., COPPLESON, L. W. and BROWN, B. W.: The rate of division of antibody-forming cells during the early primary immune response. J. Exper. Med. **127**, 983 (1968).
12. SAFIER, S., COTTIER, H., CRONKITE, E. P., JANSEN, C. R., RAI, K. R. and WAGNER, H. P.: Studies on lymphocytes. VI. Evidence showing different generation times for cytologically different lymphoid cell lines in the thoracic duct of the calf. Blood **30**, 301 (1967).
13. STERZL, J., VESELEY, J., JILEK, M. and MANDEL, L.: The inductive phase of antibody formation studied with isolated cells. *In:* Molecular and Cellular Basis of Antibody Formation. J. Sterzl (ed.). Publishing House of the Czechoslovak Academy of Science, Prague, 463 (1965).
14. SZENBERG, A. and CUNNINGHAM, A. J.: DNA synthesis in the development of antibody-forming cells during the early stages of the immune response. Nature **217**, 747 (1968).
15. TANNENBERG, W. J. K.: Induction of 19 S antibody synthesis without stimulation of cellular proliferation. Nature **210**, 41 (1966).
16. WAGNER, H. P., COTTIER, H., CRONKITE, E. P., CUNNINGHAM, L., JANSEN, C. R., and RAI, K. R.: Studies on lymphocytes. V. Short *in vivo* DNA synthesis and generation time of lymphoid cells in the calf thoracic duct after simulated or effective extracorporeal irradiation of circulating blood. Exptl. Cell Res. **46**, 441 (1967).

Composition of the Cell Life Cycle

DAVID M. PRESCOTT

Institute for Developmental Biology
University of Colorado
Boulder, Colorado

The degree of restraint operating on the proliferation of free-living cells of all types is obviously different from that normally imposed on the proliferation of cells within a multicellular organism. The reproduction of free-living cells is limited only by the general nutritional state of the environment. In the stationary phase of a culture of microorganisms, for example, inhibition of cell reproduction stems from exhaustion of one or more essential nutrients, insufficient oxygen, or similar forms of deterioration or depletion of the medium. Such an effect constitutes inhibition but not control or regulation of cell reproduction by environmental factors.

In vitro situations contrast distinctly with the limitation on cell proliferation in multicellular organisms, in which the number of cells in a particular tissue is precisely regulated by highly specific controls over cell division. Populations of different cells, all with the same genetic endowment, share the same general environment within an animal or a plant but have vastly different rates of cell reproduction, *e.g.,* the stem cell population of the erythropoietic tissue, the stem cells of various epithelia, hepatocytes, neurons, *etc.* The dynamic state of the regulatory mechanism is especially apparent with the changes in the rates of cell proliferation that occur following wounding of epithelia, partial hepatectomy, or similar disturbances to renewable tissues. Such regulation must be based on an interplay between the cells and the microenvironment, but the very precise manner with which each cell type is differentially regulated is proof that more is involved than the general, non-specific environmental factors of the type that are responsible for inhibition under *in vitro* conditions.

It is clear that the differentiation of any cell type for performance of a particular, specialized function is at the same time accompanied by differentiation of a highly characteristic regulation of the reproductive rate for that given cell type. Obviously, functional differentiation of cells can only be successful for the multicellular organism if differentiation of rates of cell reproduction is equally precise. As a part of differentiation, each cell type is believed to establish and to maintain a specific microenvironment for itself and by continuous interaction with this microenvironment achieves the appropriate regulation over cell reproduction. This hypothesis of autoregulation is usually considered to apply to all renewing cell populations but is not ordinarily extended to cells that have been permanently and irreversibly arrested as a part of differentiation, *e.g.,* neurons, skeletal muscle cells, and nucleated erythrocytes. In the latter cases differentiation provides for a complete and irreversible arrest of reproduction that apparently does not involve environmental feedback.

Most of what is known about autoregulation comes from studies on wound healing in epithelia and on liver regeneration. Each cell type is usually postulated to release into the environment a labile product that specifically interacts only with the cell type that produces it; the interaction results in arrest of the cell cycle in the G_1 stage. To explain how cell renewal in a tissue remains balanced against cell loss, it is assumed that the regulating substance is labile, that the degree of arrest of reproduction in a given cell population is dependent upon the concentration of the regulatory substance, and that concentration in the environment is proportional to cell number.

The hypothesis of autoregulation can still only be stated in such general terms and undoubtedly it is an oversimplified formulation. The phenomenon of contact inhibition observed in diploid cells in culture, for example, must certainly play some part in regulation of proliferation, but contact inhibition is not yet easily fitted together with the above outline of autoregulation.

Probably, it will not be possible to understand *in vivo* regulation of cell reproduction until the series of steps that comprises the cell life cycle has been identified and the causal relationships between steps have been defined.

It is ordinarily most convenient to mark out the cell life cycle as the period and events that extend from the completion of one cell division and the next, although other events such as the beginning of DNA synthesis could be used as markers to define the cycle. During each cycle, all of the structural elements and functional capacities of both the nucleus and cytoplasm undergo a doubling. Little can yet be said about the regulation of the production or reproduction of mitochondria, ribosomes, various membrane components, machinery for glycolysis and lipid metabolism, *etc*. Nevertheless, the increases in all of these elements must be integrated through a complex of regulatory mechanisms that assures balanced cell growth. It seems certain that the increase in each cellular element will be governed by the demand of cellular metabolism for the functional contribution of that element, and the interactions that maintain a balance in growth among cell components, therefore, must occur through the functions of the components.

All of the growth activities of a proliferating cell are ultimately geared directly or remotely to the nuclear cycle of chromosome replication and segregation. These activities of the chromosomes define the four periods of the nuclear cycle, *i.e.*, G_1, S, G_2, and D, and govern the progress of the cell's reproductive cycle. Control, regulation, or inhibition of cell reproduction all are achieved by interruption of the nuclear cycle. The sections to follow review some of the available information on the composition and continuity of the nuclear cycle.

The G_1 Period

At least the very terminal part of G_1 is generally assumed to contain known or postulated preparations for DNA synthesis, *e.g.*, the synthesis of DNA duplicase and enzymes needed to produce deoxynucleoside triphosphates. For example, in liver tissue caused to renew cell proliferation by partial hepatectomy, a DNA polymerase and enzymes for the synthesis of thymidine triphosphate increase dramatically before the bulk of DNA synthesis is initiated (6, 7, 15). Similar rises in DNA polymerase and thymidine kinase coincide with the beginning of DNA synthesis in newly explanted mammalian kidney cells (1, 26). In such cases, however, the cells in question have been arrested in G_1 for a very long time, and it is not surprising that enzymes concerned with DNA synthesis have largely disappeared. In at least some cell types undergoing continuous proliferation, however, thymidine kinase synthesis occurs at the onset of DNA synthesis (39, 43). In contrast, in other cell types in continuous proliferation, kinases (40) and DNA polymerase (27) are present throughout the G_1 period and show no detectable increase in relation to the beginning of S. The presence of these enzymes throughout G_1 (presumably left over from DNA synthesis in the previous cell cycle) is some of the evidence that rules out the hypothesis that synthesis of these enzymes forms the primary basis for the presence of a G_1 phase or for the control of DNA synthesis. The explanation for G_1 existence needs to be sought in other events.

A variety of experiments have demonstrated that both RNA and protein synthesis are necessary for cell progress through G_1 (see for example: 22, 2, 46, 31); synthesis of new protein is apparently required until a very short time before DNA synthesis begins if not to the very end of G_1. Blockage in G_1 by such drastic measures as inhibition of RNA and protein synthesis may not be unexpected, but the requirement of protein synthesis so shortly before DNA synthesis suggests that the transition from G_1 to S is brought about by synthesis of a particular protein just before the transition point. The observation is in line with the hypothesis discussed below that synthesis of a protein initiator of chromosome replication is the final event of G_1.

Granted that a particular protein synthesis immediately before S brings about the initiation of S, the major part of G_1 in continuously proliferating cells remains unexplained. Killander and Zetterberg (21) have presented rather clear evidence that the length of G_1 in L cells is mass dependent; the greater the mass of a cell when it begins G_1, the shorter the G_1 period. The observation indicates that the rate of accomplishment of G_1 events is dependent upon the amount of general metabolic machinery; this might be interpreted to mean that G_1 is primarily a period of cell growth and that it perhaps does not contain a tightly coupled chain of molecular events directly connecting nuclear division and the next chromosome replication.

With such cells as hepatocytes, kidney cells, or small lymphocytes, which are normally arrested in G_1 for very extended periods, the return to proliferation is marked by a long interval (G_1) between application of the proliferative stimulus and the initiation of the first S period. In subsequent cycles G_1 is much shorter (4). These observations support the idea that a long arrest in G_1 leads to deterioration of metabolic machinery or intracellular conditions specifically required for continuous cell reproduction. The quantitative relationship between the duration of G_1 arrest and the time required to reinitiate DNA synthesis can be demonstrated with cells in culture; the longer a cell population is allowed to remain in stationary phase (in G_1 arrest), the longer the time required for the initiation of DNA synthesis when the cells are returned to culture conditions that permit reproduction (unpublished results).

Another striking property of G_1 is its elasticity. The variation in individual cell cycle times (generation times) for proliferating cells in culture is due to variation in the length of G_1 usually with little or no change in S, G_2, or D (41). When cells grown *in vitro* show an increased generation time because of a change in culture conditions (except temperature), the increased generation time is accounted for largely and often entirely by an expansion of the G_1 phase with little or no increase in the duration of S, G_2, or D. An extreme extension occurs in the stationary phase during which all of the cells in the culture are arrested in the G_1 state. The observation has been made on a wide variety of cell types including bacteria, fungi, protozoa, and mammalian cells.

A similar behavior is present in cell populations within the multicellular organism, although a longer generation time may in certain situations include some elongation of S or G_2. In general, S plus G_2 plus D of progenitor cells occupies a relatively fixed period in renewing cell populations. In different epithelia of the alimentary tract of the mouse, Cameron and Greulich (9) found average generation times that varied between 17 hours (ileum) and 181 hours (esophagus), but $S + G_2 + D$ remained virtually constant at roughly 10 hours. Similar data have been reported for other mammalian tissues.

Data of this type strongly suggest that the regulation of the cell's renewal rate in each particular tissue is achieved by extending or contracting the length of the G_1 phase. Such regulation of G_1 length is obviously a tissue specific property developed as a part of differentiation. The different regulator substances specific for the different tissues may, nevertheless, all exercise their effects ultimately on the same G_1 stage or G_1 event within the nucleus. In a manner analogous to cells in stationary phase culture *in vitro*, cells *in vivo* that have ceased proliferation (reversibly, but for an extended time; or permanently, *e.g.*, neurons and striated muscle cells), retire from the cell cycle in the G_1 phase.

A breakdown in the control of cell proliferation within a renewing tissue presumably stems from a loss of sensitivity of G_1 events to the regulator substances produced by the tissue or failure of a stem cell product to differentiate the appropriate sensitivity during its maturation. A variety of evidence points to a genetic basis for such loss or failure of sensitivity; usually, there are extensive karyotype changes although not necessarily. Gateff and Schneiderman (personal communication) have recently discovered a mutation in Drosophila located on the second chromosome that leads to the development in the larva of a transplantable, lethal, malignant brain tumor when present in the homozygous condition. Thus, a mutation at a specific well-defined locus has been shown to lead to neoplastic growth in a given tissue at a given time during its differentiation.

Although these various observations do not explain the basis for G_1, they give rise to the important generalization that control of cell proliferation is exercised through some event(s) in G_1. This applies whether the arrest is 1. due to presumably rather non-specific causes in the environment as in the case of stationary phase cultures of microorganisms or transformed mammalian cells, 2. a consequence of the somewhat more specific contact inhibition of mammalian cells in culture (33), or 3. mediated by highly tissue specific agents presumed to be present in the micro-environment of each renewing tissue in multicellular organisms.

Further insight into the significance of G_1 stems from two additional discoveries: 1. a number of cell types normally have no measurable G_1 period during active proliferation, *e.g.*, several protozoa, a slime mold, various bacteria; 2. cells may grow without a measurable G_1 phase under certain conditions and have a distinct G_1 phase under others. During cleavage stages of embryogenesis, the cell cycle usually has no measurable G_1 (16, 19). A G_1 period appears early in development (19) presumably as the need arises for differential regulation of cell reproduction in connection with tissue formation. Bacteria that normally have no measurable G_1 evidence a distinct G_1 when forced into a long generation time by a change in carbon source (23), and at least one line of mammalian cells can be grown *in vitro* without a detectable G_1 (37). The latter is a Chinese hamster cell line that stemmed ultimately from a cell population in which G_1 was presumably a constant feature. What cellular change underlies the elimination of a measurable G_1 is not known, but it could well be genetic. All of these findings demonstrate that virtually all of G_1 is expendable as a time period with respect to maintenance of continuity of the cell life cycle. This expendable nature of G_1 suggests the possibility that it is normally a period of intracellular hesitation or indecision brought about by the temporary interruption of the direct causal connection between mitosis and initiation of S. Such a view fits well with the fact that regulation of cell reproduction is normally achieved by delay or prevention of an expeditious transition from mitosis to S.

Even in the absence of a measurable G_1 period the unknown events that initiate DNA synthesis are still present in some very small fragment of time between mitosis and DNA synthesis and might reasonably still be called G_1 events.

The G_1 to S Transition

Currently the strongest hypothesis for the control of initiation of the S phase states that an initiator protein is produced that brings about the interaction between DNA and DNA duplicase necessary for DNA synthesis. A specific protein initiator is produced for initiation of each DNA replicon. The hypothesis was originally formulated to account for the behavior of a mutant F factor (a DNA episome in *E. coli*) whose replication had become temperature sensitive (18). The mutant F factor could replicate its DNA at 30°C but was unable to do so at 42°C unless a second, normal F factor was present in the same cell. Presumably the normal F factor released into the bacterial cytoplasm an initiator substance that could initiate DNA replication in both the mutant and normal F factor. The mutation apparently is expressed as a temperature sensitivity of the initiator itself or of its synthesis. While the temperatures involved suggest that the sensitive element is a protein, much stronger evidence for an initiator protein has come from studies of the bacterial chromosome (see 24). The experiments are too extensive to review here, but in essence the initiation of a new replication of the bacterial chromosome requires the new synthesis of a protein with each cell cycle. The postulated initiator protein is presumed to be labile or expended since new synthesis is required with each cell cycle. Production of initiator is apparently controlled at the transcription level since RNA synthesis is required for its synthesis. The bacterial chromosome is envisaged to possess normally only one site of initiation of replication and to consist, therefore, of only one replicon. Once initiated, DNA synthesis in the replicon proceeds to completion independently of further production of RNA or protein.

Application of the initiator protein hypothesis and replicon concept to larger cells appears reasonable in spite of the more complicated nature of their chromosomes and the presence of chromosome multiplicity.

The presence of an initiator of DNA synthesis in the cytoplasm of cells in the S period is suggested by nuclear transplantation in several cell types. In *Amoeba proteus* transfer of a nucleus from a cell in the G_2 phase to a cell in S results in a new DNA synthesis in the G_2 nucleus (36). Transfer of a nucleus from an S phase cell into a G_2 cell results in a sharp diminishment of DNA synthesis, presumably because the cytoplasm of a G_2 cell lacks the appropriate initiators to maintain the sequence of replicon replications. The latter interpretation invokes the concept that the nuclei of a larger cell contain many different replicons whose replication is controlled individually or in groups in a sequential pattern rather than with simultaneous replication of all replicons.

Additional evidence of cytoplasmic initiators stems from injection of various types of nuclei into the cytoplasm of amphibian eggs (17). Such nuclei, including those from adult erythrocytes, are induced to undergo DNA synthesis in the new cytoplasmic environment. Neither this experiment nor the one on ameba excludes the possibility that the situation is based on the presence in the cytoplasm of an inhibitor during G_1 (in the amphibian experiment) or in G_2 (in the ameba experiment) and on its absence during S. The interpretation that initiators are present in S and absent during other parts of the cycle is preferable because of the findings for bacterial events. In addition, however, fusion of two Stentor, one in S and the other in non-S, does not inhibit the S nucleus but leads to new synthesis in the non-S nucleus (12). These results are more compatible with an initiator hypothesis than one based on active inhibition.

Granting that the production of an initiator protein (whose production is controlled at the transcription level) is the immediate cause of transition of a cell from G_1 to S, we are immediately presented in turn with the question of temporal regulation of the transcription for this protein.

Many of the foregoing interpretations and speculations are based on the concept of chromosome structure that is currently most strongly supported by experimental evidence. The autoradiographic studies of Taylor (see, for example, 44), and later of others, demonstrated that the larger chromosomes of certain mammals and plants must each contain at least several separate initiation sites for DNA synthesis. This was the first clear evidence that such chromosomes are multireplicons (45). Cairns' measurements (8) of the rate of DNA helix replication in HeLa cells considered against the length of the S period and the amount of DNA per average chromosome indicated a minimum of 100 separate initiation sites for DNA synthesis (replicons) per chromosome. From experiments using a combination of BUDR and tritium labeling a minimum estimate of 10^3 to 10^4 replicating sites has been made for a single complement of chromosomes in the HeLa cell (34). Taylor (personal communication) has calculated from isotope labeling experiments that there must be at least 205 replicons in the long arm of the X chromosome in the Chinese hamster. In autoradiographic studies Plaut, Nash, and Fanning (35) have identified 30 initiation sites over only 15% of the total chromosome length in the salivary glands of Drosophila.

The autoradiographic work of Taylor and subsequently of others not only pointed to the multireplicon nature of chromosomes in larger cells but showed in addition that not all replicons are replicated simultaneously. The discovery that different parts of different chromosomes within a single complement replicate according to a rather well defined temporal sequence indicates that replicons are controlled individually or at least in groups. In this sense the S period for a larger cell is a composite of many S periods for many replicons whose replications are under individual or group control. The report of Stubblefield (42) that translocation of a chromosomal segment of an autosome to a heterochromatic region of a Y chromosome in the Chinese hamster does not detectably alter the replication pattern of the translocated DNA further supports this concept of independent replicon behavior.

Although homologous chromosomes for the most part show the same sequential labeling pattern (14) as would be predicted by the initiator protein-replicon hypothesis, there are notable exceptions, e.g., the heterochromatic X in an XX cell. The reason for a different replication pattern (late replicating) in the heterochromatic portions present in one homologue of a pair of chromosomes is not at all understood.

Experiments such as those of Miller (30) on the production of multiple nucleoli in amphibian oocytes demonstrate that particular replicons may be brought into multiple rounds of DNA synthesis in the absence of, and independently of, replication of other parts of the same chromosome. A similar type of replicon amplification occurs in the giant salivary chromosome in *Chironomus* (20). These observations provide further justification for application of the replicon hypothesis for larger cells.

The S Period

Not only is protein synthesis required for the transition from G_1 to S, but it is also necessary for the maintenance of S in multichromosome cells with multi-repliconic chromosomes. Mammalian cells in S treated with inhibitors of protein synthesis show a rapid, marked decline in DNA synthesis (28, 49, 3, 5). This might mean that, unlike bacteria, DNA synthesis in larger cells requires concomitant protein synthesis, for example, histone synthesis (38). Alternatively the rapid decline in DNA synthesis may represent the completion of replication of replicons already initiated, and failure of new replicons to begin replication in the absence of protein synthesis. The latter interpretation would be consistent with what is known about the protein dependence of DNA synthesis in bacteria and the sequential pattern of DNA replication in eukaryotic cells.

Inhibition of RNA synthesis with actinomycin D in cells already in S takes much longer to affect DNA synthesis (32). Actinomycin D added to HeLa cells in early S inhibited the synthesis of some DNA, but when added later in S, the antibiotic had no detectable effect on DNA synthesis (32). The long lag between inhibition of RNA synthesis and inhibition of DNA synthesis could mean that the messenger for an initiator protein is transcribed considerably in advance of the time of action of that initiator; there are too many other possible explanations to warrant much reliance on this interpretation.

The application of the initiator protein-replicon hypothesis does not at this point require any precise knowledge of how DNA is arranged within the chromosome, but such information would undoubtedly be helpful. Enzyme digestion studies on amphibian lampbrush chromosomes (29) and giant salivary gland chromosomes (25) indicate that the linear integrity of the chromosome does not involve RNA or protein but is maintained only by DNA. This would require DNA continuity from replicon to replicon with perhaps some nucleotide sequence punctuation between adjoining replicons. Swivel action for release of helix rotations during replication and the presence or absence of polyteny become involved in deciphering the structure of the multireplicon chromosome and its replication.

There is a high degree of asynchrony within and between chromosomes with respect to completion of DNA synthesis (14). Any hypothesis on the control of DNA synthesis must consider this asynchrony as well as the fact that the DNA of each chormosome normally only replicates once during each S phase. Both observations can be accounted for, at least in a general way, by the assumption that, as in bacteria, the initiator protein for a given replicon or group of replicons is produced only once per cell cycle and is sufficiently short-lived or somehow expended to avoid causing a second initiation in the same replicons within the same cycle. It is difficult to be satisfied, even for the moment, with such a tenuously based explanation that raises, in addition, other difficult questions, *e.g.*, what mechanism guarantees the synthesis of each initiator only once per cycle, and how is the initiator used up or otherwise removed?

The G₂ Period

The G_2 period contains the events that link the end of chromosome replication with chromosome segregation. In bacteria, G_2 has not been detected, although it may exist (as a short period between completion of chromosome replication and separation of the daughter chromosomes). In some nuclei (in ameba, slime mold, the micronucleus in some ciliates) G_2 is extremely long and can be quite variable in length. G_2 in these nuclei (all of which lack a measurable G_1) may be more complex than in cells of multicellular plants and animals, where it is relatively short and of constant duration. In multicellular organisms, G_2 is usually assumed to be required for condensation of chromosomes and assembly of the mitotic apparatus. In Chinese hamster cells, actinomycin D blocks division if administered up to 1.9 hours before mitosis would have been completed (47). Succesesful mitosis requires protein synthesis at least into late G_2 (47, 11). These findings again support the idea that cycle progress is dependent upon new transcriptions and synthesis of new protein (in this case to set up the mitotic apparatus). The discovery by Gelfant (13) that some cells in the epithelium of the mouse normally remain in G_2 for many hours will have to be accommodated in any comprehensive explanation of the period.

The mechanics of chromosome segregation in larger cells involve a series of events, *i.e.,* chromosome condensation, synthesis and assembly of the mitotic apparatus, alignment of chromosomes on the apparatus, splitting of kinetochores, chromosome movements, *etc.* Little is known about the molecular causation of any of these activities or of such associated phenomena as separation, and function of mitotic centers; or how any or all of these are linked molecularly to the other components of the cell cycles.

Final Remarks

As information about the components of the cell cycle has become available, a hypothesis has gradually emerged which states that progress through the cycle is governed by and based on a temporal sequence of genetic transcriptions. The transcriptions are presumably held in sequence by a dependency of one upon the next that is mediated through protein products in a manner similar to the scheme proposed by Clever (10) for sequential gene activation initiated by ecdysone in Chironomus. More direct support for this hypothesis is provided by the observation on mammalian cells in culture that synthesis of protein in early G_2 is necessary for subsequent synthesis of RNA in early G_2 that is in turn needed for synthesis of protein in late G_2 that is in turn required for mitosis (48).

The primary task in the future will be to determine the nature of such cell cycle transcriptions and translations, their regulation and to decipher the mechanisms by which the wide diversity of component parts of cell growth are ultimately tied to the chromosome cycle of replication and segregation.

References

1. ADAMS, R. L. P., ABRAMS, R., and LIEBERMAN, I.: Rise in deoxyribonucleic acid polymerase in the absence of deoxyribonucleic acid synthesis in cultured kidney cells. Nature 206, 512 (1965).
2. BASERGA, R., ESTENSEN, R. D., and PETERSEN, R. O.: Inhibition of DNA synthesis in Ehrlich ascites cells by actinomycin D. II. The presynthetic block in the cell cycle. Proc. Natl. Acad. Sci. U.S. 54, 745 (1965).
3. BASERGA, R., ESTENSEN, R. D., PETERSEN, R. O., and LAYDE, J. P.: Inhibition of DNA synthesis in Ehrlich ascites cells by actinomycin D. I. Delayed inhibition by low doses. Proc. Natl. Acad. Sci. U.S. 54, 745 (1965).
4. BENDER, M. A., and PRESCOTT, D. M.: DNA synthesis and mitosis in cultures of human peripheral leukocytes. Exp. Cell Res. 27, 221–229 (1962).

5. BENNETT, L. L., SMITHERS, D., and WARD, C. T.: Inhibition of DNA synthesis in mammalian cells by actidione. Biochim. Biophys. Acta 87, 60 (1964).

6. BOLLUM, F. J., and POTTER, V. R.: Incorporation of thymidine into DNA by enzymes from rat tissue. J. Biol. Chem. 233, 478 (1958).

7. BOLLUM, F. J., and POTTER, V. R.: Metabolism in regenerating liver. VI. Soluble enzymes which convert thymidine to thymidine phosphates and DNA. Cancer Research 19, 561 (1959).

8. CAIRNS, J.: Autoradiography of HeLa cell DNA. J. Mol. Biol. 15, 372 (1966).

9. CAMERON, I. L., and GREULICH, R. C.: Evidence for an essentially constant duration of DNA synthesis in renewing epithelia of the adult mouse. J. Cell Biol. 18, 31 (1963).

10. CLEVER, U.: Actinomycin and puromycin: effects on sequential gene activation by ecdysone. Science 146, 794 (1964).

11. CUMMINS, J. E., BLOMQUIST, J. C., and RUSCH, H. P.: Anaphase delay after inhibition of protein synthesis between late prophase and prometaphase. Science 154, 1343 (1966).

12. DETERRA, N.: Macronuclear DNA synthesis in stentor: regulation by a cytoplasmic initiator. Proc. Natl. Acad. Sci. U.S. 57, 607 (1967).

13. GELFANT, S.: A new theory on the mechanism of cell division. In: Cell Growth and Cell Division. R. J. C. Harris (ed.). Academic Press, Inc., New York (1963).

14. GERMAN, J.: The pattern of DNA synthesis in the chromosomes of human blood cells. J. Cell. Biol. 20, 37 (1964).

15. GIUDICE, G., KENNEY, F. T., and NOVELLI, G. D.: Effect of puromycin on deoxyribonucleic acid synthesis by regenerating rat liver. Biochim. Biophys. Acta 87, 171 (1964).

16. GRAHAM, C. F., and MORGAN, R. W.: Changes in the cell cycle during early amphibian development. Devel. Biol. 14, 439 (1966).

17. GRAHAM, C. F., ARMS, K., and GURDON, J. B.: The induction of DNA synthesis by frog egg cytoplasm. Devel. Biol. 14, 349 (1966).

18. JACOB, R., BRENNER, S., and CUZIN, F. On the regulation of DNA replication in bacteria. Cold Spring Harbor Sym. on Quant. Biol. 28, 329 (1963).

19. KAUFFMAN, S. L.: An autoradiographic study of the generation cycle in the ten-day mouse embryo neural tube. Exp. Cell Res. 42, 67 (1966).

20. KEYL, H. G., and HAGELE, K.: Heterochromatinproliferation an den Speicheldrüsenchromosomen von Chironomus melanotus. Chromosoma 20, 223 (1966).

21. KILLANDER, D., and ZETTERBERG, A.: A quantitative cytochemical investigation of the relationship between cell mass and initiation of DNA synthesis in mouse fibroblasts in vitro. Exp. Cell Res. 40, 12 (1965).

22. KISHIMOTO, S., and LIEBERMAN, I.: Synthesis of RNA and protein required for the mitosis of mammalian cells. Exp. Cell Res. 36, 92 (1964).

23. LARK, C.: Regulation of deoxyribonucleic acid synthesis in Escherichia coli: dependence on growth rates. Biochim. Biophys. Acta 119, 517 (1966).

24. LARK, K. G.: Regulation of chromosome replication and segregation in bacteria. Bact. Reviews 30, 3 (1966).

25. LEZZI, M.: Die Wirkung von DNase auf isolierte Polytän-chromosomen. Exp. Cell Res. 39, 289 (1965).

26. LIEBERMAN, I., ABRAMS, R., HUNT, N., and OVE, P.: Levels of enzyme activity and deoxyribonucleic acid synthesis in mammalian cells cultured from the animal. J. Biol. Chem. 238, 3955 (1963).

27. LITTLEFIELD, J. W., McGOVERN, A. P., and MARGESON, K. B. Changes in the distribu-

tion of polymerase activity during DNA synthesis in mouse fibroblasts. Proc. Natl. Acad. Sci. U.S. **49**, 102 (1963).

28. LITTLEFIELD, J. W., and JACOBS, P. S.: The relation between deoxyribonucleic acid and protein synthesis in mouse fibroblasts. Biochim. Biophys. Acta **108**, 652 (1965).

29. MACGREGOR, H. C., and CALLAN, H. G.: The actions of enzymes on lampbrush chromosomes. Quant. J. Microscop. Sci. 103(2), 173 (1962).

30. MILLER, O. L.: Structure and composition of peripheral nucleoli of salamander oocytes. *In*: The Nucleolus, Its Structure and Function. Natl. Cancer Inst. Monograph **23** (1966).

31. MUELLER, G. C., KAJIWARA, K., STUBBLEFIELD, E., and RUECKERT, R. R.: Molecular events in the reproduction of animal cells. I. The effect of puromycin on the duplication of DNA. Cancer Res. **22**, 1084 (1962).

32. MUELLER, G. C., and KAJIWARA, K.: Actinomycin D and p-fluorophenylalanine, inhibitors of nuclear replication in HeLa cells. Biochim. Biophys. Acta **119**, 557 (1966).

33. NILAUSEN, K., and GREEN, H.: Reversible arrest of growth in G_1 of an established fibroblast line (2T3). Exp. Cell Res. **40**, 166 (1965).

34. PAINTER, R. B., JERMANY, D. A., and RASMUSSEN, R. E.: A method to determine the number of DNA replicating units in cultured mammalian cells. J. Mol. Biol. **17**, 47 (1966).

35. PLAUT, W., NASH, D., and FANNING, T. Ordered replication of DNA in polytene chromosomes of *Drosophila melanogaster*. J. Mol. Biol. **16**, 85 (1966).

36. PRESCOTT, D. M., and GOLDSTEIN, L.: Nuclear-cytoplasmic interaction in DNA synthesis. Science **155**, 469 (1967).

37. ROBBINS, E., and SCHARFF, M. D.: The absence of a detectable G_1 phase in a cultured strain of Chinese hamster lung cell. J. Cell Biol. **34**, 684 (1967).

38. ROBBINS, E., and BORUN, T. W.: The cytoplasmic synthesis of histones in HeLa cells and its temporal relationship to DNA replication. Proc. Natl. Acad. Sci. U.S. **57**, 409 (1967).

39. SACHSENMAIER, W., FOURNIER, D. V., and GURTLER, K. F. Periodic thymidine kinase production in synchronous plasmodia of *Physarum polycephalum*: inhibition by actinomycin and actidione. Biochem. Biophys. Res. Comm. **27**, 655 (1967).

40. SHOUP, G. D., PRESCOTT, D. M., and WYKES, J. R.: Thymidine triphosphate synthesis in tetrahymena. I. Studies on thymidine kinase. Jour. Cell Biol. **31**, 295 (1966).

41. SISKEN, J. E., and KINOSITA, R.: Timing of DNA synthesis in the mitotic cycle in vitro. Exp. Cell Res. **9**, 509–518 (1961).

42. STUBBLEFIELD, E.: Mammalian chromosomes in vitro. XIX. Chromosomes of Don-C, a Chinese hamster fibroblast strain with a part of autosome 1b translocated to the Y chromosome. J. Natl. Can. Inst. **37**, 799 (1966).

43. STUBBLEFIELD, E., and MURPHREE, S.: Synchronized mammalian cell cultures. II. Thymidine kinase activity in colcemid synchronized fibroblasts. Exptl. Cell Res. **48**, 652–655 (1967).

44. TAYLOR, J. H.: Asynchronous duplication of chromosomes in cultured cells of Chinese hamster. J. Biophys. Biochim. Cytol. **7**, 455 (1960).

45. TAYLOR, J. H.: DNA synthesis in relation to chromosome reproduction and reunion of breaks. J. Cell Comp. Physiol., Suppl. 1, **62**, 73 (1963).

46. TERASIMA, T., and YASUKAWA, M.: Synthesis of G_1 protein preceding DNA synthesis in cultured mammalian cells. Exp. Cell Res. **44**, 669 (1966).

47. TOBEY, R. A., PETERSEN, D. F., ANDERSON, E. C., and PUCK, T. T.: Life cycle analysis of mammalian cells. III. The inhibition of division in Chinese hamster cells by puromycin and actinomycin. Biophysical J. **6**, 567 (1966).

48. Tobey, R. A., Anderson, E. 'C., and Petersen, D. F.: RNA stability and protein synthesis in relation to the division of mammalian cells. Proc. Natl. Acad. Sci. U.S. **56**, 1520 (1967).

49. Young, C. W.: Inhibitory effects of acetoxycycloheximide, puromycin, and pactamycin upon synthesis of protein and DNA in asynchronous populations of HeLa cells. Molecular Pharmacology **2**, 50 (1966).

Discussion

Methods and Criteria of Mammalian Cell Synchrony *

Warren K. Sinclair

Division of Biological and Medical Research
Argonne National Laboratory
Argonne, Illinois

The sequence of events occurring between one cell division and the next, *i.e.*, during the cell generation cycle, and the relationship between these different events is of primary importance to our understanding of the proliferation process in cells and perhaps also to the distinctions between normal and malignant cells.

In the case of mammalian cells much of the information presently available concerning the cell cycle has been obtained from cells *in vitro* and, apart from observations on single cells, primarily as a result of the study of synchronized populations of cells. The use of synchronized populations has become the major way of studying events and responses which depend upon the position of the cell (*i.e.*, its age) within the cell cycle. For this reason, I intend to devote my discussion to a survey of synchrony methods currently in use with mammalian cells and to the criteria that may be employed to assess the degree of synchrony in a given procedure.

Methods

A number of useful methods for obtaining synchronous (unmodified) or synchronized (modified) populations of mammalian cells *in vitro* have been developed during the past decade. None of these methods is ideal and each has different advantages and disadvantages which must be considered in relation to the purpose of the investigation.

The principles of most of the methods in current use are apparent from Fig. 1. These may be grouped into three main categories involving, first, blocking of cells

---

* Work supported by the U.S. Atomic Energy Commission.

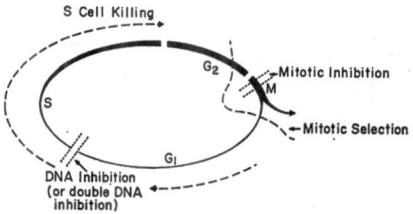

Fig. 1. Methods of cell synchrony

at some point in the cell cycle usually either in DNA synthesis or mitosis; second, killing of cells during a portion of the cycle, usually S; and third, selection of specific groups of cells usually at or near mitosis.

(a) Blocking of cells in the cell cycle. Metabolic alterations resulting from cooling (12), starvation (11) or serum deprivation (28) appear to result in a block often in G_1. However, more generally applicable are specific agents which block DNA synthesis. DNA inhibition (17, 30, 27, 8, 18) results in one group of cells (Fig. 2a) being piled up at the end of G_1, while another group, those spread throughout S at the time the agent was added, are essentially arrested at that point. When the block is released, cells progress in the cycle in two groups, those spread throughout S and those originally blocked at G_1; thus a single application of a DNA inhibitor will not produce very good synchrony (Fig. 2b). A second application (15, 3, 13) appropriately timed can be much more effective in producing synchrony. If a time equal to or greater than S is allowed to elapse after the first release, all cells will at least have reached G_2 (Fig. 2b). The total interval must not be greater than $T - S$ (*i.e.*, generation time T minus the S period) before the inhibitor is added for a second time. Then all cells will pile up at the end of G_1 (Fig. 2c). When the block is released for the second time these cells move through S in a single cohort. The individual cells of the cohort are not, however, all alike; some have been blocked twice and for varying lengths of time at the end of G_1, while others were initially blocked in S. In all cases inhibition is specifically concerned with beginning or continuing DNA synthesis only. Other processes, *e.g.*, RNA and protein synthesis, continue to a greater or less degree; consequently the cell population is unbalanced and this may influence its subsequent

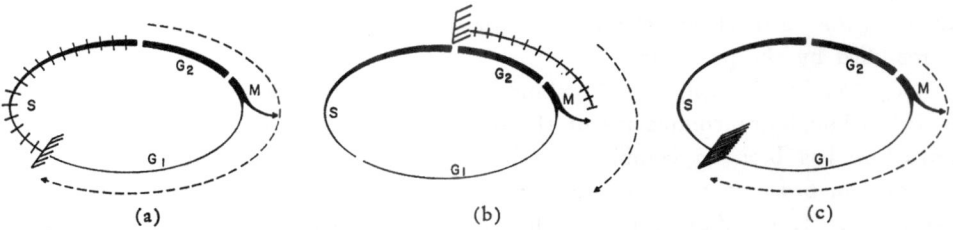

(a) (b) (c)

Fig. 2. (a) Cell distribution when DNA inhibitor is added. (b) Cell distribution when DNA inhibition is released and cells pass through S. (c) Cell distribution when a second application of the DNA inhibitor is made.

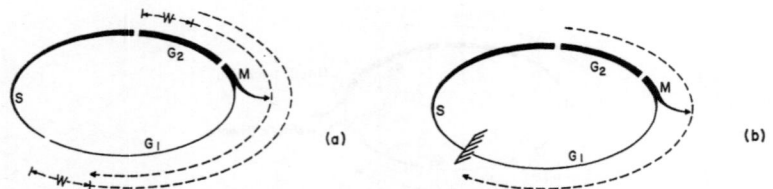

Fig. 3. (a) Cell progression during S cell killing without inhibition of DNA synthesis. (b) Cell progression during S cell killing with inhibition of DNA synthesis.

performance or response. Therefore, independent tests must be applied, to insure that the responses are indeed representative of normal unmodified cells.

(b) Killing of cells in DNA synthesis. The killing of cells during the S period with high specific activity tritiated thymidine (HSA-[3]HTdR) (29) is an interesting method. Cells in S and those moving into S take up lethal quantities of tritium so that if the agent is kept on for a period almost equal to $T - S$, *i.e.*, $T - S - W$, where W is a window width, all cells except those in this window will have taken up a lethal amount of the radioactive precursor and are moribund (Fig. 3a). The window may be made as narrow as the properties of the cell line will allow, the smaller the window the better the synchrony. The presence of the moribund cells, while unimportant for assays such as colony formation, is an almost insurmountable handicap for cytological or biochemical assays however.

(c) Mitotic selection. The simplest and in many respects the most suitable method, applicable with some modifications in technique to most cell lines, is that of mitotic selection (25, 23, 22, 16) which involves the selective detachment of mitotic cells which are poorly attached as a result of the cell rounding up during mitosis (Fig. 4). The period during which cells are rounded up is quite brief, ~30 minutes altogether in Chinese hamster cells, or only 5 percent of a cell cycle of 10 hours. Not more than a few percent of other interphase cells are usually obtained. This method is limited only by the yield it is possible to obtain from most cultures of normal size. However, even this problem has been overcome in HeLa cells by culturing in Blake bottles using a low calcium concentration in the medium (16). The method also has the advantage that inoculated cells of this mitotic population are at the beginning of a cell cycle rather than part way through, as with methods involving DNA inhibition. An additional important advantage is that these cells are essentially synchronous and their responses are unmodified by the procedure.

(d) Combined techniques. Combinations of the above methods have also proved useful although the complexity of the technique is increased. For example a useful procedure has been to combine S cell killing using HSA-[3]HTdR, with mitotic selection in order to eradicate the population of S cells during other parts of the cycle (21, 5). In addition DNA inhibition together with S cell killing (19, 20), a property of hydroxyurea, especially in Chinese hamster cells, has resulted in a neat method (Fig. 3b) which, except for the presence of moribund cells, appears

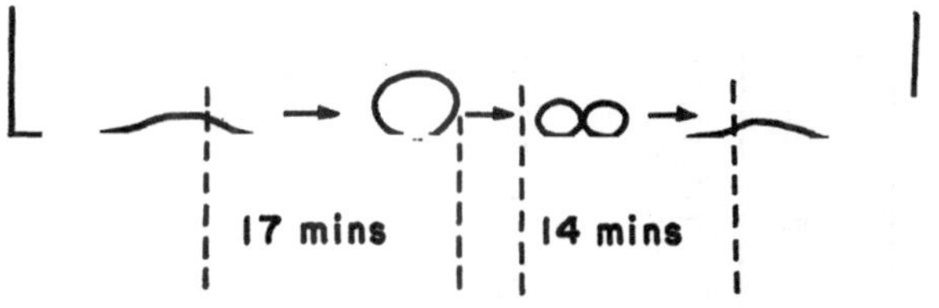

Fig. 4. Diagrammatic sketch of cells growing on surface of plastic petri dish. Time lapse photomicrography has shown that the cells remain flattened during interphase, but round up an average of 17 minutes before division and stay rounded up for a further 14 minutes after division. The total time represents about 5% of the generation cycle.

superior to the double DNA inhibition technique. Inhibition of mitosis has not, on its own, proved very useful because of the toxicity of most of the agents providing the blocking and the length of time for which it must be maintained. However, it has proved useful in combination with the method of mitotic selection, either to provide a larger number of wanted cells (24) or to remove a larger number of unwanted cells (1, 9, 14).

The main features of these methods are summarized in Table 1.

The provision of independent methods to test whether or not a given method of synchrony has modified the normal response of the cells presents some difficulty. Comparison of responses in populations synchronized by different independent methods is helpful. A necessary condition is also that the responses obtained must be consistent with those observed in asynchronous populations making appropriate allowance for the age-distribution of the cells.

Criteria of Synchrony

Appropriate criteria of synchrony are needed not only for the purpose of judging the success of a given technique but also for comparing one experiment with another. In view of the many cell cycle parameters which it may be desired to have in phase at any given instant, no single ideal criterion exists. Furthermore, a description of the various features of a nominally synchronized cell population at the instant of its selection is possible usually only with difficulty. A special case is the selection of mitotic cells where indeed the cytological criterion of a high initial mitotic index or the cell size distribution may be useful guides (22). The mitotic index is often no more than a guide however, since unless this index is actually 100 percent it does not describe the state of the remaining, nonmitotic cells. If these other cells are very close to mitosis, synchrony may be quite good even though the mitotic index is not high (*e.g.*, ref. 22, Fig. 6, response for 30 percent to 70 percent initial mitotic index).

Since a static description of the starting population is lacking in most cases, experimental criteria are usually derived from the subsequent performance of the population as it progresses in time. It is well known that the generation time of a population is not the same for all cells but is the average of a distribution with

TABLE 1

METHODS OF SYNCHRONIZING MAMMALIAN CELLS

Method	Agent	Initial stage	Advantages	Disadvantages	References
Metabolic alterations, cooling, starvation, serum deprivation	None	early G_1?	Simple	Not generally applicable.	(12, 11, 28)
DNA Inhibition	Amethopterin FudR Excess TdR and others	early S	Many cells available. Simple	Two groups of cells present; properties may be modified.	(17, 30, 27, 8, 18)
Double DNA Inhibition	Excess TdR	early S	Many cells available.	Cell properties may be modified.	(15, 3, 13)
S Cell Killing (suicide)	HSA-³HTdR	late G_1	Cell properties unmodified. Cell yield adequate.	Moribund cells present. Synchrony inversely related to yield.	(29)
Mitotic Selection	None	mitosis	Simple. No modification of properties. No other cells present.	Yields limited in most cases.	(25, 23, 16, 22)

Mitotic Selection and S cell killing	None HSA-^{3}HTdR	mitosis	Especially good synchrony in G_1, G_2, mitosis.	Some moribund cells present. Technique more complex.	(21, 5)
DNA Inhibition S cell killing	Hydroxyurea	early S	Good synchrony. Many cells available. Properties recovered rapidly.	Moribund cells present.	(19–20)
Mitotic Inhibition and Selection	Colcemid and selection	mitosis	Good synchrony and yield.	Possible modification of cell properties.	(24)
	Vinblastine and selection	early G_1	Cell properties unmodified. Yield adequate.	Technique more complex. Cell synchrony inversely related to yield.	(1, 14, 9)

a standard deviation in the range 10–20 percent (10). An example is shown in Fig.
5a for the V79 line of Chinese hamster cells. The existence of this distribution
means that a population will rapidly lose synchrony with time, the rate of loss
depending upon the breadth of the distribution. Knowing the breadth of the
distribution, one can predict the decay of synchrony with time (6). Even in the
first cycle, substantial loss of synchrony occurs, as shown in Fig. 5b, where an
initially well-synchronized Chinese hamster cell population selected at mitosis shows
a broad spread of cycle stages (some cells in S, G_2, M and G_1) by the time G_2 is
reached. The situation is worse in cell lines for which the distribution of generation
times is broader.

Criteria of synchrony are usually confined to events and performance during
the first generation cycle after synchronization. Some of the parameters that have
been used include growth, cytological criteria (mitotic index), identification of
DNA synthesis by ^{3}HTdR incorporation, and cell sizing.

(a) Growth. Asynchronous (log phase) cells grow and divide at a constant
rate. Synchronous cells proceed through a cell cycle until the division point is
reached. If they were perfectly in phase, the cohort of synchronized cells would
then divide within a time no greater than that required for the division process
itself. In practice the time over which division occurs is greater and its duration
can be used as a measure of synchrony. Three similar indices have been developed,

(1) percent phasing (Zeuthen, 31, Burns, 4) is simply

$$= \frac{T/2 - D\frac{1}{2}}{T/2} \times 100$$

where T is the generation time and $D\frac{1}{2}$ the time for half the cells to divide
($D\frac{1}{2}$ is used because often 100% of the cells do not divide)

(2) an index developed by Blumenthal and Zaler (2) denoted

$$F = \frac{N_2}{N_1} - 2^{\frac{t_2 - t_1}{T}}$$

where N_1 is the number of cells at t_1
where N_2 is the number of cells at t_2

(3) a graphical method based on the rate of cell division described by Engelberg
(7) [the rate of cell division is plotted as a function of time and the fractional
excess of this rate over the rate for an asynchronous population (Ru) is the
percent synchrony].

Obviously each of these indices is zero for an asynchronous population and
approaches 100 percent for perfect synchrony.

In synchronized populations there is usually little difference between these three
indices. For example (Fig. 6) in the growth curve of survivors in a Chinese hamster
cell population synchronized by hydroxyurea, there was no cell division for about
5½ hours after removal of the agent, then cells divided over a period of about

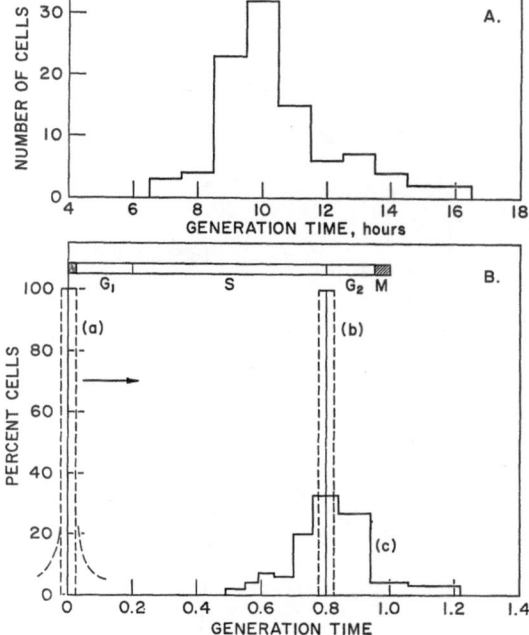

Fig. 5. (a) Distribution of generation times in a log-phase population of V79 Chinese hamster cells, determined by time lapse cinemicrography. (b) Effect of desynchronization of a population of synchronous Chinese hamster cells. Initially these cells are spread over only about 5% of the cycle (a). By the time G₂ is reached (0.8T) the distribution would be (b) if there was no desynchronization, but in fact it is like (c).

NOTE: The flare at the foot of distribution (a) is to indicate that some cells are spread beyond 5% of the cycle and from labeling with ⁸HTdR it is believed that about 5% of the cells selected may be randomly distributed through the cycle.

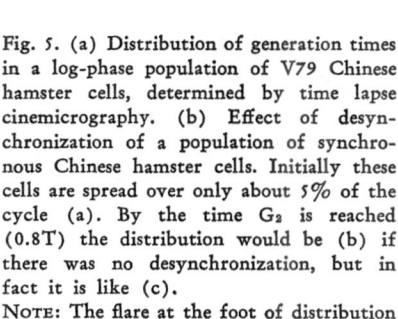

3 hours. The generation time in the control population was 11 hours. This yields a percent phasing of 73 percent, a Blumenthal and Zaler index of 79 percent and an Engelberg percent synchrony of 75 percent. In another example for HeLa cells (26) synchronized by selection (Fig. 7) the three indices are 41 percent, 40 percent, and 41 percent. This example illustrates that even when these indices are below 50 percent, the synchrony evident in the population is quite marked.

Since these indices agree so well, the simple indices such as percent phasing or or the Blumenthal and Zaler index, especially the latter, are usually quite adequate. They are simple to calculate and the extra labor involved in computing the Engelberg percentage synchrony is not often rewarding. The Engelberg procedure appears, however, to be of particular value when the percentage synchrony is low and there may be a question whether a given population is truly asynchronous or not.

(b) Cytological. The degree of synchrony can be determined also by plotting the mitotic index as a function of time during the division period. An example is shown in Fig. 8 for Chinese hamster cells synchronized by selection. Curve A is for a well-synchronized population and the mitotic index rises to a value of 34 percent at 10.5 hr whereas curve B is for a less well-synchronized population and rises only to 14½ percent at this time. The index could be made more quantitative, but the procedure requires large samples, is relatively tedious and is not too useful as a general index.

(c) DNA synthesis. The limited duration of DNA synthesis during the cell cycle is useful as a measure of synchrony. Pulse labeling for 15 minutes at various

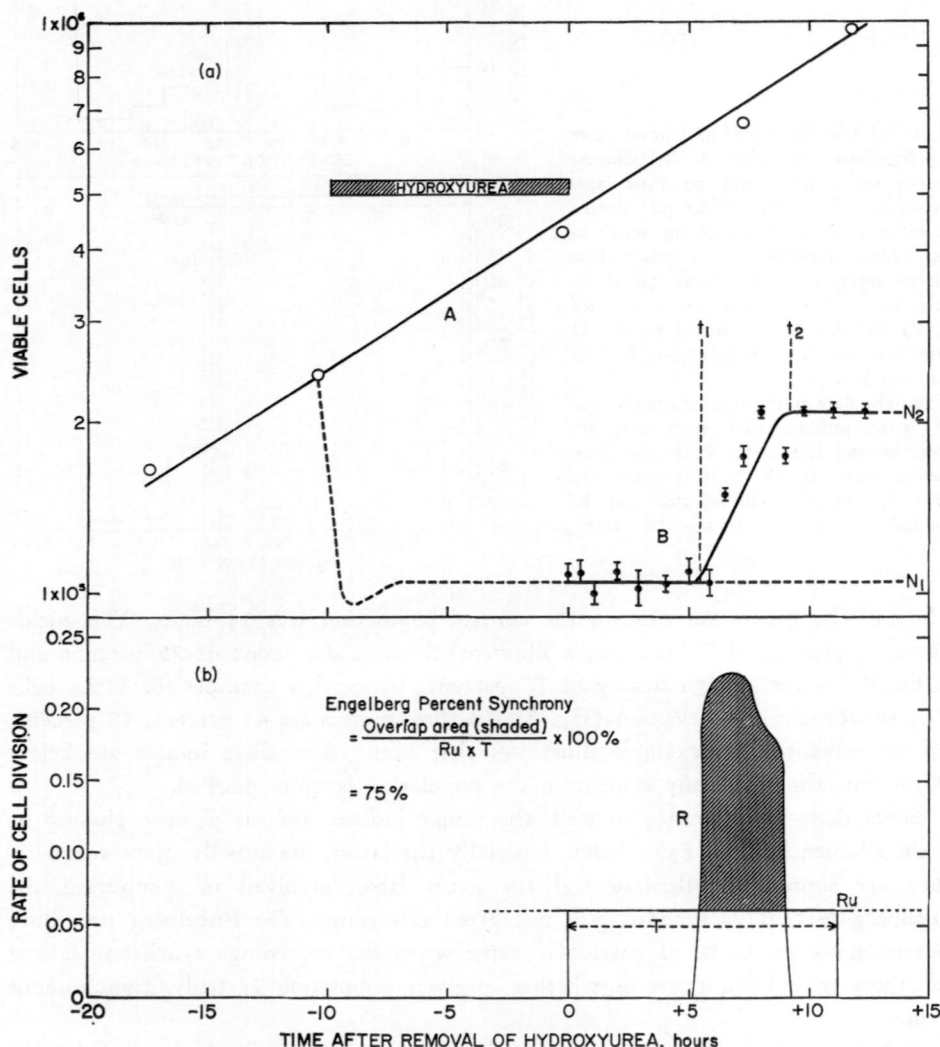

Fig. 6. (a) Growth of survivors of an asynchronous Chinese hamster cell population exposed to hydroxyurea (1mM for 10 hours), curve B, compared with untreated cells, curve A. (b) Rate of cell division (fractional change in population per hour) as a function of time. Derivation of Engelberg percent synchrony (7); Ru is the rate for an asynchronous population. [Sinclair (20)].

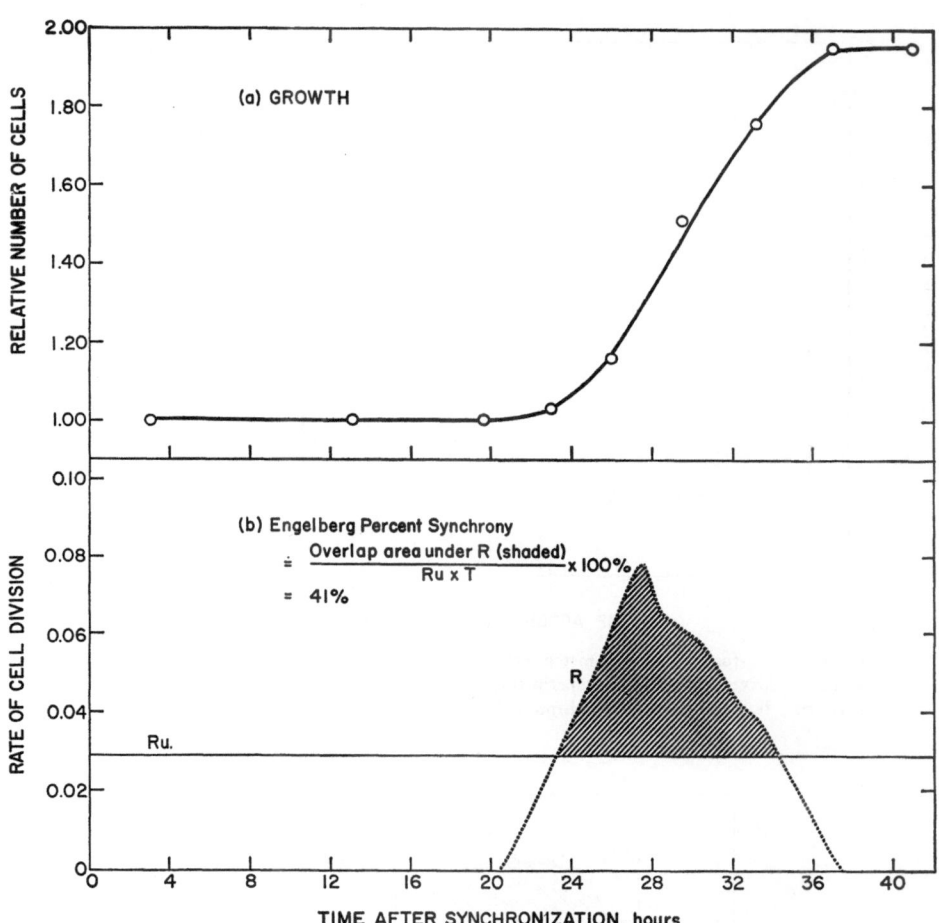

Fig. 7. (a) Growth of HeLa cells synchronized by selection, Terasima and Tolmach (26). (b) Rate of cell division and derivation of Engelberg percent synchrony.

times through the cell cycle yields the data (from autoradiography) shown in Fig. 9 for a Chinese hamster cell population synchronized by selection. If the population were asynchronous, the result would have been a straight line at about 65 percent. As an index of synchrony, we (22) have used a labeling index, the difference between L max and L min. In a good experiment this will be high, 75 percent or more (Fig. 9); in a poor experiment it will be lower. Other ways of handling the data can also be used; for example, if synchrony were perfect, all cells would enter and leave the S period at the same time yielding the rectangle shown. The actual number of cells in this region in Fig. 9 (shaded) is 85 percent, an arbitrary measure of synchrony. Furthermore, outside the box there are 15 percent labeled cells, indicating that, for this population, 100 percent of the cells incorporated the label and none failed to do so. A disadvantage of this procedure is that the results are not available immediately.

(d) Cell sizing. Another qualitative and potentially quantitative indication of

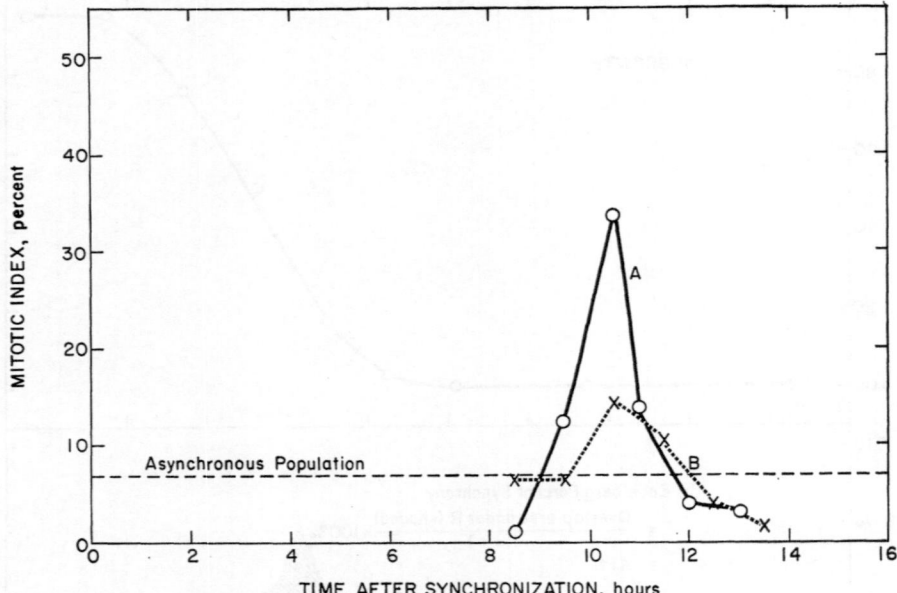

Fig. 8. Mitotic index for Chinese hamster cells synchronized by selection at mitosis during the following division. Curve A, from one experiment, represents very good synchrony and curve B, from another experiment, less satisfactory synchrony. (Data obtained by C. K. Yu)

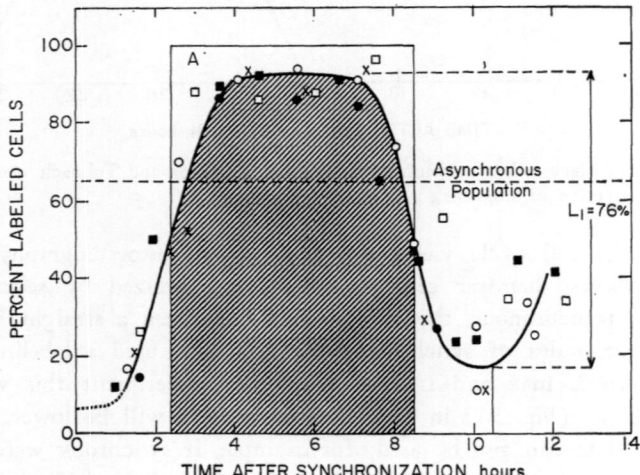

Fig. 9. Pulse labeling with ^{3}HTdR for 15 minutes, populations of Chinese hamster cells synchronized by selection. Each set of points represents a separate experiment in each of which the degree of synchrony and the rate of progression through the cycle vary slightly. The labeling index L_1 for the average smooth curve is 76%. The line at 65% indicates the expected result for an asynchronous population.

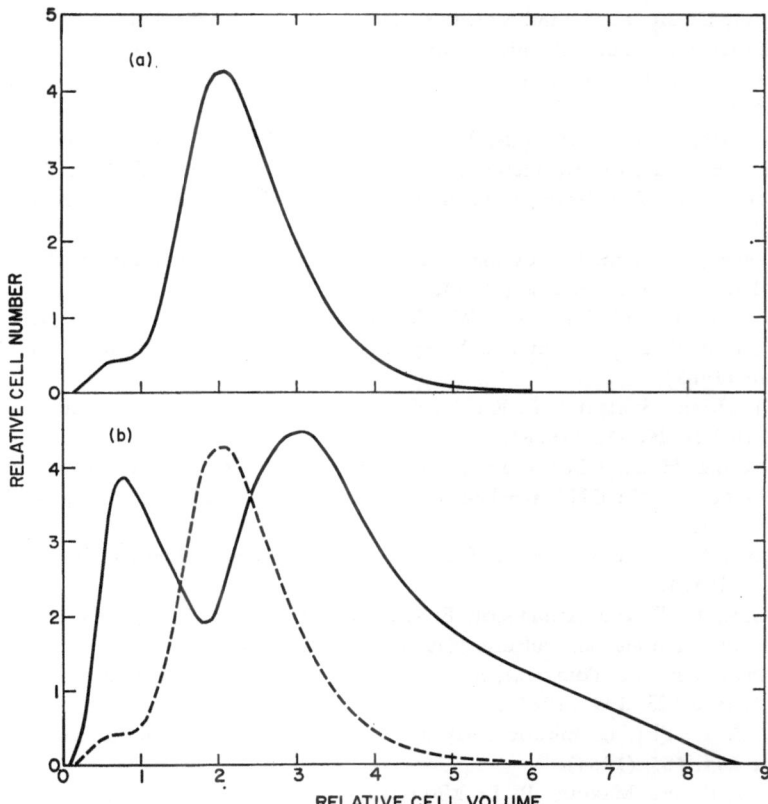

Fig. 10. (a) Size distribution for asynchronous Chinese hamster cells. (b) Size distribution of Chinese hamster cells synchronized by selection at mitosis. (Data obtained by A. Han)

synchrony is obtained from cell sizing using an electronic counter. Fig. 10 panel A shows the distribution of cell sizes (volumes) in an asynchronous population of Chinese hamster cells. Panel B shows the bimodal distribution of cell volumes obtained when a synchronous population close to mitosis is selected (the distribution of the asynchronous population of A is dotted in). The peak due to large cells is for those not yet divided and the peak due to small cells is for those just divided. A quantitative measure could be developed by comparing the cells outside the asynchronous region with those inside it when equal numbers of cells are involved. This procedure is rapid, requires only a small sample and yields an immediate result.

References

1. BELLI, J. A.: Effect of temperature on the radiation response of synchronous mammalian cells in culture. Rad. Res. 25, 174 (1965).
2. BLUMENTHAL, L. K. and ZALER, S. A.: Index for measurement of synchronization of cell populations. Science 135, 724 (1962).

3. BOOTSMA, D., BUDKE, L. and VOS, O.: Studies on synchronous division of tissue culture cells initiated by excess thymidine. Exp. Cell Res. 33, 301 (1964).
4. BURNS, V. W.: Cell division synchronization. Progr. Biophysics and Biophysic. Chem. 12, 1 (1962).
5. DJORDJEVIC, E. and TOLMACH, L. J.: X-ray sensitivity of HeLa S3 cells in the G_2 phase: Comparison of two methods of synchronization. Biophys. 7, 77 (1967).
6. ENGLEBERG, J.: The decay of synchronization of cell division. Exp. Cell Res. 36, 647 (1964).
7. ENGLEBERG, J.: A method of measuring the degree of synchronization of cell populations. Exp. Cell Res. 23, 218 (1961).
8. ERIKSON, R. L. and SZYBALSKI, W.: Molecular radiobiology of human cell lines. IV. Variation in ultraviolet light and X-ray sensitivity during the division cycle. Rad. Res. 18, 200 (1963).
9. KIM, J. H. and STAMBUK, B. K.: Synchronization of HeLa cells by vinblastine sulfate. Exp. Cell Res. 44, 631 (1966).
10. KUBITSCHEK, H. E.: Discrete distributions of generation-rate. Nature 195, 350 (1962).
11. LITTLEFIELD, J. W.: DNA synthesis in partially synchronized L cells. Exp. Cell Res. 26, 318 (1962).
12. NEWTON, A. A. and WILDY, P.: Parasynchronous division of HeLa cells. Exp. Cell Res. 16, 724 (1959).
13. PETERSEN, D. F. and ANDERSON, E. C.: Quantity production of synchronized mammalian cells in suspension culture. Nature 203, 642 (1964).
14. PFEIFFER, S. E. and TOLMACH, L. J.: Selecting synchronous populations of mammalian cells. Nature 123, 139 (1967).
15. PUCK, T. T.: Phasing, mitotic delay and chromosomal aberrations in mammalian cells. Science 144, 565 (1964).
16. ROBBINS, E. and MARCUS, P. I.: Mitotically synchronized mammalian cells: A simple method of obtaining large populations. Science 144, 1152 (1964).
17. RUECKERT, R. R. and MUELLER, G. C.: Studies on unbalanced growth in tissue culture. I. Induction and consequences of thymidine deficiency. Cancer Res. 20, 1584 (1960).
18. SCHINDLER, R.: Biochemical studies of the division cycle of mammalian cells: Evidence for the premitotic period. Biochem. Pharmacol. 12, 533 (1963).
19. SINCLAIR, W. K.: Hydroxyurea: Differential lethal effects on cultured mammalian cells during the cell cycle. Science 150, 1729 (1965).
20. SINCLAIR, W. K.: Hydroxyurea: Effects on Chinese hamster cells grown in culture. Cancer Res., Part I, 297 (1967).
21. SINCLAIR, W. K. and MORTON, R. A.: X-ray sensitivity during the cell generation cycle of cultured Chinese hamster cells. Rad. Res. 29, 450 (1966).
22. SINCLAIR, W. K. and MORTON, R. A.: X-ray and ultra-violet sensitivity of synchronized Chinese hamster cells at various stages of the cell cycle. Biophys. J. 5, 1 (1965).
23. SINCLAIR, W. K. and MORTON, R. A.: Variations in X-ray response during the division cycle of partially synchronized Chinese hamster cells in culture. Nature 199, 1158 (1963).
24. STUBBLEFIELD, E. and KLEVECZ, R.: Synchronization of Chinese hamster cells by reversal of colcemid inhibition. Exp. Cell Res. 40, 660 (1965).
25. TERASIMA, T. and TOLMACH, L. J.: Growth and nucleic acid synthesis in synchronously dividing populations of HeLa cells. Exp. Cell Res. 30, 344 (1963).
26. TERASIMA, T. and TOLMACH, L. J.: Variations in several responses in HeLa cells to X-irradiation during the division cycle. Biophys. J. 3, 11 (1963).

27. TILL, J. E., WHITMORE, G. F. and GULYAS, S.: Deoxyribonucleic acid synthesis in individual L-strain mouse cells. II. Effects of thymidine starvation. Biochim. Biophysica Acta **72**, 277 (1963).

28. WHITFIELD, J. F. and YOUDALE, T.: Synchronization of cell division in suspension cultures of L-strain mouse cells. Exp. Cell Res. **38**, 208 (1965).

29. WHITMORE, G. F. and GULYAS, S.: Synchronization of mammalian cells with tritiated thymidine. Science **151**, 691 (1966).

30. XEROS, N.: Deoxyriboside control and synchronization of mitosis. Nature **194**, 682 (1962).

31. ZEUTHEN, E.: Artificial and induced periodicity in living cells. Advances Biol. and Med. Physics **6**, 37 (1958).

Susceptibility of Intestinal Crypt Epithelium to Hydroxyurea and Other Antitumor Agents *

Frederick S. Philips, Stephen S. Sternberg, and Luigi Lenaz

Pharmacology Division
Sloan-Kettering Institute for Cancer Research
New York, New York

The outstanding limitation in the effective use of most antitumor agents is selective damage in normal cell renewal systems *in vivo*. These systems contain undifferentiated or partially differentiated precursors of various mature cells such as leukocytes, erythrocytes, villar epithelium of intestine, sperm, and non-germinal components of epidermis. Normally the systems operate to maintain a steady balance between the birth of differentiated descendants and their continuous loss from the organism (6). The susceptibility of two of the cell renewal populations, that is, hematopoietic tissues and digestive tract epithelium, commonly determines the upper limit of doses of antitumor drugs. It is likely that lesions in the digestive tract are the major determinant of maximal dosage since these give rise to distressing symptoms such as oropharyngitis, nausea, and abdominal cramps and cause alarming signs of intoxication such as diarrhea and ulceration of pharyngeal and intestinal mucosa.

We have in the past described the intestinal lesions induced in experimental animals by such diverse cancer chemotherapeutic agents as the 4-amino substituted derivatives of folic acid, aminopterin and amethopterin (15), 6-mercaptopurine (13), actinomycin D (11), 0-diazoacetyl-L-serine, azaserine (21), alkylating agents, mechlorethamine and busulfan (22), mitomycin C (10), and hydroxyurea (14). The primary site of cytotoxic action of each of the agents has been the epithelial cells of crypts; changes in villar epithelium and structure, when they occur, are presumably secondary manifestations of prolonged failure of proliferative activity in the crypts. In this respect the intestinal effects of the above chemical agents closely resemble those of x-radiation (9).

Cell damage can develop rapidly in crypt epithelium and may account for the nausea and emesis which frequently appear within a few hours after giving antitumor drugs and after x-irradiation of the abdominal region. At such early times, abundant numbers of degenerating crypt cells have been seen in laboratory animals receiving x-irradiation (9, 1, 23) or antitumor agents such as methotrexate (15), actinomycin D and mitomycin C (18), hydroxyurea (14), and cytosine arabinonucleoside (4).

In an effort to gain some understanding of the nature of the acute cell degenera-

* Aided by Grant CA-08748 from the National Cancer Institute, USPHS.

tion caused by antitumor agents, we have been studying the cytotoxic effects of hydroxyurea. We have shown that the agent induces cell death in intestinal crypts, bone marrow, and germinal centers of all lymphoid tissues within a few hours after injection into rats. Its cytotoxicity is limited to these highly proliferative tissues. In organs containing such tissues, the agent causes an immediate, selective inhibition of DNA-synthesis that precedes mitotic inhibition and cell necrosis. The actions of hydroxyurea are rapidly terminated by biotransformation and renal excretion and the block in DNA synthesis is correspondingly transient, lasting only so long as effective concentrations of the agent are present in tissues. The pathologic process is also of short duration and tissue defects are rapidly repaired (14).

The cell death observed in proliferating tissues of rats given hydroxyurea has been presumed to result from the metabolic imbalance induced by selective arrest of DNA synthesis (14). The effect is considered comparable to the loss of reproductive capacity in bacteria (3) and in mammalian cells in culture (17) when these are specifically deprived of the capacity to synthesize thymidylic acid. We have also proposed that the lethal effects of hydroxyurea *in vivo* are restricted in mitotic tissues to those cells which are in the DNA synthetic stage (S phase) of the generation cycle. Cells in other phases of the mitotic cycle escape injury and serve to repopulate the proliferating tissues after disappearance of the agent. A similar mechanism has been offered to account for the loss of reproductible capacity caused by hydroxyurea in Chinese hamster cells in culture (20).

We have obtained evidence consistent with the proposal that S phase cells are in fact uniquely susceptible to hydroxyurea *in vivo* (12). Epithelium in the crypts of mouse duodenum was used as the object for study since the kinetics of proliferation in this tissue are well known and readily analyzed by radioautographic technics after labeling with tritiated thymidine (16, 8). After injection of effective doses in mice, mitosis is sharply inhibited and degenerating cells appear in crypts within 2 hours. The necrotic cells consist of condensed, fragmented, basophilic, Feulgen positive material surrounded by a halo of structureless, eosinophilic cytoplasm. Basophilic, Feulgen positive debris is scattered throughout the adjacent region. In time of onset, duration, and appearance the karyorrhectic process resembles that produced by x-irradiation in mouse duodenal crypts (19). The production of necrotic cells is maximal at about 4 hours; thereafter, dead cells and debris are steadily removed and mitoses return. By 24 hours the crypts are essentially normal. The disturbance's duration in the generative crypt region is sufficiently brief and recovery so rapid that there is no histologically obvious reduction in size of villi.

Study of the response of the crypt epithelium to single injections of varying amounts of drug reveals that damage is produced by minimally effective doses as low or even lower than those commonly used in treatment of experimental or clinical tumors. Doses, severalfold larger than minimal, produce a maximal effect. Factors contributing to the plateau in responsiveness may include 1. the rapid termination in action of hydroxyurea due to its metabolic inactivation and renal excretion (14), 2. the highly reversible nature of the inhibition of DNA synthesis caused by the agent (24), and 3. the restriction of cytotoxic susceptibility to that fraction of the proliferating epithelium which is in the DNA synthetic period (S phase) of the mitotic cycle (20, 12). Evidence obtained in the mouse in support of these suggestions includes the demonstration that cell death in crypts is produced by doses of hydroxyurea sufficient to maintain blood concentrations above 10^{-4} M for more than 1 hour. Such concentrations are known to inhibit DNA synthesis in mammalian cells in culture by more than 50 percent (24). In mice receiving cytotoxic doses, followed at varying intervals by pulse doses of tritiated thymidine, the number of labeled crypt cells is reduced to negligible levels for at least one hour after injection. Labeling of epithelial cells resumes, thereafter, in step with the decrease of blood concentrations below 10^{-4} M. The degenerating cells which appear are not labeled. Doses which are not cytotoxic cause only a transient decrease in number of labeled cells during the first half-hour after injection.

In spite of prompt inhibition of uptake of tritiated thymidine in crypt cells mitoses are present in normal numbers during the first half-hour after injection of maximally cytotoxic doses. Thereafter, mitotic cells decrease and in 2 hours none are present. This is the result to be expected if cells in G_2 and M are unaffected by hydroxyurea; for the maximum duration of G_2 and M in mouse crypt cells has been found to be 2 hours (8). Mitoses do not reappear in damaged crypts until about six hours have elapsed from the time tritiated thymidine labeling is resumed. A similar interval is required for normal duodenal crypt cells to advance through the entire S and G_2 phases of the mitotic cycle (8). The fact that the two intervals are alike is consistent with the supposition that all or most of the S compartment is destroyed by maximally effective doses while G_1 cells are undamaged and movement of cells into S begins promptly after the inhibition of DNA synthesis is relieved.

Other evidence for the selective susceptibility of S-phase cells has been obtained by pulse labeling with tritiated thymidine immediately before injection of cytotoxic amounts of hydroxyurea. Most of the degenerating cells which appear in the crypts of these animals are labeled. Finally it should be mentioned that the maximal number of degenerating cells found after single doses of hydroxyurea does not exceed the number of crypt cells which are labeled by labeled thymidine in untreated mice.

The results which have been obtained in analyzing the cytotoxic effects of hydroxyurea in intact animals are consistent with the proposal that cell death is the consequence of selective interruption of DNA synthesis. Additional support for this proposal has been obtained from studies with another selective inhibitor of DNA synthesis, 1-β-D-arabinosylcytosine, ara-C (2) and with its 5-fluoro derivative, ara-FC (5). Both ara-C and ara-FC have been shown to induce rapid and marked inhibition of DNA synthesis in mouse small intestine; this action is followed within a few hours by the appearance of degenerating cells in crypt epithelium (4, 7). We have also found ara-FC to induce equally marked and prompt inhibition of DNA synthesis in other proliferating systems of mice such as spleen and thymus. Minimal numbers of necrotic cells are found in duodenal crypts after doses of ara-FC which are sufficient to inhibit DNA synthesis by more than 90 percent for one to two hours. After giving minimally cytotoxic doses synthesis returns to normal within 4 to 6 hours. Doses three- to tenfold greater induce maximal numbers of degenerating cells. As in mice receiving hydroxyurea the lesion is most prominent at 4 hours after injection; thereafter, necrotic cells disappear from crypts and by 24 hours there are few or none remaining. Changes in mitotic rates are seen in crypts similar to those described above in animals treated with hydroxyurea. Two hours elapse before mitoses disappear completely in mice given maximally cytotoxic doses of ara-FC. No mitoses are seen for the next 6 hours; thereafter, they return to control levels.

In view of the similarity of the cytotoxic responses to hydroxyurea and the cytosine arabinonucleosides it is reasonable to anticipate that any agent capable of inducing selective inhibition of DNA synthesis in crypt epithelium will cause necrosis of a portion of the proliferating cell population. For reasons advanced above the susceptible fraction may consist exclusively of S-phase cells. There is no satisfactory explanation at present for the rapid development of injury when DNA synthesis is arrested in such cells. Suggestions that cell death is due to a metabolic imbalance induced by selective inhibition of DNA synthesis are only restatements of experimental findings (3, 17). Clearly further work is needed to elucidate the nature of the instability that develops in proliferating cells when these, in the face of a commitment to complete the mitotic cycle, are unable to replicate DNA.

It would be a gross oversimplification to leave the impression that the cytotoxic effects of antitumor agents in cell renewal systems *in vivo* have been in all instances unambiguously associated with selective inhibition of DNA synthesis. For example, we have previously described the lesions induced in proliferating tissues by actinomycin D (11, 18). This agent, generally considered to have as its primary action the inhibition of DNA-dependent RNA synthesis, induces degeneration of crypt epithelium in rat small intestine within a few hours after injection. The lesion is not preceded by measurable inhibition of DNA synthesis (18). Recently an inhibitor of protein synthesis, puromycin, has been shown to cause extensive necrosis in duodenal crypts of mice. This effect is preceded by an early depression of protein synthesis which is accomplished by an equally marked, simultaneous inhibition of DNA synthesis (4). Possibly future clarification of the mechanism alluded to above by which S-phase cells break down, when acted upon by selective inhibitors of DNA synthesis like hydroxyurea and ara-FC, will also provide understanding of the susceptibility of dividing cells to inhibitors of the synthesis of other kinds of macromolecules.

References

1. BLOOM, W.: Histopathology of Irradiation from External and Internal Sources. McGraw-Hill, New York (1948).
2. COHEN, S. S.: Introduction to the biochemistry of D-arabinosyl nucleotides. Progr. Nucleic Acid Res. **5**, 1 (1966).
3. COHEN, S. S. and BAHNER, H. D.: Studies on unbalanced growth in Escherichia coli. Proc. Natl. Acad. Sci. **40**, 885 (1954).
4. ESTENSEN, R. D. and BASERGA, R.: Puromycin-induced necrosis of crypt cells of the small intestine of mouse. J. Cell. Biol. **30**, 13 (1966).
5. KIM, J. H., EIDINOFF, M. L. and FOX, J. J.: Action of 1-β-D-arabinosyl-5-fluorocytosine on the nucleic acid metabolism and viability of HeLa cells. Cancer Res. **26**, 1661 (1966).
6. LEBLOND, C. P. and WALKER, B. E.: Renewal of cell populations. Physiol. Rev. **36**, 255 (1956).

7. LENAZ, L., STERNBERG, S. S. and PHILIPS, F. S.: unpublished observations.

8. LESHER, S., FRY, R. J. M. and KOHN, H. I.: Age and generation time of the mouse duodenal epithelial cells. Exp. Cell Res. 24, 334 (1961).

9. PATT, H. M. and QUASTLER, H.: Radiation effects on cell renewal and related systems. Physiol. Rev. 43, 357 (1963).

10. PHILIPS, F. S., SCHWARTZ, H. S. and STERNBERG, S. S.: Pharmacology of mitomycin C.I. Toxicity and pathologic effects. Cancer Res. 20, 1354 (1960).

11. PHILIPS, F. S., SCHWARTZ, H. S., STERNBERG, S. S. and TAN, C. T. C.: The toxicity of actinomycin D. Ann. N.Y. Acad. Sci. 89, 348 (1960).

12. PHILIPS, F. S., STERNBERG, S. S., CRONIN, A. P., VIDAL, P. M. and SCHWARTZ, H. S.: Hydroxyurea (HU): selective susceptibility of S-phase cells in vivo. Proc. Am. Assoc. Cancer Res. 8, 54 (1967).

13. PHILIPS, F. S., STERNBERG, S. S., HAMILTON, L. and CLARKE, D. A.: The toxic effects of 6-mercaptopurine and related compounds. Ann. N.Y. Acad. Sci. 60, 283 (1954).

14. PHILIPS, F. S., STERNBERG, S. S., SCHWARTZ, H. S., CRONIN, A. P., SODERGREN, J. E. and VIDAL, P. M.: Hydroxyurea. I. Acute cell death in proliferating tissues in rats. Cancer Res. 20, 1354 (1967).

15. PHILIPS, F. S., THIERSCH, J. B. and FERGUSON, F. C.: Studies of the action of 4-amino-pteroylglutamic acid and its congeners in mammals. Ann. N.Y. Acad. Sci. 52, 1349 (1950).

16. QUASTLER, H. and SHERMAN, F. G.: Cell population kinetics in the intestinal epithelium of the mouse. Exp. Cell Res. 17, 420 (1959).

17. RUECKERT, R. R. and MUELLER, G. C.: Studies on unbalanced growth in tissue culture. I. Induction and consequences of thymidine deficiency. Cancer Res. 20, 1584 (1960).

18. SCHWARTZ, H. S., STERNBERG, S. S. and PHILIPS, F. S.: Pharmacology of mitomycin C. IV. Effects in vivo on nucleic acid synthesis; comparison with actinomycin D. Cancer Res. 23, 1125 (1963).

19. SHERMAN, F. G. and QUASTLER, H.: DNA synthesis in irradiated intestinal epithelium. Exp. Cell Res. 19, 343 (1960).

20. SINCLAIR, W. K.: Hydroxyurea: Differential lethal effects on cultured mammalian cells during the cell cycle. Science 150, 1729 (1965).

21. STERNBERG, S. S., PHILIPS, F. S.: Azaserine: pathological and pharmacological studies. Cancer 10, 889 (1957).

22. STERNBERG, S. S., PHILIPS, F. S. and SCHOOLER, J.: Pharmacological and pathological effects of alkylating agents. Ann. N.Y. Acad. Sci. 68, 811 (1958).

23. WILLIAMS, R. B., JR., TOAL, J. N., WHITE, J. R. and CARPENTER, H. M.: Effect of total body x-radiation from near threshold to tissue-lethal doses on small bowel epithelium of the rat. I. Changes in morphology and rate of cell division in relation to time and dose. J. Natl. Cancer Inst. 21, 17 (1958).

24. YOUNG, C. W. and HODAS, S.: Hydroxyurea: inhibitory effect on DNA metabolism. Science 146, 1172 (1964).

Discussion

Mammalian Cell Killing by Inhibitors of DNA Synthesis

G. F. Whitmore, J. Borsa, S. Bacchetti and F. Graham

University of Toronto and
Ontario Cancer Institute
Toronto, Canada

During the course of his discussion this afternoon, Dr. Philips mentioned two agents, hydroxyurea and cytosine arabinoside which appeared to bring about rapid destruction of the cells of the intestinal lining. Like a number of other groups we have been interested in the effects of these compounds and others on mammalian cells in tissue culture. In agreement with the observation of Dr. Philips and others (1, 2, 3) we have observed that with these two compounds there is a class of cells which are rapidly killed by the compounds and these are cells in the S phase. There is, however, a second mode of killing which is not restricted to cells in the S phase and which is not apparent until much later times in the cell cycle, times which are approximately equal to the times required for a cell to pass from the beginning of S through S and G_2 and into mitosis (2, 3, 4). After this length of exposure to the drug there appears to be a rapid and almost exponential decline in the fraction of viable cells. This paper presents some data and questions which we feel bear on the nature of these two types of killing.

The nature of the types of survival curves we are talking about can be seen in the first two figures. Figure 1 shows the survival of mouse L cells as a function of time in the presence of hydroxyurea at a concentration of 10^{-2} M. It is obvious that immediately upon the addition of the compound there is a rapid drop in the survival to about 50 percent. There is considerable evidence from our own studies and those of Sinclair (1, 2) and Kim *et al.* (3) that this rapid decline in survival is due to the killing of S phase cells. Following this initial decline there is a long plateau lasting perhaps as long as 10 or 12 hours during which there is little or no change in the level of survival. Following this interval there is a rapid and almost exponential loss of surviving cells. It would appear therefore that there are two distinct modes of cell killing operational here—one reserved for cells in the S phase and another, probably quite distinct, reserved for cells in other phases of the cell cycle.

Figure 2 shows similar types of survival curves for mouse L cells in the presence of various concentrations of cytosine arabinoside. For a concentration of 1 μgm/ml the initial burst of killing is absent although there may be some evidence of killing after about five hours; but there is a phase of rapid cell killing beginning about 15

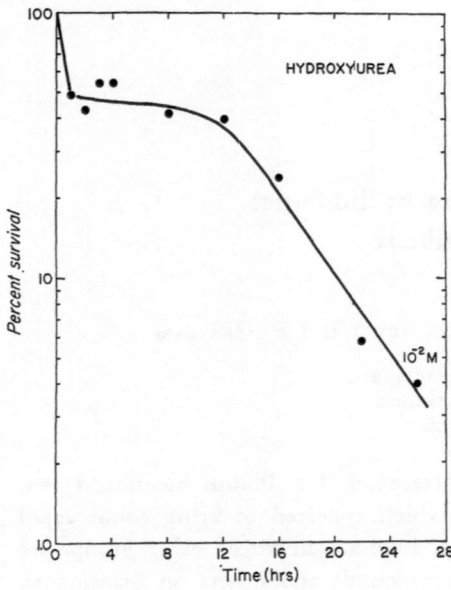

Fig. 1. Survival of mouse L-cells as a function of time in the presence of 10^{-2} hydroxyurea.

hours after the addition of the compound. With a concentration of 1 μgm/ml there is an initial rapid drop, a plateau lasting about ten hours and then the final exponential decline. For a concentration of 100 μgm/ml there is the initial rapid decline followed by a very short plateau and then a very rapid decay of survival extending over approximately three decades. Here again there would appear to be at least two modes of cell death involved, one responsible for the delayed cell killing observed at 1 and 10 μgm/ml and the other responsible for the rapid decline observed at early times in concentrations of 10 and 100 μgm/ml and perhaps for the secondary decline observed after four hours in the presence of 100 μgm/ml. This latter curve is highly reminiscent of the type of survival curve observed for L cells continuously exposed to very high concentrations of tritiated thymidine. This might suggest that at high concentrations cytosine arabinoside is somehow being incorporated into DNA.

While the hypothesis that cytosine arabinoside is being incorporated into DNA would not seem unreasonable it must be pointed out that under the conditions used in the experiments with hydroxyurea and cytosine arabinoside the rate of DNA synthesis was rapidly inhibited (3, 4, 5, 6, 7, 8). Therefore any incorporation of cytosine arabinoside must occur under conditions where very little DNA is being synthesized.

This lack of DNA synthesis and the appearance of the second mode of cell killing apparent after long exposures to hydroxyurea and cytosine arabinoside leads us to some observations made in our laboratory using the compound methotrexate, a known inhibitor of DNA and RNA synthesis. The inhibition of DNA synthesis comes about because of a double inhibition of thymidylate synthesis and purine synthesis under the influence of the drug whereas the inhibition of RNA synthesis is due to the inhibition of purine synthesis. One of the problems which interested us was the role played by each of these inhibitions in determining the amount of cell killing. The

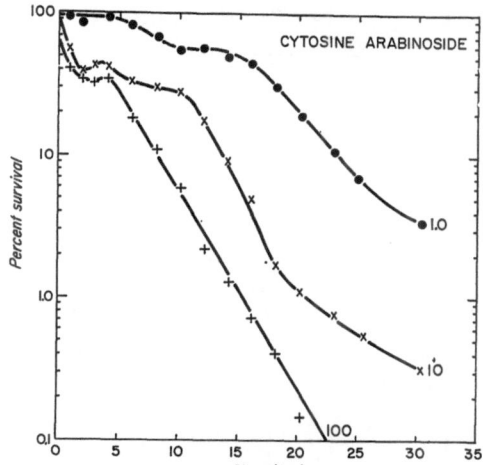

Fig. 2. Survival of mouse L-cells as a function of time in the presence of 1, 10 and 100 μgms cytosine arabinoside per ml.

results of the experiments clearly indicate that cell death is primarily a consequence of the suppression of DNA synthesis. The experiments also indicate that if RNA synthesis is inhibited at the same time as DNA synthesis this will to some extent protect the cells against the killing effect due to lack of DNA synthesis.

All of the experiments to be described here were carried out on L60T cells, a subline of Earle's L cells (9). These were grown in suspension culture in medium C.M.R.L. 1066 (10) from which the nucleosides and coenzymes were omitted. The medium was supplemented with 10% V/V dialysed fetal calf serum. In all cases cell survival was measured by the ability to form colonies in the Puck and Marcus assay (11) and total cell counts were determined by means of an electronic cell counter.

The experiments to be described here deal with a separation of the effects of the inhibition of thymidylate and purine synthesis. The approach used to achieve this is as follows. Initial experiments carried out with methotrexate had indicated that the effects of the compound can be completely reversed or prevented by the addition of suitable concentrations of both thymidine and deoxyadenosine or adenosine as a source of purines (12). Hence it must follow that whatever inhibitory effects methotrexate exhibits on L cells in our growth medium must arise from the inhibition of either or both of the thymidylate or purine synthetic pathways. The effects on the pathways can be separated however by growing cells in growth medium supplemented in such a way that only one of the folate requiring pathways must be functional in order for the cells to grow. Thus methotrexate inhibition of cells in growth medium supplemented with thymidine will reveal the effects of the methotrexate suppression of purine synthesis whereas the inhibition of cells in growth medium supplemented with purines will reveal the effects of the methotrexate inhibition of thymidylate synthesis.

Making use of the procedure outlined above we have tested separately the effect on viability of each block produced by methotrexate. When cells in the exponential phase growth, in growth medium, were exposed to 10^{-6} gm methotrexate per ml for a period of 72 hours in the presence of various concentrations of thymidine the re-

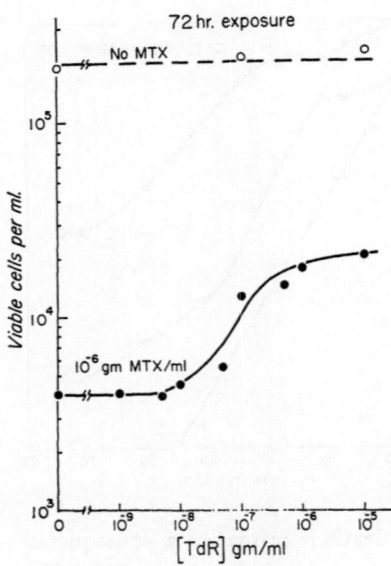

Fig. 3. Effect of thymidine concentration on the survival of L-cells during a 72-hour period in the absence or presence of methotrexate (10^{-6} gm/ml). Initial cell concentration 1×10^5 cells/ml.

sults shown in Figure 3 were obtained. From the figure it can be seen that thymidine concentrations above 10^{-8} gm/ml result in increasing levels of survival until a maximum is reached at a concentration between 10^{-6} and 10^{-5} gm/ml. However, even when this maximum survival is reached there is still considerable cell killing, amounting in most experiments to approximately 50 percent of the cells initially present.

Figure 4 shows the results of a similar experiment in which cells were exposed to the same concentration of methotrexate in the presence of various concentrations of deoxyadenosine over a period of 72 hours. Here, in contrast to the data obtained with thymidine, the addition of increasing amounts of deoxyadenosine results in enhanced

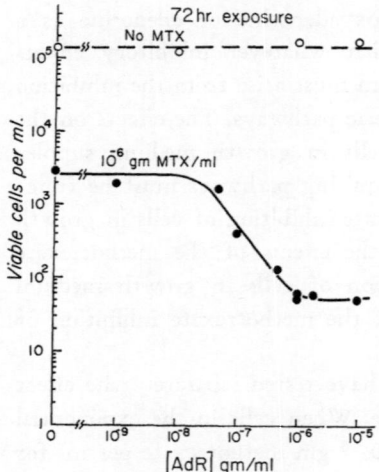

Fig. 4. Effect of deoxyadenosine concentration on the survival of L-cells during a 72-hour period in the absence or presence of methotrexate (10^{-6} gm/ml). Initial cell concentration 1×10^5 cells/ml.

cell killing which ultimately reaches a maximum value when the deoxyadenosine concentration is approximately 10^{-6} gm/ml.

From the data presented in Figures 3 and 4 it is apparent that cell killing is more efficient in the absence of thymidine than in its presence and therefore it can be concluded that the methotrexate induced suppression of thymidylate synthesis tends to foster cell killing. In contrast it is apparent that in the absence of thymidine cell killing occurs more efficiently in the presence of deoxyadenosine than in its absence. Therefore it can be concluded that the methotrexate induced inhibition of purine synthesis tends to protect against the cell killing brought about by the methotrexate induced inhibition of thymidylate synthesis. Thus it can be seen that the two effects of the compound are antagonistic to one another and that when both inhibitions are operational the one tends to protect against the effects of the other.

Figure 5 gives the results of a similar experiment in which cells were exposed to methotrexate for 72 hours in the presence of various concentrations of Leucovorin, a specific reversing agent for methotrexate. The upper part of the figure shows the increase in cell number over the 72 hour interval as a function of the Leucovorin

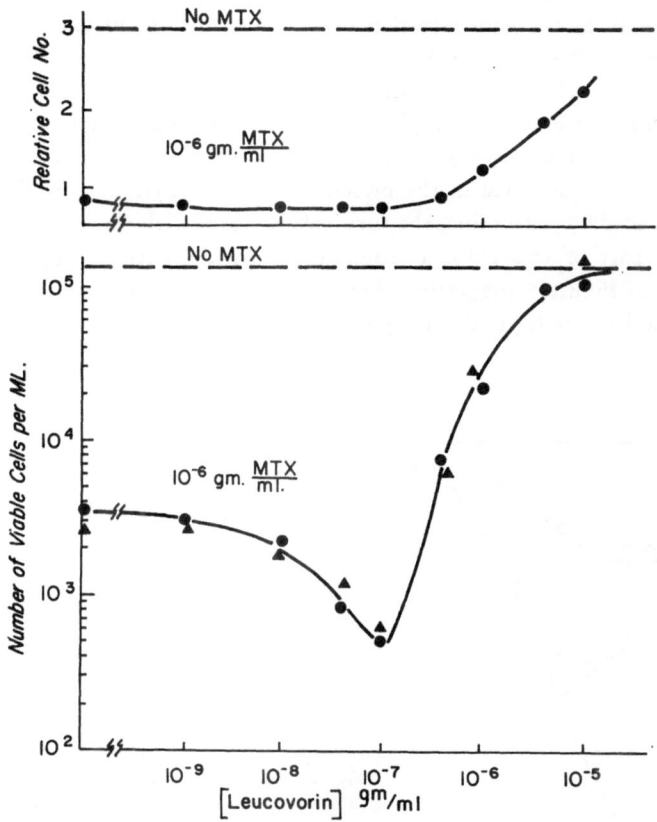

Fig. 5. Effect of Leucovorin concentration on growth of L-cells (upper curve) and on cell viability (lower curve), both over a 72-hour interval. The upper curve shows the ratio of the cell number at the end of 72 hours to that present at time zero.

concentration. In this figure unity corresponds to the cell number present at the beginning of the growth experiment. The lower part of the figure shows the survival of colony forming ability as a function of Leucovorin concentration over the same interval. In this figure it can be seen that there is a distinct minimum in the cell survival for a concentration of 10^{-7} gm/ml. At this concentration the upper curve indicates that cell growth is still completely inhibited. Concentrations of Leucovorin greater than 10^{-7} gm/ml result in increasing levels of cell survival and cell growth. It should be noted that the two sets of symbols in the figure come from completely separate experiments, both of which clearly show the existence of the minimum.

Having obtained the data shown in Figure 5 it seemed necessary to propose a model to account for the minimum in the curve of survival versus Leucovorin concentration. The model which we proposed (12) is that at low concentrations of Leucovorin both DNA and RNA synthesis are inhibited and that the inhibition of DNA synthesis results in a certain amount of cell killing. However, because RNA synthesis is also inhibited the killing is not as efficient as it might be in the presence of purine synthesis. However, as the concentration of Leucovorin is increased the purine synthetic block is lifted, some RNA synthesis takes place and this enchances the killing. Finally as the concentration of Leucovorin is increased even further the synthesis of both DNA and RNA resumes and ultimately the survival becomes indistinguishable from the control. There are several ways of testing the above model but we will limit ourselves to one piece of evidence which is shown in Figure 6. In addition to repeating the curve of Figure 5 this curve shows the effect of Leucovorin concentration on cell survival in the presence of either thymidine or deoxyadenosine. In the presence of deoxyadenosine, the survival increases with increasing concentration and the upper part of this curve is essentially identical with the upper part of the survival curve of Figure 5 suggesting that for Leucovorin concentrations above 10^{-7} gm/ml it is the lack of thymidylate synthesis which is the major determinant of cell killing.

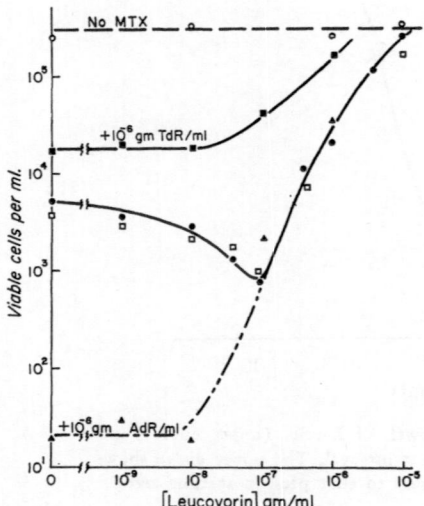

Fig. 6. Effect of Leucovorin together with 10^{-6} gm/ml of either thymidine or deoxyadenosine during a 72-hour exposure to methotrexate (10^{-6} gm/ml). Initial cell number, 1×10^5 cells/ml.

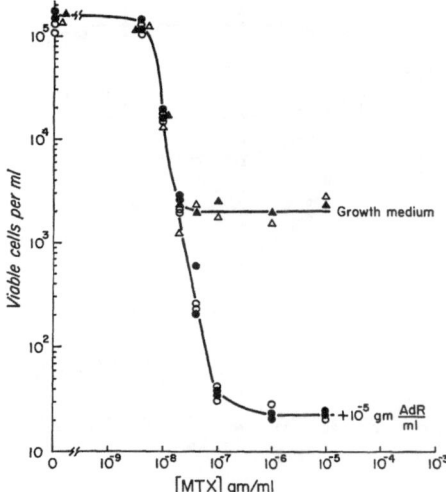

Fig. 7. Influence of the concentration of methotrexate on L-cell viability during a 72-hour exposure. Suspension cultures were treated wither with the indicated concentration of methotrexate alone or together with 10^{-5} gm deoxyadenosine/ml. Initial cell concentration 1×10^5 cells/ml.

All of the methotrexate experiments which we have discussed so far have been carried out with a methotrexate concentration of 10^{-6} gm/ml. The data of Figure 7 indicate the effect of changing the concentration of methotrexate on cell survival measured over a 72-hour interval. The experiment was carried out in the presence of methotrexate alone, and in the presence of methotrexate plus deoxyadenosine. In growth medium the maximum cell killing is reached for a concentration of between 2 and 4×10^{-8} gm/ml and higher concentrations do not result in increased killing. In the presence of excess deoxyadenosine the maximum cell killing is reached for a concentration of about 10^{-7} gm/ml and as has been seen earlier the survival level is far below that found in the absence of deoxyadenosine.

The experiments detailed above have served to illustrate the effect of various conditions on the efficiency of methotrexate induced cell killing over a fixed interval of time. From the point of view of our discussion today it is especially pertinent to determine the variation in survival as a function of time in methotrexate. The results of some experiments which bear on this question are shown in Figure 8. In the absence of methotrexate the viable cell number increased approximately threefold in a time of thirty hours. In the presence of methotrexate alone the viable cell number remained approximately constant for about 10 to 12 hours and then declined to approximately 10 percent of the starting value. In the presence of methotrexate plus thymidine the cell number again remained constant for about 10 hours and then declined to approximately 25 percent of the starting value. Finally in the presence of methotrexate plus deoxyadenosine the survival remained constant for about 10 hours and then fell rapidly over the next 60 hours to a value of less than 0.1 percent of the starting value.

The important feature of Figure 8 would appear to be that in no instance did cell killing commence in less than 10 to 12 hours after the addition of the drug suggesting that inhibition of DNA synthesis must continue over long periods of time before it can possibly induce cell killing. Therefore it would appear that the imme-

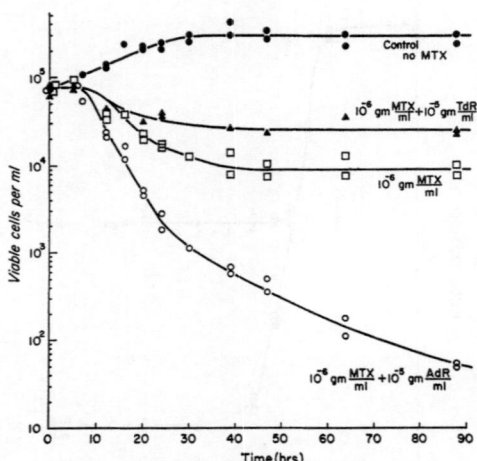

Fig. 8. The time course of L-cell killing by 10^{-6} gm. methotrexate per ml under various conditions.

diate cell killing effects observed with hydroxyurea and with cytosine arabinoside on cells in the S phase are not due simply to a cessation of DNA synthesis, although there is a rapid decrease of DNA synthesis in the presence of both of these compounds. Also the fact that at a cytosine arabinoside concentration of 1.0 μgm/ml the rate of DNA synthesis is reduced to less than 2 percent of control in less than three hours and yet there is no cell killing until 16 hours would also argue that immediate cell killing is not due simply to an inhibition of DNA synthesis.

Therefore it would appear that there are at least two modes of cell death induced by inhibitors of DNA synthesis. There is the immediate cell death restricted to cells in the S phase. This is observed with hydroxyurea, cytosine arabinoside, and probably with high concentrations of FUdR (9). There is also the much slower developing cell death seen with methotrexate, low concentrations of FUdR and cytosine arabinoside and with hydroxyurea. This immediately poses the question as to the mechanisms of or reasons for the two kinds of death. Does the rapid killing of cells in the S phase indicate incorporation of the drug or some reaction product of the drug or does it represent degradation or alteration of DNA molecules which have been rendered sensitive by the fact that the cells are in the S phase? Also what is the mechanism responsible for the less rapidly developing cell death? Does it appear only in cells which by some time scale or measured by the accumulation of some critical compound have reached the stage of mitosis without synthesizing a new complement of DNA? Does it occur in cells which have been held up in any part of the cycle too long? If it is the former why does it not occur sooner in methotrexate treated cells some of which must have been in late S phase when DNA synthesis was halted and therefore should have been ready for mitosis soon after?

To the best of our knowledge the answers to these questions are not available and it is therefore obvious that a great deal of work remains to be done before we will understand the mechanisms of cell killing.

Finally it seems pertinent to make one additional observation which would seem to apply to all of the compounds which have been mentioned today. This is the observation that in each case there appears to be an efficient and rapid mode of cell killing which is to some extent and for part of the population inhibited by a secondary effect of the compound. For example, with hydroxyurea and cytosine arabinoside their ability to inhibit DNA synthesis prevents the entry of cells into the most sensitive phase of the cell cycle, namely S. For methotrexate the concomitant inhibition of RNA synthesis prevents the efficient killing of cells due to a lack of DNA synthesis. For this reason all of these compounds would appear to be less than ideal chemotherapeutic agents and these observations may to some extent explain why tumors almost always exhibit some degree of refractoriness to these compounds.

References

1. SINCLAIR, W. K.: Hydroxyurea: Differential lethal effects on cultured mammalian cells during the cell cycle. Science 150, 1729 (1965).
2. SINCLAIR, W. K.: Hydroxyurea: Effects on Chinese hamster cells grown in culture. Can. Res. 27, 297 (1967).
3. KIM, J. H., GELBARD, A. S., and PEREZ, A. G.: Action of hydroxyurea on the nucleic acid metabolism and viability of HeLa cells. Can. Res. 27, 1301 (1967).
4. PFEIFFER, S. J., and TOLMACH, L. J.: Inhibition of DNA synthesis in HeLa cells by hydroxyurea. Can. Res. 27, 124 (1967).
5. YOUNG, C. W., SCHOCHETMAN, G., and KARNOFSKY, D. A.: Hydroxyurea-induced inhibition of deoxyribonucleotide synthesis: Studies in intact cells. Can. Res. 27, 526 (1967).
6. YOUNG, C. W., and HODAS, S.: Acute effects of cytoxic compounds on incorporation of precursors into DNA, RNA and protein of HeLa monolayers. Biochem. Pharmacol. 14, 205 (1965).
7. CHU, M. Y., and FISCHER, G. A.: A proposed mechanism of action of 1-B-D-arabinofuranosylcytosine as an inhibitor of the growth of leukemic cells. Biochem. Pharmacol. 11, 423 (1962).
8. DOERING, A., KELLER, J., and COHEN, S. S.: Some effects of D-arabinosyl nucleosides on polymer syntheses in mouse fibroblasts. Can. Res. 26, 2444 (1966).
9. TILL, J. E., WHITMORE, G. F., and GULYAS, S.: Deoxyribonucleic acid synthesis in individual L-strain mouse cells. II. Effects of thymidine starvation. Biochem. Biophys. Acta 72, 277 (1963).
10. PARKER, R. C.: Methods of tissue culture, 3rd Ed. Paul B. Hoeber, New York (1961).
11. PUCH, T. T., and MARCUS, P. I.: A rapid method for viable cell titration and clone production with HeLa cells in tissue culture: The use of X-Irradiated cells to supply conditioning factors. Proc. Nat. Acad. Sci. U.S. 41, 432 (1955).
12. BORSA, J., and WHITMORE, G. F.: Studies relating to the mode of action of methotrexate. I. Cell killing studies on L-cells in vitro. (In press.)

The Growth of Tumor Cells
Under Normal and Fasting Conditions *

RENATO BASERGA and FRIEDRICH WIEBEL †

Fels Research Institute and Department of Pathology
Temple University,
Philadelphia, Pennsylvania

The growth rate of a tumor depends upon a number of kinetic factors that can be grouped under three headings: 1. the length of the cell cycle, that is, the interval between completion of mitosis and completion of the subsequent mitosis in one or both daughter cells; 2. the growth fraction (14), that is, the fraction of cells that participate in the proliferating process; and 3. cell loss, that is, the number of tumor cells that are lost through death, exfoliation or metastasis. The last parameter, whose importance has been discussed by Steel *et al.* (20), has thus far received little attention, and the available quantitative data are too few for a critical analysis. The first two parameters have been studied extensively, and have already been adequately reviewed in previous studies (13, 2, 10, 5). Some of the conclusions offered by these studies can be summarized here very briefly: 1. the length of the cell cycle of tumor cells is not necessarily shorter than the cell cycle of some normal adult tissues (4). This is true both in laboratory animals and in man (2); 2. when a tumor is compared to its tissue of origin, the length of the cell cycle is usually, but not always, shorter in tumors than in their normal counterparts (see review by Baserga and Wiebel (5). However, this does not solve the problem of selective anti-tumor therapy, at least not in those situations in which the therapeutic target is the cell machinery that synthesizes DNA. Since some normal cells, notably the epithelial cells lining the crypts of the small intestine and cells of the bone marrow, have, as mentioned above, a shorter cell cycle than most tumor cells, inhibitors of cell proliferation will be as effective on some normal cells as on tumor cells; 3. the growth rate of transplantable tumors in experimental animals generally decreases with time after transplantation. Some tumors accomplish such a decrease in growth rate by decreasing the growth fraction, while keeping the length of the cell cycle unchanged (8). In other tumors, on the contrary, the decrease in growth rate is accomplished by a lengthening of the cell cycle, while the growth fraction does not change (12); 4. the length of the S phase is not constant, neither in normal nor in tumor cells. Somehow, the mistaken notion that the length of the S phase is con-

---

* This work was supported by Research Grant E-400 from the American Cancer Society.
† Recipient of a Damon Runyon Memorial Fund Fellowship (DRF-431AT).

stant has become so ingrained, that some investigators still feel compelled to report variable S phases, a finding which, they believe, will cast doubts on the dogma of the constancy of the S phase. There is no such dogma, and if there ever was one, it was consigned to oblivion some years ago (see review by Baserga (2)). In fact, the S phase is so variable that it varies in the same tumor with time after transplantation (12) or with the sex of the animal (5); 5. the length of G_2 also varies, both in normal and tumor cells, but its variations show an interesting tendency. Figure 1 shows a distribution of T_{G_2} in normal adult tissues, tumor tissues and cells in cultures. The *in vivo* data refer mostly to mice and rats. It is evident that T_{G_2} has a tendency to be longer in tumors and in cells in cultures than in normal adult tissues (5).

Although a precise rule cannot be formulated from these data, the tendency to a longer T_{G_2} in tumor cells may have some interest, both for the cell biologist who wishes to probe the cell's life processes, and for the clinician, always on the lookout for a vulnerable point in the tumor's defenses. We shall then deal, in the rest of this paper, with an experimental manipulation, *i.e.*, fasting, that has a marked effect on the length of the G_2 period of Ehrlich ascites tumor cells.

The advantages of restricted caloric intake were known to both Greeks and Romans. Celsus (about 100 A.D.) stated: "Neque ulla res magis adiuvat laborantem quam tempestiva abstinentia" (To a sufferer nothing is more advantageous than a timely abstinence) (7). In more recent times (1909) and in the field of tumors, it was shown by Moreschi (15) that underfeeding retards the growth of transplanted tumors, and his observations have been subsequently confirmed by Rous (18), Sugiura and Benedict (21) and many others. The effect of restricted caloric intake on the genesis and growth of tumors has been discussed by Tannenbaum and Silverstone (22), and an excellent review of the literature on underfeeding's effect on transplantation and growth of tumors can be found in White (26). We refer the reader to these reviews for further details. From the clinician point of view, we may notice that Tannenbaum and Silverstone (22) also reviewed the insurance

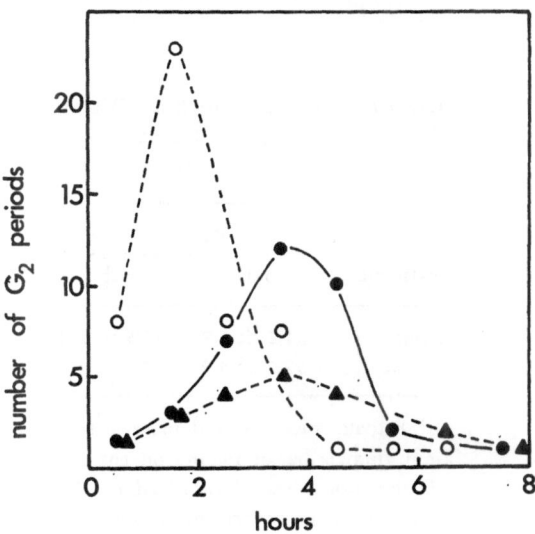

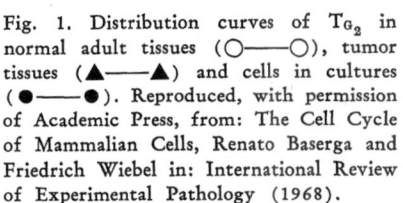

Fig. 1. Distribution curves of T_{G_2} in normal adult tissues (○——○), tumor tissues (▲——▲) and cells in cultures (●——●). Reproduced, with permission of Academic Press, from: The Cell Cycle of Mammalian Cells, Renato Baserga and Friedrich Wiebel in: International Review of Experimental Pathology (1968).

companies' statistics and found that, for most cancers, mortality increased with increasing body weight. Also pertinent to clinical interest is a recent observation by Gropper and Shimkin (9) on the growth of mammary carcinoma induced in female rats by oral 3-methylcholanthrene. These authors found that the best inhibition of growth without mortality was obtained by a combination of ovariectomy with food restriction. On the basis of these well-known studies, we have investigated the effect of fasting on the cell cycle of Ehrlich ascites tumor cells growing in the peritoneal cavity of female mice.

Materials and Methods

Female A mice, 4–5 months old, weighing approximately 30 g. and bred in our laboratory were inoculated intraperitoneally with 0.1 cc of Ehrlich ascites tumor, corresponding to 12–14 × 10⁶ tumor cells. The animals were fasted in metabolic cages; all food was withdrawn but they were allowed water *ad libitum*. The total number of tumor cells per mouse was determined by counting an aliquot of the tumor suspension in a hemocytometer. For studies of the cell cycle and its phases, thymidine-methyl-³H (New England Nuclear Corporation, Boston, Massachusetts), 6.7 Ci/mmole, was injected intraperitoneally, 0.03 μCi/g. body wt., dissolved in 0.2 cc of sterile water. The animals were sacrificed by cervical dislocation, and smears of Ehrlich ascites tumor cells were autoradiographed as previously described (1). The percentage of labeled tumor cells was determined, on each smear, on 2,000 cells; the percentage of labeled mitoses on 100 mitoses. The mitotic index is expressed as the number of mitoses per 1,000 cells.

Results and Discussion

Table I shows the effect of a 48-hour fasting on body weight and total number of tumor cells per mouse. The animals lose about one-fourth of their weight in two

TABLE I

EFFECT OF FASTING ON BODY WEIGHT AND TOTAL NUMBER OF TUMOR
CELLS IN MICE CARRYING AN INTRAPERITONEAL GROWTH
OF EHRLICH ASCITES TUMOR *

| | Body wt. in g. on day | | | Total number of |
Treatment	5th	6th	7th	tumor cells × 10⁻⁶
None	31.5 ± 1.7	32.9 ± 1.8	34.5 ± 2.0	500 ± 39
Fasted	32.7 ± 4.2	27.8 ± 4.4	23.6 ± 3.3	393 ± 74

* Female mice injected intraperitoneally with 12 × 10⁶ tumor cells. The fasted animals began fasting on the 5th day and the total number of tumor cells per mouse was determined on 7th day after inoculation. Six mice per group; values given are mean and standard deviations.

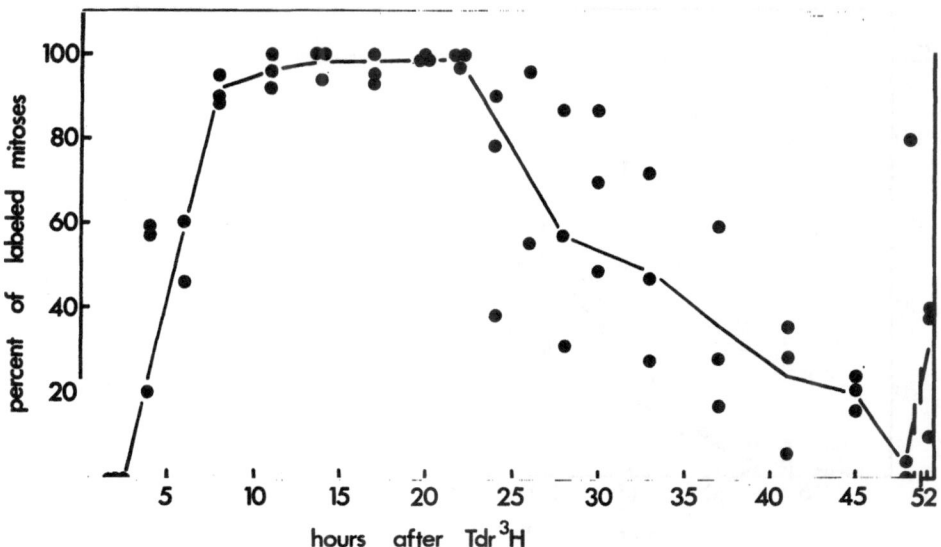

Fig. 2. Curve of the percentage of labeled mitoses, at various times after a single injection of thymidine-³H, of Ehrlich ascites tumor cells on the 5th day after inoculation into the peritoneal cavity of female mice. Each closed circle represents one animal.

days, and tumor growth is retarded. It may be noted here, incidentally, that a 72-hr. fast does not produce irreversible illness in mice. When fed after a 72-hr. fast, the animals survive and return to apparently normal behavior in 24 hrs. Longer fasting (96 hrs. or more) results in sickness, from which a majority of animals are incapable of recovering despite feeding.

Figure 2 gives the percentage of labeled mitoses, at various times after a single administration of thymidine-³H, of Ehrlich ascites tumor on the 5th day after intra-peritoneal inoculation into female A mice. The cell cycle times, estimated from this curve by the method of Quastler and Sherman (17), are as follows: $T_C = 47$ hrs., $T_S = 26.5$ hrs., $T_{G_2} = 5.5$ hrs., T_M (from the mitotic index) $= 1$ hr., and T_{G_1} (by subtraction) $= 14$ hrs. It may be added at this point that the growth fraction of Ehrlich ascites tumor on the 5th day after inoculation is 0.97. The cell cycle times obtained in this experiment differ slightly from those obtained with the same tumor 3 years ago, when, for instance, T_C was 36 hrs. (3).

Figure 3 shows the percentage curve of labeled mitoses of Ehrlich ascites tumor from animals that were fasted for 48 hrs. and then given thymidine-³H on the 5th day of growth. The curve is so irregular that reliable estimates cannot be made. However, a few things are clearly apparent. In mice fasted for 48 hrs., the G_2 period of Ehrlich ascites tumor cells is prolonged, from 5.5 hrs. to 20–24 hrs. The duration of the S phase (the 50 percent points of the ascending and descending limbs) is of the same magnitude as in control animals, somewhere between 24 and 28 hrs. T_C cannot be measured from this curve, but is presumably longer than in control mice, since $T_{G_2} + T_S$ in fasting animals is equal to T_C in control mice. Assuming a growth

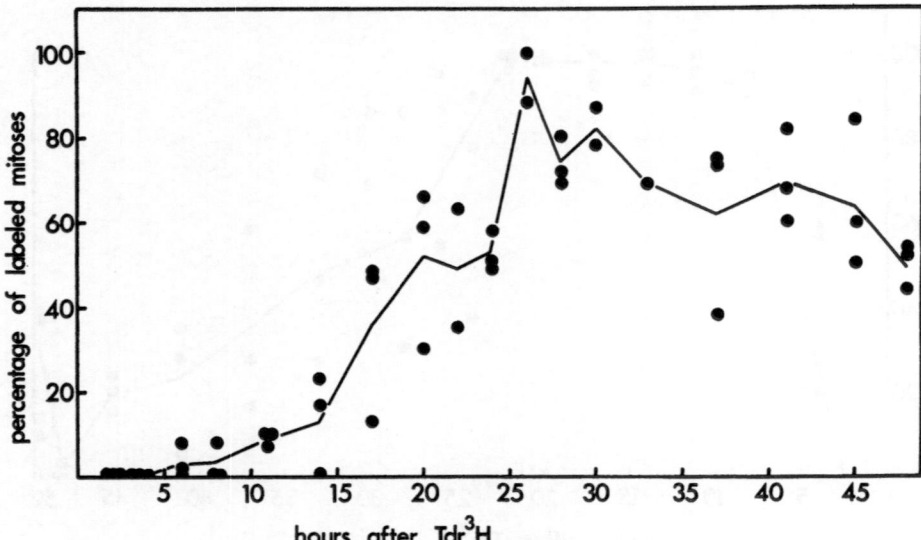

Fig. 3. Curve of the percentage of labeled mitoses, at various times after a single injection of thymidine-³H, of Ehrlich ascites cells on the 5th day after inoculation into the peritoneal cavity of female mice. The animals were fasted for 48 hrs. prior to the injection of thymidine-³H. Each closed circle represents one animal.

fraction near 1.0, and with a thymidine index (see Table II) of 37.2 percent, one can calculate a T_C of 70 hrs. for cells from fasted mice. This estimate, however, is purely conjectural.

Table II shows the effect of various periods of fasting on the thymidine and mitotic indices of Ehrlich ascites cells, on the 7th day after intraperitoneal inoculation. The thymidine index is affected by fasting, but only modestly for the first 24 hrs., and markedly afterwards. A 72-hr. fasting produces a 50 percent decrease in the number of cells in DNA synthesis. The mitotic index decreases in the first 17 hrs., but then it increases and, after a 72-hr. fast, it reaches a figure of 58.7, a very high value for the Ehrlich tumor, especially on the 7th day of growth. Since tumor growth is retarded in fasting animals, the high mitotic index at 72 hrs. probably represents a metaphase block. This was confirmed in one experiment, in which feeding of the fasting animals promptly reduced the mitotic index from 50 to 15 within 1 hr. and to 4.0 within 2 hrs.

Table III shows the marked effect that fasting has on T_{G_2} of Ehrlich ascites cells, the effect becoming apparent even after only 12 hrs. of fasting. It seems thus that the G_2 period of Ehrlich ascites cells is extremely sensitive to restricted caloric intake.

The effect of a 48-hr. fasting on the flow of cells from G_1 to S was studied by the method described by Baserga et al. (3). Both control and fasted mice were injected with thymidine-³H, and, after 30 min. a sample of tumor was aspirated from the peritoneal cavity for autoradiography. Six hours after the first injection, the mice were given a second injection of thymidine-³H and killed 30 minutes later.

TABLE II

EFFECT OF FASTING ON THE THYMIDINE AND MITOTIC
INDICES OF EHRLICH ASCITES TUMOR CELLS GROWING
IN THE PERITONEAL CAVITY OF FEMALE MICE *

Length of fasting (in hrs.)	Thymidine index † mean (range)	Mitotic index ‡ mean (range)
Controls	502 (456–552)	4 (2–6)
16.5	480 (462–516)	4 (0–6)
17	453 (370–502)	1.8 (0–3)
24	466 (430–506)	9.3 (4–18)
42	398 (364–430)	10.5 (6–12)
48	372 (310–415)	13.4 (7–25)
72	263 (245–287)	58.7 (34–82)
96	264 (73–362)	8.5 (0–23)
120	48 (0–118)	11.7 (1–29)

* All mice were killed on the 7th day after inoculation of tumor.

† The thymidine index is the number of labeled cells per 1,000 tumor cells 30 min. after injection of thymidine-^{3}H. Each point represents the mean of 3 animals, except for controls and 42 and 48 hrs., where 6 animals were used.

‡ Number of mitoses per 1,000 tumor cells.

In control mice, the percentage of labeled tumor cells rose from 48.4 after the first injection to 55.3 after the second injection, an increase of 14.2 percent. The corresponding figures for the fasted animals were 41.9, 46.7 and 11.5 percent. This indicates that the G_1 flow may be slowed down, but modestly. Since cells flow into S, and yet the thymidine index is decreased, they must leave the S phase at a normal or only slightly reduced rate. This confirms that the delays shown in Fig. 3 and Table III are G_2 delays, and not due to a block at the end of the S phase.

An attempt was made to determine whether the G_2 block could be released by appropriate manipulations. The most direct approach was to feed the fasted mice, but this procedure was not satisfactory. Not all mice began eating promptly after food was introduced, and in any case recovery was slow and irregular. We then tried another procedure, namely, the transplantation of tumor cells from fasted animals into normally fed mice. Transplantation of Ehrlich ascites tumor cells results in a dramatic shortening of the cell cycle and its phases, as demonstrated by Lala and Patt (12) and confirmed by us (unpublished results). When the tumor is transplanted from normally-fed to normally-fed mice and when thymidine-^{3}H is given at the time of transplantation, the cell cycle times (as measured by the method of Quastler and Sherman (17) are as follows: $T_C = 21.5$ hrs., $T_S = 16$ hrs., $T_{G_2} = 4$ hrs., $T_M = 0.5$ hr., $T_{G_1} = 1$ hr. When tumor cells from mice fasted for 48 hrs. were transplanted into normally-fed recipient mice, T_{G_2} decreased from 20–

TABLE III

Effect of Fasting on the Length of the G_2
Phase of Ehrlich Ascites Tumor Cells Growing
in the Peritoneal Cavity of Female Mice *

Hrs. of fasting (prior to TdR³H inj.)	Hrs. after TdR³H inj. †			
	4	6	8	11
	Percentage of labeled mitoses			
Control	51	97	99	99
12	6		15	
16	5		19	
20	0		19	
24	0	0	0	28
48	0	3	2	9

* All mice were injected with TdR³H on the 5th
day after intraperitoneal inoculation with 0.2 cc of
Ehrlich ascites tumor. There were at least 3 animals
per point. The variability of the figures can be evaluated from Figs. 2 and 3.

† Thymidine-³H injection.

24 hrs. to 12 hrs. (Table IV). Although the block is partially released by transplantation into normally-fed mice, T_{G_2} is still much longer than in control mice injected
with cells from normally-fed donors, i.e., 4 hrs. Similar results were obtained when
T_{G_2} was measured at 4, 8 and 12 hrs. after transplantation. In this experiment, the
percentage of labeled mitoses was determined at 4 and 8 hrs. after thymidine-³H,
but thymidine-³H was injected at different times after transplantation of tumor cells
from fasted into normally-fed mice. The results, shown in Table V, confirm that the
G_2 block persists for some time after transplantation into normally-fed animals.

In conclusion, these experiments show that the cell cycle of Ehrlich ascites tumor
cells, growing in the peritoneal cavity of female mice, is severely disrupted by a
48-hr. fasting. The G_2 period is most severely affected, and a marked delay in G_2
becomes apparent even after a fasting of only 12 hrs. In 1964, Cameron and Cleffmann (6) studied the effect of starvation and refeeding on the cell cycle of the
gut and esophagus of chicken. They concluded from their results that cells of the
small intestine normally stop in G_1, while those of the esophagus normally stop in
G_2. Our impression is that an arrest or delay in G_2 during fasting reflects an abnormal rather than a normal condition. It would be of interest now to follow up
these studies from both points of view, the one of the cell biologist and the clinician's.
For the cell biologist, it would be of interest to study the metabolic events occurring
in fasted cells when transplanted to normally-fed mice, and thus to gain further
insight into the chemistry of the G_2 period, which has been the object of only a very

TABLE IV

RELEASE OF THE G_2 BLOCK OF EHRLICH ASCITES CELLS
GROWING IN THE PERITONEAL CAVITY OF FASTED MICE *

	Hrs. after Tdr-^{3}H inj.				
	2	4	6	8	12
	Percentage of labeled mitoses				
Controls	0	30	60	92	100
Fasted mice	0	0	3	3	9
Fasted to normally-fed	0	0	4	29	53

* Control mice and mice fasted for 48 hrs. were injected
with Tdr-^{3}H on the 5th day after inoculation. Another
group of mice fasted for 48 hrs. were killed on the 5th day,
the tumor was pooled and 1 cc inoculated into normally-fed
recipient mice. Immediately after inoculation, recipients were
injected with Tdr-^{3}H.

TABLE V

EFFECT OF TRANSPLANTATION OF FASTED CELLS ON THE LENGTH OF THE G_2 PHASE *

Treatment	Tdr-^{3}H inj. (hrs. after transpl.)	Hrs. after Tdr-^{3}H	Percent of lab. mitoses	M.I.†
Normally-fed to normally-fed	0 hrs.	4 hrs.	52	11
Normally-fed to normally-fed	0 hrs.	8 hrs.	99	15
Normally-fed to normally-fed	12 hrs.	4 hrs.	56	10
Normally-fed to normally-fed	12 hrs.	8 hrs.	98	14
Fasted to normally-fed	4 hrs.	4 hrs.	0	20
Fasted to normally-fed	4 hrs.	8 hrs.	53	9
Fasted to normally-fed	8 hrs.	4 hrs.	3	5
Fasted to normally-fed	8 hrs.	8 hrs.	70	9
Fasted to normally-fed	12 hrs.	4 hrs.	10	8
Fasted to normally-fed	12 hrs.	8 hrs.	59	14

* Normally-fed recipient mice were injected with 1 cc of Ehrlich ascites tumor either from
normally-fed donors (normally-fed to normally-fed) or from donor mice fasted for 48 hrs.
(fasted to normally-fed). Thymidine-^{3}H (Tdr-^{3}H) was injected at different intervals after
transplantation and the recipient mice were killed at 4 or 8 hrs. after thymidine-^{3}H.

† Mitotic Index.

few reports (11, 25, 24, 23, 19, 16). For the clinician, the next question is whether a therapeutic attack may be more effective on the G_2 period or on the S phase. The first step would be of course to determine the sensitivity of the G_2 period of normal cells to a variety of manipulations, *in vivo*.

Summary

Fasting greatly affects the cell cycle of Ehrlich ascites tumor cells growing in the peritoneal cavity of mice. The G_2 period is markedly prolonged after a 48 hr. fasting, and even a 12-hr. fasting produces a delay in G_2. Other phases of the cell cycle are less affected by fasting.

References

1. BASERGA, R.: Autoradiographic Methods. *In*: Methods in Cancer Research. Vol. 1. H. Busch (ed.). Academic Press, New York, 45 (1967).
2. BASERGA, R.: The relationship of the cell cycle to tumor growth and control of cell division: A Review. Cancer Res. **25**, 581 (1965).
3. BASERGA, R., ESTENSEN, R. D., and PETERSEN, R. O.: Inhibition of DNA synthesis in Ehrlich ascites cells by actinomycin D. II. The presynthetic block in the cell cycle. Proc. Natl. Acad. Sci. **54**, 1141 (1965).
4. BASERGA, R., and KISIELESKI, W. E.: Comparative studies of the kinetics of cellular proliferation of normal and tumorous tissues with the use of tritiated thymidine. I. Dilution of the label and migration of labeled cells. J. Natl. Cancer Inst. **28**, 331 (1962).
5. BASERGA, R., and WIEBEL, F.: The cell cycle of mammalian cells. *In*: Intern. Rev. Exp. Path. Vol. 7. G. Richter (ed.). Academic Press, New York (1968).
6. CAMERON, I. L., and CLEFFMANN, G.: Initiation of mitosis in relation to the cell cycle following feeding of starved chickens. J. Cell Biol. **21**, 169 (1964).
7. CELSUS, AULUS CORNELIUS: De Medicina II, 16 (I Cent. A.D.).
8. FRINDEL, E., MALAISE, E. P., ALPEN, E., and TUBIANA, M.: Kinetics of cell proliferation of an experimental tumor. Cancer Res. **27**, 1122 (1967).
9. GROPPER, L., and SHIMKIN, M. B.: Combination therapy of 3-methylcholanthrene-induced mammary carcinoma in rats: Effect of chemotherapy, ovariectomy, and food restriction. Cancer Res. **27**, 26 (1967).
10. HOFFMAN, J., and POST, J.: Replication and 5-Iodo-2′-deoxyuridine-^{3}H incorporation by tumor and normal cells. Cancer Res. **26**, 1313 (1966).
11. KISHIMOTO, S., and LIEBERMAN, I.: Synthesis of RNA and protein required for the mitosis of mammalian cells. Exp. Cell Res. **36**, 92 (1964).
12. LALA, P. K., and PATT, H. M.: Cytokinetic analysis of tumor growth. Proc. Natl. Acad. Sci. **56**, 1735 (1966).
13. MENDELSOHN, M. L.: Cell proliferation and tumor growth. *In*: Cell Proliferation. L. F. Lamerton and R. J. M. Fry (eds.). Blackwell Scientific Publications, Oxford (1963).
14. MENDELSOHN, M. L.: Autoradiographic analysis of cell proliferation in spontaneous breast cancer of C3H mouse. III. The Growth Fraction. J. Nat. Cancer Inst. **28**, 1015 (1962).
15. MORESCHI, C.: Beziehungen zwischen Ernährung und Tumorwachstum. Ztschr. Immunitätsforsch. **2**, 654 (1909).
16. PALME, G., LISS, E., and WIEBEL, F.: Autoradiographische Untersuchungen über den

Einfluss alkylierender Zytostatika auf den Generationszyklus normaler Wechselgewebe und Aszitestumorzellen. Nuch. Med. Sup. 3, 39 (1965).

17. QUASTLER, H., and SHERMAN, F. G.: Cell population kinetics in the intestinal epithelium of the mouse. Exp. Cell Res. 17, 420 (1959).
18. ROUS, P.: The influence of diet on transplanted and spontaneous mouse tumors. J. Exp. Med. 20, 433 (1914).
19. SISKEN, J. E., and WILKES, E.: The time of synthesis and the conservation of mitosis-related proteins in cultured human amnion cells. J. Cell Biol. 34, 97 (1967).
20. STEEL, G. G., ADAMS, K., and BARRETT, J. C.: Analysis of the cell population kinetics of transplanted tumours of widely-differing growth rate. Brit. J. Cancer 20, 784 (1966).
21. SUGIURA, K., and BENEDICT, S. R.: The influence of insufficient diets upon tumor recurrence and growth in rats and mice. J. Cancer Res. 10, 309 (1926).
22. TANNENBAUM, A., and SILVERSTONE, H.: Nutrition in Relation to Cancer. In: Advances in Cancer Research. Vol. 1. J. P. Greenstein and A. Haddow (eds.). Academic Press, New York, 451 (1953).
23. TOBEY, R. A., ANDERSON, E. C., and PETERSEN, D. F.: RNA stability and protein synthesis in relation to the division of mammalian cells. Proc. Natl. Acad. Sci. 56, 1520 (1966b).
24. TOBEY, R. A., PETERSEN, D. F., ANDERSON, E. C., and PUCK, T. T.: Life cycle analysis of mammalian cells. III. The inhibition of division in Chinese hamster cells by puromycin and actinomycin. Biophys. J. 6, 567 (1966a).
25. TOBEY, R. A., PETERSEN, D. F., and ANDERSON, E. C.: Mengovirus replication. IV. Inhibition of Chinese hamster ovary cell division as a result of infection with mengovirus. Virology 27, 17 (1965).
26. WHITE, F. R.: The relationship between underfeeding and tumor formation, transplantation, and growth in rats and mice. Cancer Res. 21, 281 (1961).

Cell Proliferation during Carcinogenesis *

ALLAN B. REISKIN

Division of Biological and Medical Research
Argonne National Laboratory, and The University of Chicago
Argonne, Illinois

Introduction

Many classical concepts about the nature of normal and neoplastic growth have a largely intuitive basis and are often proved erroneous when confronted with quantitative data. The recent development and application of sophisticated analytical methods has shown that proliferative growth is a function of many complicated interdependent parameters, all of which require careful definition. Nevertheless, it is apparent that growth and cell division are certainly among the most striking attributes of cancer.

In the last decade, a considerable quantity of data has been generated from studies of proliferation kinetics in several normal and malignant tissues. These data, which define rates of cell movement through different stages of the life cycle, the distribution of cells in proliferating and non-growing compartments, and rates of cell loss, are especially relevant to the rational use of many therapeutic agents. However, they shed little light on the pathogenesis of neoplastic disease. The established growing tumor probably represents a mosaic of inherent and acquired proliferative characteristics and therefore may be a poor system for studies of carcinogenic mechanisms compared to early tumors or preneoplastic tissues.

While few experiments in cancer literature were designed specifically to study carcinogenic mechanisms from a kinetic point of view, it is possible to obtain enough information to explore generally some pertinent questions. In particular, it would be useful to know if cell division or cell cycle dependent metabolic activity, such as DNA synthesis, is required for either the initiation or expression of neoplastic transformation. It would also be useful to know if proliferative changes during carcinogenesis reflect either tissue or agent specificity.

Cellular Proliferation and Carcinogenesis *In Vivo*. Tumors can be induced experimentally in a large number of mammalian tissues. Since the response is reasonably uniform in many of these tissues, it has been possible to study proliferative changes at specific stages of tumor development and to study tumor induction as a function of different kinetic conditions.

---

* Work supported by the U.S. Atomic Energy Commission.

McCarter and Quastler (29, 30) measured the rate of incorporation of tritiated thymidine ([3]HTdR) and cell generation times in normal and carcinogen treated hair follicles of female swiss mice. Their data indicate that from approximately 6 to 30 hours after application of the carcinogen the rate of incorporation of thymidine into DNA was reduced in the follicular epithelium. Concomitantly, the mean time for DNA synthesis in these cells was increased. A similar depression of [3]HTdR uptake was observed by Juhn and Prodi (21) in growing and regenerating rat liver when animals were injected intraperitoneally with DMBA (7,12-dimethylbenz(a)-anthracene). Shimkin et al. (41) gave Sprague-Dawley rats a single dose of DMBA by gastric intubation. The number of cells labeled by a pulse of [3]HTdR was then determined at intervals over a two-week observation period. An initial reduction in the number of cells in DNA synthesis was seen in mammary ducts and glands, in hair follicles and adrenal cortex, but not in the basal cells of the skin.

These experiments involved only a single dose of the carcinogen and where the response was followed for several days or weeks, inhibition and recovery of DNA synthetic activity were common features. Aleo (1) followed the pattern of [3]HTdR labeling in a hamster cheek pouch treated with DMBA over a 15-week period. Although absorption of the carcinogen is rapid at this site (24, 26) no change in the labeling pattern was observed during the first week. During the second week of treatment, the incidence of labeled cells increased, then dropped, probably in association with inflammatory changes, and then increased again.

Rajewsky (34) has reported changes in the livers of rats receiving chronic doses of diethylnitrosamine (DEN) in their drinking water. Some animals were given [3]HTdR and studied autoradiographically. Liver explants from others were incubated briefly in [3]HTdR, after which the specific activity of the DNA was measured. Although the labeling pattern of the non-parenchymal population remained unchanged, the number of parenchymal cells labeled by a pulse of [3]HTdR increased almost by a factor of 3 by the 20th day of DEN administration. Measurements of DNA specific activity were reported to show an initial depression in DNA synthesis at the start of DEN administration followed by recovery and an overshoot.

Dörmer et al. (12), Reiskin and Mendelsohn (37), and Reiskin and Berry (36) studied proliferation kinetics during carcinogen induced hyperplasia of mouse skin and hamster cheek pouch. In both tissues, it was observed that the mean duration of DNA synthesis during hyperplasia was the same as in untreated tissue. In each instance, however, the number of cells in synthesis was significantly increased.

It is important to stress that conclusions from these data must be drawn with great caution. The experiments are based on a broad spectrum of approaches and methods which are not, strictly speaking, comparable. Moreover, no single investigation covers the entire time course from the initiation of treatment to the production of a frankly malignant tumor. Target tissues, carcinogenic agents, routes of administration, doses and animal species and strains varied widely. Although in some cases general toxicity was apparent, this was not a consistent finding, and there is no sure way of distinguishing between effects associated directly with the carcinogenic action of each agent and effects related in some way to other types of pharmacologic activity. In some cases it is quite probable that the cell populations which were studied were heterogenous, containing normal, transformed, differentiating, dying and regenerating cell types which cannot be distinguished from one another. This factor adds considerably to the problem of analysis. In spite of these difficulties it is possible to see a pattern, namely, that chemical carcinogens do alter the proliferative behavior of cells in a variety of mammalian tissues. DNA synthesis appears to be the most consistently affected parameter and although the time scale varies, an initial inhibition of synthesis is usually followed by recovery. The net effect of treatment with these chemicals seems to be an increase of the number of cells in synthesis, resulting from either a differential slowing of the passage of cells through synthesis, a selective shortening of other phases of the cycle, an increase in the number of dividing cells or combinations of these mechanisms.

In many mammalian tissues, the rate of cell movement through the generation cycle can change spontaneously. These naturally occurring differences have been exploited in assessing the dependence of carcinogenic efficiency on proliferative activity. The increase in cell number which accompanies normal growth, depending on the tissue, can occur as the result of rapid proliferation, a large stem population, or by minimizing cell loss. In liver, for example, early growth is achieved by a combination of a large number of cells in the division cycle and a short intermitotic time. At maturity, cell division nearly stops. In other tissues, the proliferative rate may be the prime regulatory factor, although shifts in the size of stem cell populations do occur.

Unfortunately, there is very little detailed information available on the kinetics of proliferation during developmental growth. Often, where there are reliable data, as for intestine, the tissue is not a suitable experimental tool. However, carcinogenesis has been studied in skin and mucous membrane as a function of aging (14, 27). In these cases the latent period for tumor induction increases with age and the incidence of tumors declines. Although kinetic data are incomplete there seems to be a good correlation between tissue maturity and carcinogenic susceptibility.

In 1945, Mottram (28) reported finding diurnal variation in the production of tumors and since then other investigators have reported rather striking circadian changes in kinetic behavior (32, 8, 10). Although the connection between these factors requires further study, it has been suggested that some carcinogens act specifically on cells synthesizing DNA (15). Further support for this hypothesis has been put forth by Shinozuka and Ritchie (42) who found that pretreatment of mouse skin with croton oil increased the number of cells in DNA synthesis and also the number of tumors produced by a subsequent injection of urethane. However, as suggested by Tannenbaum et al. (44) experiments with croton oil are often difficult to interpret because this agent is both a carcinogen and a promoter. DNA synthetic activity has also been implicated as a necessary step for tumor induction by Bates et al. (4), who found that Actinomycin D inhibited both DNA synthesis and tumor induction in mouse skin.

There are other experimental situations which also seem to suggest that DNA synthesis or cell division is an essential part of the transformation process. Ball et al. (3) showed that glass beads and wax pellets implanted in the mouse bladder produced frequent and intense proliferative reactions enhancing the response of the tissue to subsequent treatment with urethane. Pound and Withers (33) observed an increase in the yield of skin tumors in mice injected with urethane in areas which were pretreated with a variety of irritant chemicals. Of all the irritants used, only acetone failed to augment the urethane response and only acetone failed to produce a proliferative reaction.

This relationship is not restricted to tumor induction by chemical agents. Rosen and Cole (39) and Cole and Nowell (9) reported that the incidence of renal tumors in mice following irradiation was significantly increased by unilateral nephrectomy performed prior to irradiation. The removal of one kidney effectively stimulates proliferation in the other (38, 18).

It is interesting to note that, in general, when proliferative stimuli failed to augment carcinogenic activity, stimulation occurred some time after treatment with the carcinogen (43) rather than shortly before. There are, of couse, exceptions to this pattern. Peraino and Fry (personal communication) studied the livers of rats treated with phenobarbital (which stimulates proliferation (20) and a carcinogen, acetylaminofluorine (AAF). They did not observe an enhancement of AAF carcinogenesis but this may be explained by the well-known induction of drug-metabolizing enzymes by phenobarbital (23).

In Vitro **Studies of Carcinogenesis.** At first sight, it may seem difficult to justify the use of *in vitro* systems in cancer research, particularly for studying mechanisms of carcinogenesis. It is not entirely clear that transformation in culture, spontaneous or induced, is an appropriate analog of transformation *in vivo*. Culture systems have been used for a variety of purposes largely because they offer specific operational advantages and often because it is assumed that they represent a simplified model of *in vivo* behavior. The data accumulated from these systems has made their position as simple models questionable. They continue however to offer unique technical advantages impossible with intact animals.

Spontaneous transformation is a recognized phenomenon *in vitro* (17). The first demonstrations of experimentally induced transformation of "normal" cells were reported by Vogt and Dulbecco (46) and by Sachs and Medina (40). In both cases the transforming agent was polyoma virus. Other reports have indicated that transformation can also be induced by other viruses (45, 2), by chemicals (6), and by x-irradiation (7).

Investigations of viral transformation have indicated that a close relationship exists between the action of the transforming agent and metabolic events associated with proliferation. Dulbecco, Hartwell and Vogt (13) observed that when confluent cultures of mouse kidney cells were infected with polyoma both the activities of enzymes associated with DNA synthesis and the rate of cellular DNA synthesis increased. Similar results have been reported by Kára and Weil (22, 47), Henry, Black and Oxman (19) and others. It has also been shown that polyoma virus is able to induce cellular DNA synthesis in rat and mouse embryo cultures inhibited by x-irradiation (16).

In an attempt to determine if cellular DNA synthesis was required for transformation of chick embryo cells by RSV, Bader (2) used cytosine arabinoside to stop DNA synthesis before or after infection. Inhibition immediately after infection prevented transformation while inhibition before or late in the course of infection had little effect. Todaro and Green (45) assayed for transformation in 3T3 cells infected with SV40. Confluent cultures of these cells are not induced to synthesize DNA or transform after infection. By seeding new cultures with serial dilutions of infected stock, it was possible to determine the number of cell divisions required for the infected cells to become transformed. It was concluded that the completely transformed phenotype did not appear until infected cells had been allowed to divide several times. To determine whether or not cell division was necessary to produce a heritable change, rather than just the expression of such a change, stationary cultures were infected; after 3 hours the virus-containing media were removed and replaced with depleted media in which no growth occurs. At different times between 1–14 days these cultures were diluted and resuspended in media which permitted the resumption of cell division. Inhibiting division for 2–4 days, or more, significantly reduced the transformation frequency. On the other hand, if infected cells were immediately allowed to complete one division it was possible to inhibit further growth for 12 days without reducing the number of transformed colonies. Similar results have been obtained with chemical- (5) and radiation- (7) induced transformations.

Discussion and Conclusions

This review of data on cellular proliferation kinetics and carcinogenesis, though incomplete, suggests that in reaching the transformation endpoint the relationship of the initial cell-carcinogen interaction to the timing of cell division, DNA synthesis and perhaps other cell cycle-dependent events is of prime importance. This conclusion is not derived from incontestable data and it is important to point out that most of the experimental work can be effectively challenged on one ground or another. For example, in the context of this discussion it can be argued that the *in vivo* experiments, individually as well as collectively, are incomplete. In most cases more extensive testing in more and better defined systems and with larger numbers of animals would be desirable. The acceptance of circadian patterns of proliferation is not universal and extrapolation of kinetic parameters is difficult to justify. Most carcinogenic agents have a broad range of activity and it is likely that only a small part is directly concerned with tumor induction.

In the intact animal it is not completely clear which are the cells at risk, nor is it completely clear that in any population the sensitivity to carcinogens remains constant at all stages of the life cycle or at all stages of maturation. Cell division and DNA synthesis are affected by a variety of factors unrelated to carcinogenesis, most of which are poorly defined. Some carcinogenic agents appear to be capable of creating the appropriate conditions for transformation by adding to or changing the cell genome. Others accomplish the same end result less directly by altering hormonal balance or by producing toxicity and regeneration. Some carcinogens inhibit the production of interferons (11) and interferons appear to inhibit cell division (31) in addition to inactivating viruses. It has been suggested that some tissues may have an intrinsic mechanism for discarding abnormal cells while in other tissues these cells may be retained (25). Although there is no *a priori* reason for such a mechanism it provides a rather neat explanation for varying tumor frequencies in different tissues. There is also evidence that different oncogenic agents can act in concert, and by contributing complementary actions produce a more dramatic effect than either could accomplish alone (35).

In vitro systems have made impressive contributions toward defining transformation mechanisms. However, it is important to stress caution in extrapolating these findings to the intact animal. Even at basic levels there are no assurances that extrapolations are valid and it would be difficult, at best, to predict the qualitative or quantitative changes which may occur as the result of physiological defense mechanisms.

The main reason for confidence in drawing a conclusion here is that almost all of the experimental work, using vastly different systems, materials and conditions, points in the same direction. Therefore, it appears that there is some justification for a hypothesis which: 1. relates the efficiency of carcinogenic agents *in vivo* to their ability to stimulate DNA synthesis and cell division, and 2. allows for the repair of transformation lesions in cells which are prevented from dividing for some time after they have interacted with the transforming agent.

References

1. ALEO, J. J.: DNA synthetic activity of the hamster cheek pouch following repeated applications of 9,10-dimethyl 1,2-benzanthracene. Proc. Int. Assn. Dental Res. (1962).
2. BADER, J. P.: Transformation by Rous sarcoma virus: A requirement for DNA synthesis. Science 149, 757 (1965).
3. BALL, J. K., FIELD, E. H., ROE, F. J. C., and WALTERS, M.: The carcinogenic and co-carcinogenic effects of paraffin wax pellets and glass beads in the mouse bladder. Brit. J. Virology 36, 225 (1964).
4. BATES, R. R., WORTHAM, J. S., COUNTS, W. B., DINGMAN, C. W., and GELBOIN, H. V.: Inhibition by actinomycin D of DNA synthesis and skin tumorigenesis induced by 7,12-dimethylbenz(a)anthracene. Cancer Res. 28, 27 (1968).
5. BERWALD, Y., and SACHS, L.: *In vitro* transformation of normal cells to tumor cells by carcinogenic hydrocarbons. J. Nat. Cancer Inst. 35, 641 (1965).
6. BERWALD, Y., and SACHS, L.: *In vitro* cell transformation with chemical carcinogens. Nature 200, 1182 (1963).
7. BOREK, C., and SACHS, L.: *In vitro* cell transformation by x-irradiation. Nature 210, 276 (1966).
8. BULLOUGH, W. L.: Mitotic activity in the adult mouse, Mus musculus L. The diurnal cycles and their relation to waking and sleeping. Proc. Roy. Soc. (London) Ser. B 135, 212 (1948).
9. COLE, L. J., and NOWELL, P. C.: *In*: Biological Effects of Neutron and Proton Irradiations, IAEA, Vienna, 2, 129 (1964).
10. COOPER, Z. K., and FRANKLIN, H. C.: Mitotic rhythm in the epidermis of the mouse. Anat. Rec. 78, 1 (1940).
11. DEMAEYER, E., and DEMAEYER-GUIGNARD, J.: Inhibition by 3-methylcholanthrene of interferon formation in rat embryo cells infected with Sindbeis virus. J. Nat. Cancer Inst. 32, 1317 (1964).
12. DÖRMER, P., TULINUIS, H., and OEHLERT, W.: Untersuchungen über die generationszeit,

DNA-synthesezeit und mitosedauer von zellen der hyperplastischen epidermis und des plattenepithelcarcinoms der maus nach methylcholanthrenpinselung. Zeitschrift für Krebsforschung **66**, 11 (1964).

13. DULBECCO, R., HARTWELL, L. H., and VOGT, M.: Induction of DNA synthesis by polyoma virus. Proc. Nat. Acad. Sci. U.S. **53**, 403 (1965).

14. FORBES, D. P.: Experimentally-induced neoplasms in the skin of mice. II. The influence of age on tumor induction in rhino mice. J. Invest. Derm. **44**, 399 (1965).

15. FREI, J. V., and RITCHIE, A. C.: Diurnal variation in the susceptibility of mouse epidermis to carcinogen and its relationship to DNA synthesis. J. Nat. Cancer Inst. **32**, 1213 (1964).

16. GERSHON, D., SACHS, L., and WINOCOUR, E.: The induction of cellular DNA synthesis by simian virus 40 in contact inhibited and x-irradiated cells. Proc. Nat. Acad. Sci. U.S. **56**, 918 (1966).

17. GEY, G. O.: Cytological and cultural observations on transplantable rat sarcomata produced by the inoculation of altered normal cells maintained in continuous cultures. Cancer Res. **1**, 737 (1941).

18. GOSS, R., and RANKIN, M.: Physiological factors affecting compensatory renal hyperplasia in the rat. J. Exp. Zool. **145**, 209 (1960).

19. HENRY, P., BLACK, P. H., OXMAN, M. N., and WEISMAN, S. M.: Stimulation of DNA synthesis in mouse cell line 3T3 by simian virus 40. Proc. Nat. Acad. Sci. U.S. **56**, 1170 (1966).

20. JAPUNDZIC, M., KNEZEVIC, B., DJORDJEVIC, V., and JAPUNDZIC, I.: The influence of phenobarbital-NA on the mitotic activity of parenchymal liver cells during rat liver regeneration. Exp. Cell Res. **48**, 163 (1967).

21. JUHN, S. K., and PRODI, G.: The effect of 7,12-dimethylbenz(a)anthracene on the incorporation of thymidine-H^3 into deoxyribonucleic acid in normal and regenerating liver. Experientia **21**, 473 (1965).

22. KÁRA, J., and WEIL, R.: Specific activation of the DNA-synthesizing apparatus in contact-inhibited mouse kidney cells by polyoma virus. Proc. Nat. Acad. Sci. U.S. **57**, 63 (1967).

23. KATO, R., SHOJI, H., and TAKANAKA, A.: Metabolism of carcinogenic compounds. I. Effect of phenobarbital and methylcholanthrene on the activities of N-demethylation of carcinogenic compounds by liver microsomes of male and female rats. Gann **58**, 467–469 (1967).

24. KISIELSKI, W. E., and REISKIN, A. B.: Unpublished results.

25. LIPKIN, M., and QUASTLER, H.: Cell retention and incidence of carcinoma in several portions of the gastrointestinal tract. Nature **194**, 1198 (1962).

26. MESKIN, L. H., and WOOLFREY, B. F.: Radiographic localization of labeled carcinogen. Arch. Path. **78**, 643 (1964).

27. MORRIS, A. L.: Production and histochemistry of experimental oral cancer. Ph.D. thesis, University of Rochester, 1957.

28. MOTTRAM, J. C.: A diurnal variation in the production of tumours. J. Pathol. Bacteriol. **57**, 265 (1945).

29. McCARTER, J. A., and QUASTLER, H.: Note on the effect of a carcinogenic hydrocarbon on the synthesis of deoxyribonucleic acid. Biochimica et Biophysica Acta **55**, 552 (1962).

30. McCARTER, J. A., and QUASTLER, H.: Effect of dimethylbenzanthracene on the cellular proliferation cycle. Nature **194**, 873 (1962).

31. PAUCKER, K.: Interference and cell division. *In:* Viruses, Nucleic Acids and Cancer. The Williams and Wilkins Co., Baltimore, 430 (1963).

32. PILGRIM, C., ERB, W., and MAURER, W.: Diurnal fluctuations in the number of DNA synthesizing nuclei in various mouse tissue. Nature 199, 863 (1963).
33. POUND, A. W., and WITHERS, H. R.: The influence of some irritant chemicals and scarification on tumour initiation by urethane. Brit. J. Cancer 17, 460 (1963).
34. RAJEWSKY, M. F.: Changes in DNA synthesis and cell proliferation during hepatocar-cinogenesis by diethylnitrosamine. Europ. J. Cancer 3, 335 (1967).
35. RAPP, F., BUTEL, J. S., FELDMAN, L. A., TERETHIS, S. S., and MELNICK, J. L.: The interaction of unrelated tumor viruses (SV40 and adenoviruses). In: Carcinogenesis: A Broad Critique. The Williams and Wilkins Co., Baltimore, 697 (1967).
36. REISKIN, A. B., and BERRY, R. J.: Cell proliferation and carcinogenesis in the hamster cheek pouch. Cancer Res. 28, 898 (1968).
37. REISKIN, A. B., and MENDELSOHN, M. L.: A comparison of the cell cycle in induced carcinomas and their normal counterpart. Cancer Res. 24, 1131 (1964).
38. ROLLASON, H. D.: Compensatory hypertrophy of the kidney of the young rat with special emphasis on the role of cellular hyperplasia. Anat. Rec. 104, 263 (1949).
39. ROSEN, V. J., and COLE, L. J.: Accelerated induction of kidney neoplasms in mice after x radiation (690 Rad) and unilateral nephrectomy. J. Nat. Cancer Inst. 28, 1031 (1962).
40. SACHS, L., and MEDINA, D.: In vitro transformation of normal cells by polyoma virus. Nature 189, 457 (1961).
41. SHIMKIN, M. B., GRUENSTEIN, M., THATCHER, D., and BASERGA, R.: Tritiated thymidine labeling of cells in rats following exposures to 7,12-dimethylbenz(a)anthracene. Cancer Res. 27, 1494 (1967).
42. SHINOZUKA, H., and RITCHIE, A. C.: Pretreatment with croton oil, DNA synthesis, and carcinogenesis by carcinogen followed by croton oil. Int. J. Cancer 2, 77 (1967).
43. SHUBIK, P.: Studies on the promoting phase in the stages of carcinogenesis in mice, rats, rabbits, and guinea pigs. Cancer Res. 10, 13 (1954).
44. TANNENBAUM, A., VESSELINOVITCH, S. D., and SILVERSTONE, H.: Increased induction of skin tumors by pretreatment with croton oil. Cancer Res. 24, 361 (1964).
45. TODARO, G. J., and GREEN, H.: Cell growth and the initiation of transformation by SV40. Proc. Nat. Acad. Sci. U.S. 55, 302 (1966).
46. VOGT, M., and DULBECCO, R.: Virus-cell interaction with a tumor-producing virus. Proc. Nat. Acad. Sci. U.S. 46, 365 (1960).
47. WEIL, R., MICHEL, M., and RUSCHMANN, G. K.: Induction of cellular DNA synthesis by polyoma virus. Proc. Nat. Acad. Sci. U.S. 53, 1468 (1965).

Comparison Between the Rates of Proliferation of Induced Malignancies and Their Normal Tissues of Origin

Felix D. Bertalanffy

Department of Anatomy
University of Manitoba
Winnipeg, Canada

The majority of malignant tumors manifest high proliferation rates of their constituent cells. In many instances, this ability to proliferate is not only acquired at the time a particular cell population turns malignant, but it has been an inherent activity of the normal cell population from which the neoplasms arose. Such renewing cell populations, which exist at many sites in the body, exhibit mitotic activity throughout life. Usually undifferentiated cells, such as epithelial basal or reserve cells, or primitive cell stages in hemato- and lymphopoiesis, divide continually giving rise to identical cell types. Some of them differentiate into higher cell forms that usually cease mitosis and eventually become extruded from the cell population, for instance, by exfoliating from an epithelium as fully differentiated epithelial cells (3), or by entering the circulation as mature blood cells. There exists a remarkable association between renewing cell populations and many so-called spontaneous malignancies. It appears as if the normal occurrence of mitosis in a cell community, serving renewal, enhances the probability of malignant change in the particular cell population. This phenomenon is evident from examining the cytodynamics of those cell populations that exhibit a high incidence of clinical malignancy. Table I lists the organs that are most frequently affected with neoplasia, that is, organs that contribute ten percent or more to the total cancer incidence. The percentages of cells dividing each day for cell renewal in the corresponding organs of the rat are likewise indicated. Although a relationship between this daily mitotic rate and the frequency at which neoplasms occur does not necessarily exist, it is evident that all organs with a high cancer incidence belong to the renewing cell populations. In all of them mitosis occurs normally throughout life.

It is a valid question whether a cell population, after having become malignant, exhibits a higher mitotic activity than a normal cell population of origin for renewal. If this should be the case, a further question follows, can a normal cell population, during some phase of physiological activity, attain mitotic rates equaling or exceeding that of its neoplastic state; or can it be induced to proliferate as fast, or faster than the malignancy?

136

TABLE I

DAILY MITOTIC RATES OF ORGANS WITH A HIGH CANCER INCIDENCE

Organs	Percentage daily mitotic rate (rat)
Skin	3–6
Breast	2
Large Intestine	10
Stomach—body and pylorus	16–56
Cervix Uteri	12–26 *
Rectum	16
Lung—bronchus and trachea	2–4
Esophagus	11
Oral Cavity—tongue and cheek	20–24

* Fluctuates during estrous cycle.

Table I. Organs that contribute ten percent or more to the total cancer incidence. Indicated in the right column are the percentages of cells dividing daily for cell renewal in the identical organs in the rat. All organs with a high incidence of malignancy are thus renewing cell populations, exhibiting normally mitotic activity throughout life.

Such problems were investigated in three types of cell populations: in epidermal cell populations that proliferate at slow rates, as in the renewal of interfollicular epidermis, and at exceedingly rapid rates, as the hair matrix during the growth phase of the hair cycle; on the mammary gland parenchyma, renewed normally at a slow rate, but attaining relatively high mitotic rates during pregnancy; and on the liver parenchyma that ordinarily exhibits negligible mitotic activity, but can be stimulated by partial hepatectomy to regenerate at an exceedingly rapid rate of proliferation.

The mitotic rates of the normal epidermal cell populations were determined throughout one growth cycle of hair, the mammary gland during pregnancy and lactation, and the liver following partial hepatectomy. Malignancies of these cell populations (epidermis, mammary gland, and liver) were induced by chemical carcinogens. Most of the data are expressed as 6-hour mitotic rates, that is, as the percentages of cells entering mitosis in a particular cell population during a 6-hour period, as they were arrested during that interval in the metaphase stage by colchicine. The colchicine technique is expedient in such studies as it provides information on the actual rates of mitosis (percentage mitosis), data that are most readily collated between different histophysiological phases of a cell population, or throughout tumorigenesis (2). Moreover, inasmuch as colchicine acts early during the mitotic phase, it is little or not at all affected by variations in the duration of mitosis that most likely occur during some physiological states, or carcinogenesis.

Epidermal Cell Populations

The mitotic rate of interfollicular mouse epidermis was ascertained on every second day, throughout the second hair cycle which was induced by hair plucking. In a second series of mice, the carcinogen, benzopyrene, was applied to an area of plucked dorsal skin, beginning with day zero of the second hair cycle. (4) The observations of these two series are presented graphically in Fig. 1. Each point in this graph represents the 6-hour mitotic rate (10 A.M.–4 P.M.) of interfollicular epidermis on a different day of the hair cycle, of both normal and benzopyrene treated mice. The 6-hour mitotic rate of the normal epidermis, indicated by the lower line, fluctuated moderately with the stages of the hair growth cycle; it ranged between 0.47 and 2 percent for the 6-hour period. Beginning with day 12 of the second hair cycle, benzopyrene treatment elicited consistently higher mitotic rates in the interfollicular epidermis, ranging between 1.5 and 4.2 percent for the 6-hour period. This range was maintained quite uniformly when bi-weekly benzopyrene treatment was continued for 120 days, at which time keratoacanthomas and carcinomas began to develop. Only at one point during treatment, on day 100, did the 6-hour mitotic rate approach 5 percent.

The mitotic rate of mouse hair matrix was similarly investigated, and the ob-

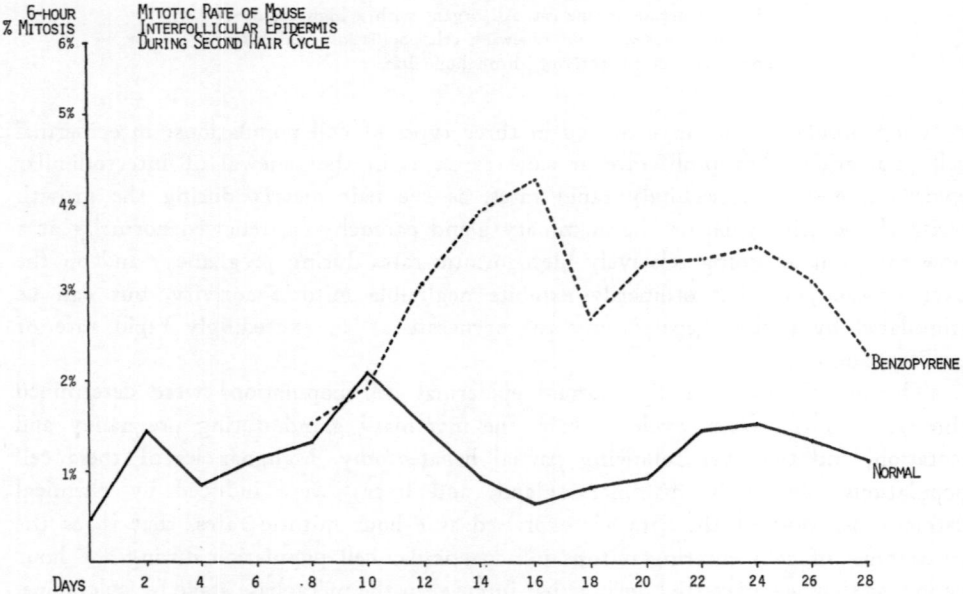

Fig. 1. Graphic representation of the mitotic rate of mouse interfollicular epidermis throughout the hair growth cycle (days 0–28) both without (lower solid line) and after benzopyrene (upper dotted line) treatment. Each point in this graph represents the 6-hour mitotic rate (10 A.M.–4 P.M.) on a different day of the hair cycle. The mitotic rate of the normal interfollicular epidermis fluctuated moderately during the hair cycle, ranging from 0.47 to 2.08 per cent for the 6-hour period. Beginning with day 12 of the hair cycle, the 6-hour mitotic rate of benzopyrene treated interfollicular epidermis was consistently higher, ranging between 1.54 and 4.20 per cent.

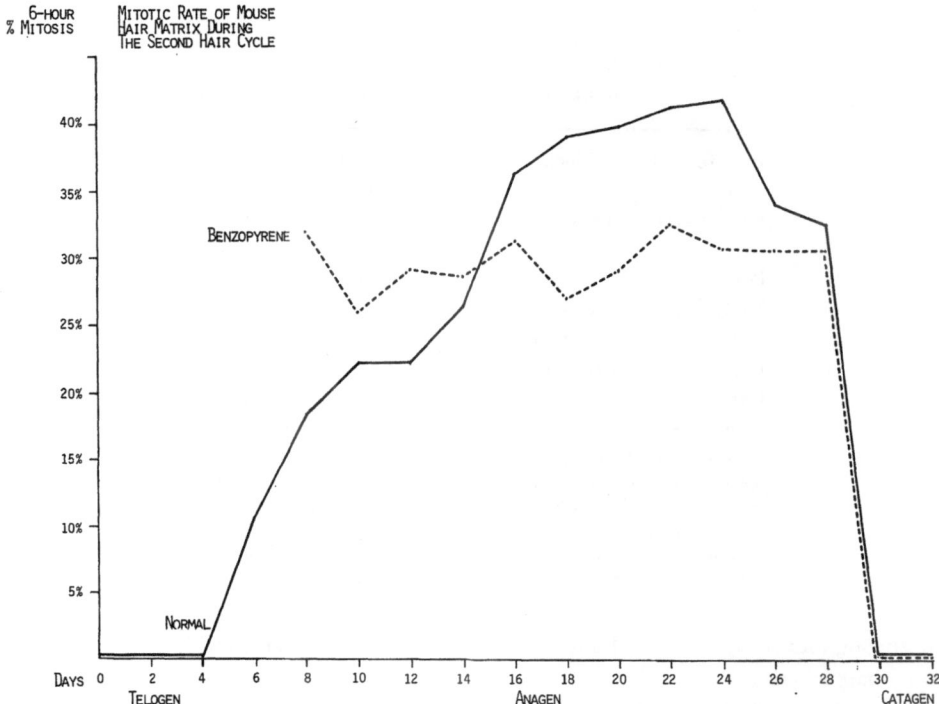

Fig. 2. Pattern of 6-hour mitotic rates of normal (solid line) and benzopyrene treated (dotted line) mouse hair matrix. Mitotic activity did not occur during the initial telogen stage (days 0–4) in the normal hair matrix. It increased rapidly during anagen (days 4–30), attaining a peak of 41.70 per cent in anagen VI (day 24). The 6-hour mitotic rate subsequently declined rapidly, and fell to zero with onset of the resting stage or catagen. This characteristic pattern of mitotic rate was abolished by benzopyrene treatment. The 6-hour mitotic rate of the carcinogen treated hair matrix remained fairly uniform throughout anagen, ranging between 27.1 and 32.6 per cent. However, the mitotic activity also of the benzopyrene treated matrix declined to zero at the beginning of catagen.

servations are presented in Fig. 2. As the graph indicates, characteristic fluctuations of the normal matrix's mitotic rate occurred throughout the hair growth cycle. Mitotic activity was absent during the initial telogen stage (days 0–4). It increased rapidly during anagen, attaining a peak of 41 percent for the 6-hour period during anagen 6 (day 24), and declined abruptly to zero at the beginning of the resting or catagen stage (day 30). During anagen, the 6-hour mitotic rate of the normal hair matrix averaged about 30 percent.

Benzopyrene treatment abolished this characteristic pattern of mitotic activity. The mitotic rate remained fairly constant throughout anagen, and the peak normally observed during anagen 6 failed to occur. It is remarkable that the mitotic activity of the benzopyrene treated matrix likewise declined to zero in catagen. This observation might indicate that mechanism controlling the hair growth was situated elsewhere, and thus remained unaffected by localized carcinogen treatment. Because of the initially higher mitotic activity of the treated matrix, the average 6-hour mitotic

TABLE II

Average 6-hour Mitotic Rates of Epidermal Cell Populations

Interfollicular epidermis	normal	1.2%
	B-treated	3.1%
Hair matrix (anagen)	normal	30%
	B-treated	30%
Follicle walls	normal	2.2%
Early keratoacanthoma		3.4%
Mature keratoacanthoma		6.5%
Regressing keratoacanthoma		4.5%
Carcinoma		5.6%

Table II. Mean 6-hour mitotic rates of normal and benzopyrene treated interfollicular epidermis and hair matrix, and normal follicle walls. The average 6-hour mitotic rates (of 40 mice) of three types of benign keratoacanthoma and squamous cell carcinoma, induced by benzopyrene application, are likewise listed.

rate throughout anagen was about 30 percent, and identical to this mean rate of normal hair matrix.

After about four months of benzopyrene treatment, epidermal tumors developed. They were classified as three types of benign keratoacanthoma and malignant squamous cell carcinoma. The mean 6-hour mitotic rates of these tumors are listed in Table II. It is evident that benzopyrene treatment soon augmented the mitotic rate of the interfollicular epidermis to a level corresponding to that of the early keratoacanthoma. The mature keratoacanthoma proliferated faster than all other tumors, including the squamous cell carcinomas. As expected, the mitotic rate of the regressing keratoacanthoma lies between the rates of the early and mature types of keratoacanthoma. It is apparent from these observations that the epidermal tumors proliferated from 3 to 5 times faster than the normal interfollicular and follicular epidermal cell populations. In contrast, during the growth phase, proliferation of the normal hair matrix was from 5 to 9 times more rapid than that of any of the tumors (8).

Mammary Gland Parenchyma

In adult female rats, the mitotic rates of the epithelial cells were determined in the ducts and secretory portions of inactive mammary glands, and in glands during pregnancy, lactation and involution (9). Mammary gland neoplasms were induced by administering to young virgin rats a single dose of 7,12-dimethylbenzanthracene by stomach tube, according to the technique developed by Huggins (10, 11).

Mitotic counts in normal mammary gland parenchyma of the virgin rat revealed that this cell population undergoes a slow continuous renewal of its constituent cells. The mitotic rate fluctuated quite characteristically with the stages of the estrous cycle. This is also true of most cell populations lining the female genital tract (5). The pattern of mitotic rate throughout the estrous cycle is demonstrated in Fig. 3; the daily mitotic rate of the mammary gland parenchyma is lowest, 0.08 percent, in proestrus, increases during estrus to its peak of 3 percent in diestrus I, and declines again in diestrus II to a little more than 1 percent. The mitotic rate per 6-hour period thus ranges between 0.02 percent in proestrus to 0.8 percent in diestrus I.

The mitotic activity is considerably augmented soon after the onset of pregnancy (Fig. 4). On day 4 of pregnancy, the 6-hour mitotic rate was still relatively low, somewhat less than 0.5 percent. However, by day 7 it had increased to 4 percent, and to 4.4 percent by day 12, the most active development period of the mammary gland parenchyma. The 6-hour mitotic rate declined subsequently to 2 percent by day 14, and to 1 percent by day 18.

The mitotic rate declined further after parturition, and on the second day of lactation was merely about 0.5 percent for the 6-hour period (Table III). It apparently maintained this level, and after three weeks of weaning, the 6-hour mitotic rate was still only 0.7 per cent in the involuting mammary gland.

Administration of dimethylbenzanthracene resulted in the development of a fair variety of mammary gland neoplasms, such as infiltrating lobular and medullary adenocarcinomas (9). Prior to performing the mitotic counts, the tumors were

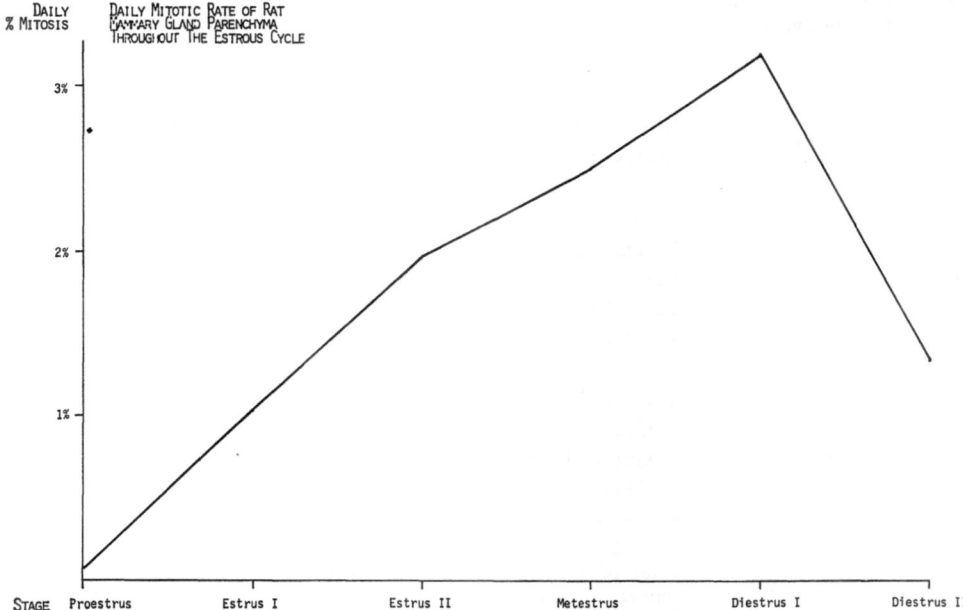

Fig. 3. Pattern of daily mitotic rates of mammary gland parenchyma of adult virgin rats during the estrous cycle. The daily mitotic rate was lowest (0.08%) during proestrus, increased steadily during estrus and metestrus to a peak of 3.20 per cent in diestrus I. It declined subsequently to 1.38% in diestrus II.

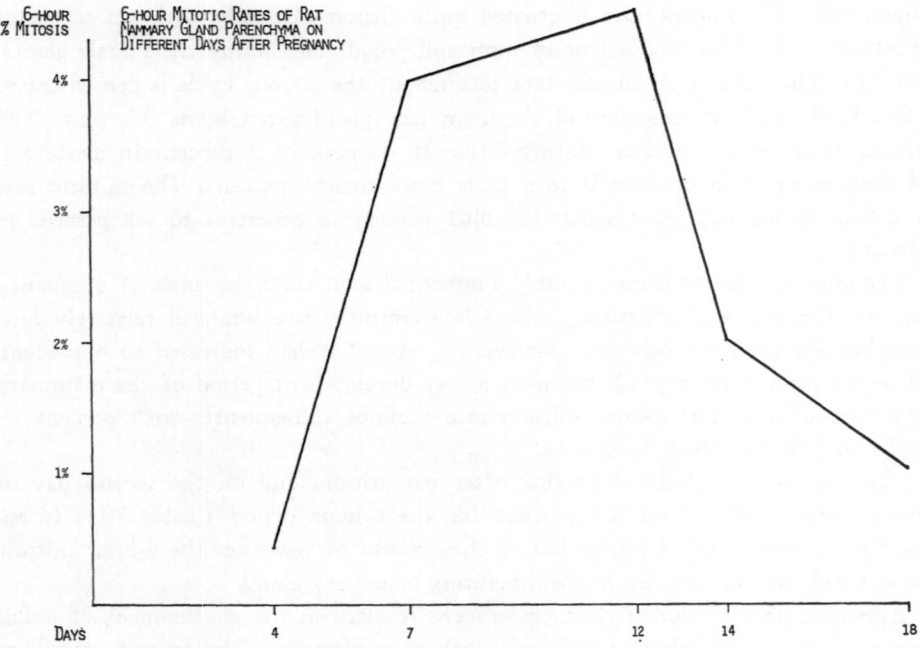

Fig. 4. Six-hour mitotic rates of rat mammary gland parenchyma on different days of pregnancy. On the fourth day of pregnancy, the 6-hour mitotic rate was still low (0.43%). It increased rather steeply to 3.99 per cent by day 7, and still further to 4.35 per cent by day 12 of pregnancy. The mitotic rate reclined subsequently to 2.01 per cent on day 14, and still further to 1.02 per cent on day 18 of pregnancy.

TABLE III

6-HOUR MITOTIC RATES OF RAT MAMMARY GLAND PARENCHYMAL CELL POPULATIONS

Virgin rat	0.02–0.8%
Pregnancy	0.43–4.4%
Lactation	0.51%
Involution	0.73%
DMBA Carcinoma	
Grade I–II	0.5–1.8%
Grade II–III	2.2–3.1%
Grade III–IV	5.2–8.4%

Table III. Mean 6-hour mitotic rates of rat mammary gland parenchyma in different phases of activity. The range of mitotic rates of the different grades of mammary gland adenocarcinoma, induced by administration of 7,12-dimethylbenzanthracene, were ascertained from 19 tumor-bearing rats.

classified by the conventional morphological criteria into Grades I to IV. The 6-hour mitotic rates of these tumor grades are also presented in Table III.

The vast majority were Grade I to III neoplasms. Less than 10 percent were anaplastic Grade III to IV tumors. Most of the malignancies proliferated at 6-hour mitotic rates ranging from 0.5 to about 3 percent. The significance of this observation lies in the fact that although most malignant tumors proliferated more rapidly than the normal and lactating mammary gland parenchyma, the mitotic rates of the vast majority of neoplasms were lower than that of the normal mammary gland when developing during pregnancy. In other words, the developing mammary gland during the first half of pregnancy attains a mitotic rate higher than that of many malignant mammary gland tumors (1).

Liver Parenchyma

The cells comprising the normal hepatic parenchyma do not belong to the renewing cell populations. A very minimal mitotic activity persists, however, contributing to a slight growth of this organ throughout life. In our series of experiments, less than 0.1 percent of the liver cells divided during a 24-hour period in the normal adult rat. In contrast to renewing cell populations, the cells newly formed in the liver do not replace other cells that become simultaneously lost.

Despite this almost negligible mitotic activity that normally occurs, the liver cells possess a tremendous potentiality for proliferation. This becomes apparent when loss of liver tissue occurs due to necrosis or surgical removal, but malignant transformation also increases the rate of proliferation. Both liver regeneration and hepatic neoplasia are characterized by relatively high mitotic activity.

Following surgical removal of about 70 to 75 percent of the rats' liver, the mitotic rates were ascertained throughout the course of hepatic regeneration (7), and compared to those of malignant hepatomas induced by 4-dimethylaminoazobenzene (6).

The pattern of mitotic rate of regenerating liver parenchyma cells is presented in Fig. 5. The rate did not increase appreciably during the first day after partial hepatectomy. By 30 hours, it became elevated and during the following six hours increased sharply to attain a peak of 16 percent for the 6-hour period at 36 hours after hepatectomy. The rapid proliferation occurring at this point is equivalent to a daily mitotic rate of more than 60 percent. The 6-hour mitotic rate subsequently declined gradually to fall again to zero after 8 days when liver regeneration was complete.

The range of the 6-hour mitotic rates of malignant hepatomas, induced in rats by dimethylaminoazobenzene, is indicated by a dotted line on the left margin of Fig. 5. Grading these tumors into two categories revealed average 6-hour mitotic rates of 4.5 percent of the Grade II hepatomas, and 7 percent of the Grade III and IV neoplasms. None of the malignant hepatomas came even close to the 16 percent of the regenerating liver at 36 hours after hepatectomy. These observations signify that a normal liver cell population, in the course of regeneration, attains levels of

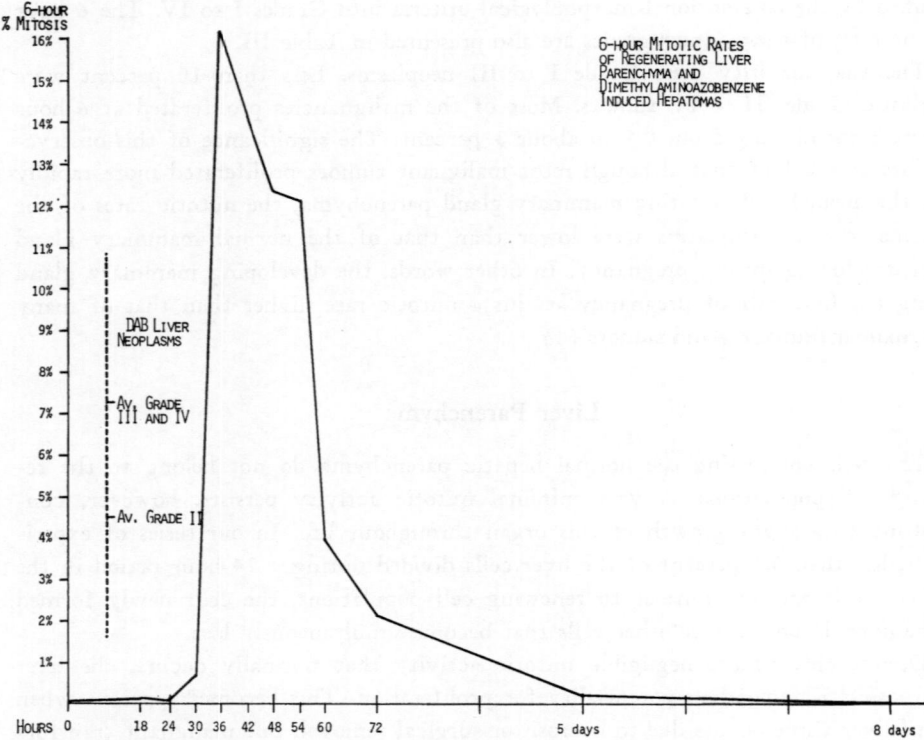

Fig. 5. Pattern of 6-hour mitotic rates of rat liver parenchyma at different intervals after partial hepatectomy throughout liver regeneration. The mitotic activity of regenerating liver did not increase appreciably during the first day after partial hepatectomy. It became augmented to 0.70 per cent by 30 hours, and during the following six hours increased steeply to a peak of 16.16 per cent at 36 hours after partial hepatectomy. The 6-hour mitotic rate declined subsequently, and fell to zero by 8 days after hepatectomy, when liver regeneration was accomplished. These data are the composite of 92 hepatectomized rats.

mitotic rate exceeding considerably those of malignant tumors induced by dimethyl-aminoazobenzene.

In conclusion, the mitotic rates of three types of cell populations, epidermis, mammary gland and liver parenchyma, were determined during various physiological activity or regeneration, and compared with those of malignancies that arose from these cell communities. The principal observations are summarized in Table IV.

It is evident that the malignant cell populations, in general, proliferated faster than the normal tissues of origin for cell renewal. Both benign and malignant tumors exhibited mitotic rates from about three to five times higher than the normal inter-follicular epidermis or follicle walls; the latter are usually regarded as being the site of origin of such tumors. Similarly, most of the mammary gland carcinomas pro-liferated considerably faster than the normal mammary gland parenchyma of the virgin rat. In contrast, at times the mitotic rates of normal cell populations exceed, often considerably, those of the malignant tumors, particularly during certain cyclic physiological activities. This is true for the hair matrix during the growth phase, anagen, or of the mammary gland during the first half of pregnancy. Moreover, some cell populations can be induced to regenerate with mitotic rates exceeding those of neoplasms that had developed from similar cell communities; for example the liver during regeneration.

TABLE IV

COMPARISON BETWEEN SIX-HOUR MITOTIC
RATES OF NORMAL AND NEOPLASTIC
CELL POPULATIONS

Cell population	Mean six-hour percentage of mitosis
Epidermis (mouse)	
NORMAL	
Interfollicular and	
follicular wall epidermis	1.2–2.2
Hair Matrix	29.8
TUMORS	
Keratoacanthoma	3.4–6.5
Carcinoma	5.6
Mammary Gland (rat)	
NORMAL	
Virgin, lactation, involution	0.4–0.7
Pregnancy	0.4–4.4
TUMORS	
Adenocarcinoma	0.4–8.4
	(Ave. 2.2)
Liver (rat)	
NORMAL	0.02
REGENERATION	0.7–16.2
HEPATOMA	1.6–10.8

Table IV. These data illustrate that the epidermal and mammary gland malignancies proliferated generally faster than the normal cell populations of origin for cell renewal. Yet, during some physiological activities, the mitotic rates of normal cell populations become augmented to exceed those of malignant tumors of such cell communities (hair matrix; mammary gland during pregnancy). Similarly, although normally exhibiting negligible mitotic activity, the liver parenchyma attains mitotic rates during hepatic regeneration exceeding those of malignant hepatomas.

References

1. Bertalanffy, F. D.: Comparison of mitotic rates in normal renewing and neoplastic cell populations. *In:* Canadian Cancer Conference. Vol. 7. Pergamon Press, New York and Toronto, 65 (1967).
2. Bertalanffy, F. D.: Tritiated thymidine *versus* colchicine technique in the study of cell population cytodynamics. Lab. Invest. 13, 871 (1964).
3. Bertalanffy, F. D.: Aspects of cell formation and exfoliation related to cytodiagnosis. Acta Cytol. 7, 362 (1963).
4. Bertalanffy, F. D., and Chivers, B. R.: Unpublished data (1968).
5. Bertalanffy, F. D., and Lau, C.: Mitotic rates, renewal times, and cytodynamics of the female genital tract epithelia in the rat. Acta Anat. 54, 39 (1963).
6. Bertalanffy, F. D., and Ozohan, M. L.: Unpublished data (1968).
7. Bertalanffy, F. D., and Parrott, J. C. W.: Unpublished data (1968).
8. Chivers, B. R.: Rates of cell division during epidermal carcinogenesis in the mouse. M.Sc. Thesis. University of Manitoba, Winnipeg (1967).
9. Grahame, R. E.: Rates of cell division in normal and malignant mammary gland tissue in the rat. M.Sc. Thesis. University of Manitoba, Winnipeg (1966).
10. Huggins, C., and Fukunishi, R.: Mammary and peritoneal tumors induced by intra-peritoneal administration of 7,12-dimethylbenz(a)anthracene in new born and adult rats. Cancer Res. 23, 786 (1963).
11. Huggins, C., and Fukunishi, R.: Cancer in the rat after single exposures to irradiation or hydrocarbons. Age and strain factors: Hormone dependence of mammary cancers. Rad. Res. 20, 493 (1963).

The Use of Three-Dimensional
Matrix Tissue Culture for Bioassay of Cancer:
A Progress Report *

JOSEPH LEIGHTON, GERALD JUSTH, and RAYMOND MARK

Department of Pathology, University of Pittsburgh
Pittsburgh, Pennsylvania

Cancer bioassay implies the capacity to predict the clinical behavior of a neoplasm as a result of studying a specimen of it as living tissue in the laboratory. There are at least two behavioral qualities about which prognostic information is desirable. First, we should like to be able to differentiate between tumors that are probably cured after surgery or radiation and those that are likely to recur as metastases. Second, we should like to recognize those tumors that will respond favorably to chemotherapeutic agents or irradiation and those that will be resistant to such treatments. Ideally, the definition and measurement of specific biochemical parameters that can be correlated with future clinical behavior would be desirable. None has yet been found. At the present stage of our understanding, we think it unlikely that well-defined biochemical indices will soon be found in view of the complex physiologic events already identified as being involved in the phenomena of malignancy, and the indication that still other factors await adequate description as well as reproducible experimental manipulation.

Inherent in our approach to bioassay is the laboratory examination of behavioral characteristics of living tumor tissue. Many qualities of behavior are potentially subject to examination, such as interaction between cells in the tumor tissue itself, and interaction between cells of the tumor tissue and of a standardized laboratory host. The laboratory host might be an intact animal of the kind usually employed in heterotransplantation. On the other hand, a standardized population of normal cells *in vitro* can serve as a "host" in a feeder capacity and can also act in direct associative interactions with cells of the tumor. The idea of bioassay of tumors in the laboratory is an old one from the point of view of both heterotransplantation and tissue culture. Reasonable *a priori* arguments can be offered in favor of either a tissue culture system or a transplantation system. In either case, however, the tumor tissue must live in order to express its behavior.

---

* This work was supported by Grant DRG-950 from the Damon Runyon Memorial Fund for Cancer Research and by Grant #CA-10412 from the National Cancer Institute. It was also supported in part by Grant #P-442 from the American Cancer Society, as well as by research grant (GM-10269) and Training Grant (GM-135) from the National Institute of General Medical Sciences.

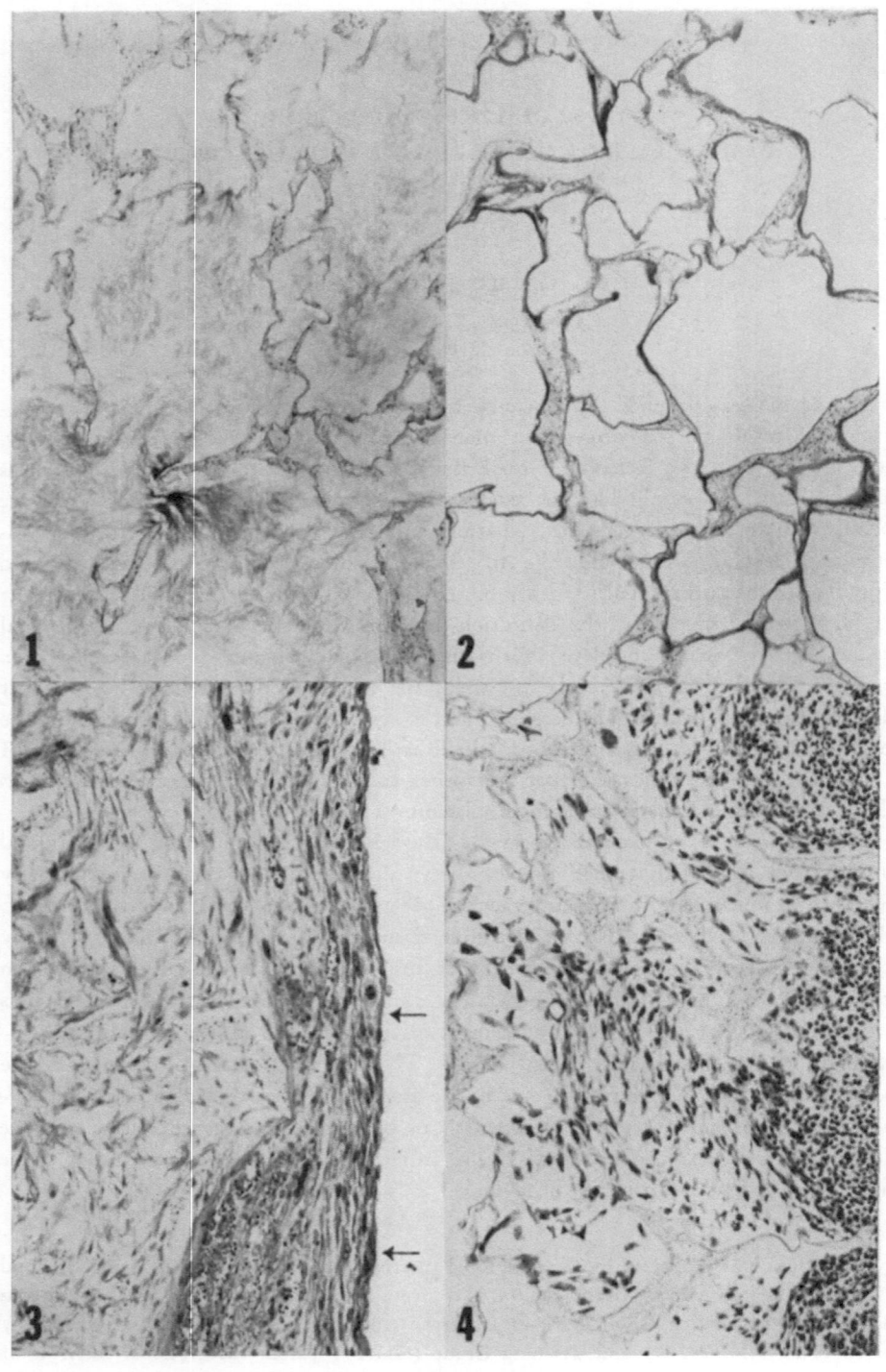

In our laboratory we are interested in both types of model systems. In the case of heterotransplantation, we have placed human as well as rodent tumors on the chorioallantois of a chick embryo (1). In the case of tissue culture, our major tool has been a three dimensional matrix as a substrate for supporting cell outgrowth (2, 3). Today's presentation deals with the matrix system.

If the surgical pathologist is to adequately avail himself of the potential of tissue culture methods in the study of his patients' tumors, in-vitro methods must permit him to study the tumor tissue within the conceptual perspective of histopathology, and with the general methods of histology. He must be able to study both the explant and its outgrowth as three-dimensional tissue using relatively routine histologic techniques, methods similar to those used in studying the original surgical specimens from which the cultures themselves were made. When outgrowth from tissue explants takes place in the interstices of a sponge, an opportunity is afforded to examine the phenomena of cell interaction, association, and the formation of organized tissue units in a three dimensional context.

Since the fall of 1966, we have used collagen coated cellulose as our matrix for tissue culture (4). We have succeeded in cultivating a variety of chick embryonic tissues and rodent carcinomas in this three-dimensional setting, and have found that histologic identity is retained in both the explant and the outgrowth (5). We are now examining the viability and growth patterns of a number of human tumors in order to obtain some indication of the potential usefulness of collagen coated sponge for studying the behavioral characteristics of clinical cancers (6). This report summarizes our experience with human tumors in the collagen coated sponge system up to December 31, 1967.

Materials and Methods

Preparation of Collagen Coated Sponge. Pieces of dry, fine pore, cellulose sponge (DuPont) measuring approximately 12 x 8 x 1 mm. were cut with a single edged razor blade and thoroughly washed in both glass distilled water and fat solvents (2). After the sponges were dried they were impregnated with a 1 percent dispersion of collagen (Ethicon). The histologic appearance of such a sponge stained for collagen

---

PLATE 1

Fig. 1. Microscopic section of a cellulose sponge fixed immediately after impregnation with liquid collagen dispersion (Ethicon). The interstices of the sponge are irregularly filled with fine fibers of collagen. Masson trichrome, ×150.

Fig. 2. Microscopic section of a cellulose sponge fixed after the dispersing medium has evaporated. Collagen fibers have matted and are deposited on the surface of the cellulose sponge trabeculae, resulting in a collagen-coated cellulose sponge. Masson Trichrome, ×150.

Fig. 3. Ten-day-old culture of a combination of a pulmonary fibrosarcoma and chick embryonic lung. Neoplastic fibroblasts appear predominately on the surface of the sponge (arrows); embryonic connective tissue is seen in the left half of the figure in the interstices of the sponge. Hematoxylin and Eosin, ×150.

Fig. 4. Eight-day-old culture of a pleural mesothelioma. Cells from the explant on the right have migrated into the interstices of the sponge, producing a distinct connective tissue pattern. Hematoxylin and Eosin, ×150.

fibers is seen in PLATE 1, Fig. 1. Here the fine collagen fibers are seen distributed irregularly in the interstices of the sponge.

Following impregnation with collagen dispersion, the sponges were permitted to dry at room temperature overnight. During the drying process, the collagen fibers mat and adhere to the trabeculae of cellulose sponge as seen in PLATE 1, Fig. 2. The details of preparation of the collagen coated sponge have been published (4).

Media. The volume and frequency of feeding were selected to maintain a pH range in the medium of 7.2 to 7.6. The medium was usually replenished every one or two days. All our cultures were grown in large flat culture tubes (7) and were usually incubated at 36°C. For the first 1 or 2 days of incubation the cultures remained at rest on a rack; for the subsequent period of cultivation the tubes were placed on a rocker for gentle agitation (Bellco Company).

The medium consisted of 30 percent calf's serum in Eagle's Minimal Essential Medium made up in Hanks' Balanced Salt Solution. Each ml. of the medium was supplemented with 50 units of penicillin and of streptomycin mixture (Microbiological Associates) as well as 100 units of mycostatin (Squibb). When the cultures became acid overnight, half of the Hanks' BSS in the replenishing medium was replaced with Earle's BSS.

Solid Tumor Tissue. The tumor inoculum consisted either of discrete explants approximately 1 mm. in diameter or of a very fine mince depending upon the physical consistency of the individual specimen. Tough fibrous tumors were cut into explants, soft mushy tumors reduced to a fine mince.

Effusion Tumors. Fluid containing tumor cells, taken from the peritoneal or pleural cavity, was provided in aliquots of 500 ml. or more. In some samples spontaneous clotting of the effusion had occurred, in others clotting was averted by the addition of heparin to the collecting container at the time the serous cavity was tapped. The formed elements of the effusion were concentrated by centrifugation in 250 ml. centrifuge bottles, and the sediment used as an inoculum. Where a spontaneous clot was found the clot was minced. The fragments that were finally obtained were greatly reduced in volume as fluid left the clot by syneresis. Fine fragments of clot were inoculated on the surfaces of slices of collagen coated sponge.

Normal Tissues. In some experiments paired small series of sponges were inoculated, one group with tumor tissue only, the other with a mixture of tumor and chick embryonic tissue. In the case of young embryos, less than eight days old, a mince of the entire embryo was generally used. For older embryos the tissue was selected more precisely and consisted of either chick embryonic heart, lung, ovary, intestine, or mesonephros. In one experiment, ovarian tissue from the same patient was inoculated in association with explants of carcinoma of the breast.

Inoculation of the Sponges. For tumor tissues providing discrete explants, a diagonal row of four to six explants was placed on the flat surface of each sponge

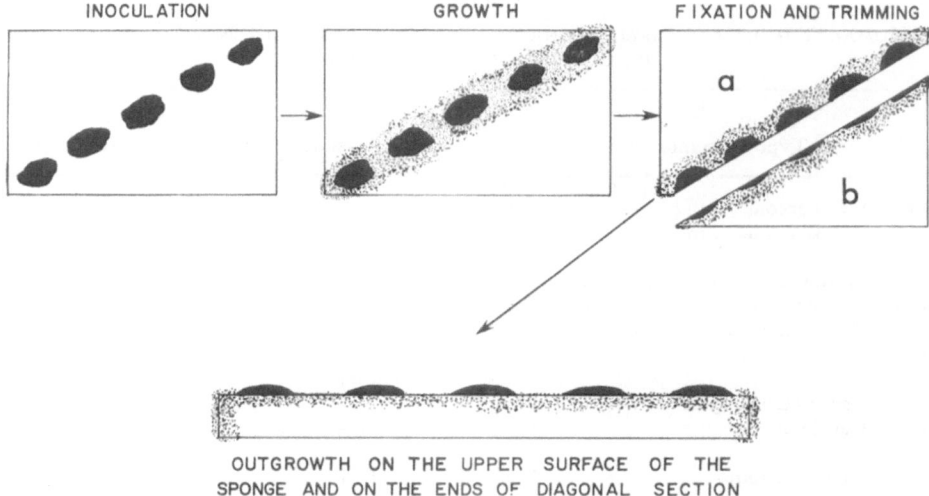

OUTGROWTH ON THE UPPER SURFACE OF THE
SPONGE AND ON THE ENDS OF DIAGONAL SECTION

Fig. 1

(Fig. 1). Where normal tissue accompanied the tumor, fragments of normal tissue were placed on the sponge after the tumor was in place so that each fragment of tumor made some peripheral contact with a fragment of embryonic tissue. Following inoculation, each sponge was placed in a large, flat tube and 2 or 3 ml. of medium was added so that the surface of the sponge exposed to the atmospheric air in the tube was just barely bathed by tissue culture medium. As mentioned above, the choice of tissue culture medium was determined by our desire to maintain a pH range from 7.6 to 7.2 on a schedule of feeding every two days.

Cultures of different tumors were kept for varying lengths of time, some for nearly two weeks, but most for a briefer period, usually 3 or 4 days (see Table 1).

Histologic Preparation. At the time of fixation the sponges were placed in Stieve's fixative and on subsequent days, after several changes of 80 percent alcohol, the sponges were trimmed for further preparation. The pattern of trimming is indicated in Fig. 1. The larger portion of sponge (labeled a) containing the explant areas and much of the adjacent zones of outgrowth was embedded on edge with the explants down, *i.e.*, toward the microtome knife. In this way, serial sections through this part of the sponge provided a view of both the explants and the outgrowth in relation to the gradient established by the air medium interphase. In some experiments the smaller triangular pieces of sponge (labeled b) were embedded flat and complete serial sections were prepared. In cultures inoculated with effusion tumors, the entire sponge in some cases was embedded flat, and serial sections made.

Observations

Thirty specimens of tumor have been cultured as listed in Table 2. Survival of tumor cells was seen in most of the specimens. Migratory outgrowth of cells onto

TABLE 1

Human Tumors Cultured Alone or with Supplementary Normal Tissue in Collagen-Coated Sponge

Exp. #	Type of tumor	Supplementary tissue	No. of cultures	Days in culture	Figure
67x11	Fibrosarcoma, lung	None	5	10	—
67x11	Fibrosarcoma, lung	Lung, 12-day chick embryo	2	10	3
67x125	Fibrous Mesothelioma, pleura	None	6	8	4
67x110	Papillary carcinoma, thyroid	None	8	4–7	5
67x116	Carcinoma, lung	None	1	6	—
67x116	Carcinoma, lung	Lung and intestine, 13-day chick embryo	4	6	6
67x7	Carcinoma, larynx	None	4	2–7	—
67x7	Carcinoma, larynx	Lung, 13-day chick embryo	4	2–7	7
67x106	Neuroblastoma	Lung, 11-day chick embryo	4	6	8
67x94	Carcinoma, breast	None	3	1–5	—
67x94	Carcinoma, breast	Mesonephros, 10-day chick embryo	6	1–5	9
67x133	Carcinoma, breast (bone metastasis)	None	8	5	10
67x124	Carcinoma, breast (mucinous)	None	4	8	11
67x96	Carcinoma, breast	None	6	2–4	—
67x96	Carcinoma, breast	Autologous ovary	6	2–4	12
66x127	Carcinoma, colon	None	4	7–13	—
66x127	Carcinoma, colon	Intestine, 11-day chick embryo	4	7–13	13
67x121	Carcinoma, colon	Intestine, 11-day chick embryo	3	5–8	14
67x95	Carcinoma, colon (rectum)	Viscera, 9-day chick embryo	3	6	15, 16
67x12	Ascites, carcinoma of stomach	None	2	2–7	—
67x12	Ascites, carcinoma of stomach	Viscera, 13-day chick embryo	10	2–7	17
67x51	Ascites, carcinoma of breast	None	5	4–8	—
67x51	Ascites, carcinoma of breast	Mesonephros and adjacent tissues, 8-day chick embryo	4	4–8	18
67x30	Pleural effusion, primary unknown	Mince, 6-day chick embryo	10	2–7	19
67x44	Ascites, carcinoma of ovary	None	5	4–9	—
67x44	Ascites, carcinoma of ovary	Mesonephros and adjacent tissues, 8-day chick embryo	5	4–9	20

the collagen coated matrix was noted in about half of the cases. PLATES 1–5, Figs. 3 through 20, with accompanying legends, illustrate and describe the microscopic appearance of seventeen specimens in matrix culture. The number of sponges inoculated, the duration of cultivation, and the addition of normal tissue are summarized in Table 2.

TABLE 2

Survey of Human Cancer in Collagen-Coated
Cellulose Sponge

Solid tumors	Number of patients
Carcinoma of the breast	7
Carcinoma of the colon	3
Carcinoma of the larynx	1
Carcinoma of the lung	1
Fibrosarcoma of the lung	1
Malignant mesothelioma	1
Papillary carcinoma of thyroid	1
Renal cell carcinoma	1
Wilms' tumor	1
Neuroblastoma	1
Melanotic progonoma	1
	19

Effusion tumors	
Carcinoma of the breast	5
Carcinoma of the stomach	1
Carcinoma of the ovary	1 (2 specimens)
Carcinoma, site unknown	1 (3 specimens)
	8

From the limited data available, we can make no generalizations about the growth characteristics of individual types of cancer on collagen coated sponge. However, considering the solid tumors as a group we readily obtained preparations in which explant and outgrowth were easily identified. The histotypic character of individual neoplasms was maintained in the explant itself. Furthermore, where migratory outgrowth occurred the new tissue usually had the essential architectural features of the neoplastic tissue in the original explant.

Explants of Solid Tumors. Almost all explants of four of the solid tumors remained completely viable in culture. The fragments of papillary carcinoma of the thyroid were free of necrosis, and the microscopic architecture of the tumor *in vitro* was essentially identical to that of the original tissue (PLATE 2, Fig. 5). There was a slight migration of low cuboidal epithelium on the trabeculae of the sponge. The carcinoma of the larynx and the fibrosarcoma of the lung were inoculated alone and with embryonic tissue. When cultured alone there was minimal outgrowth from these two tumors. On the other hand, when grown in association with embryonic tissue, extensive migration of tumor cells from the explants was noted

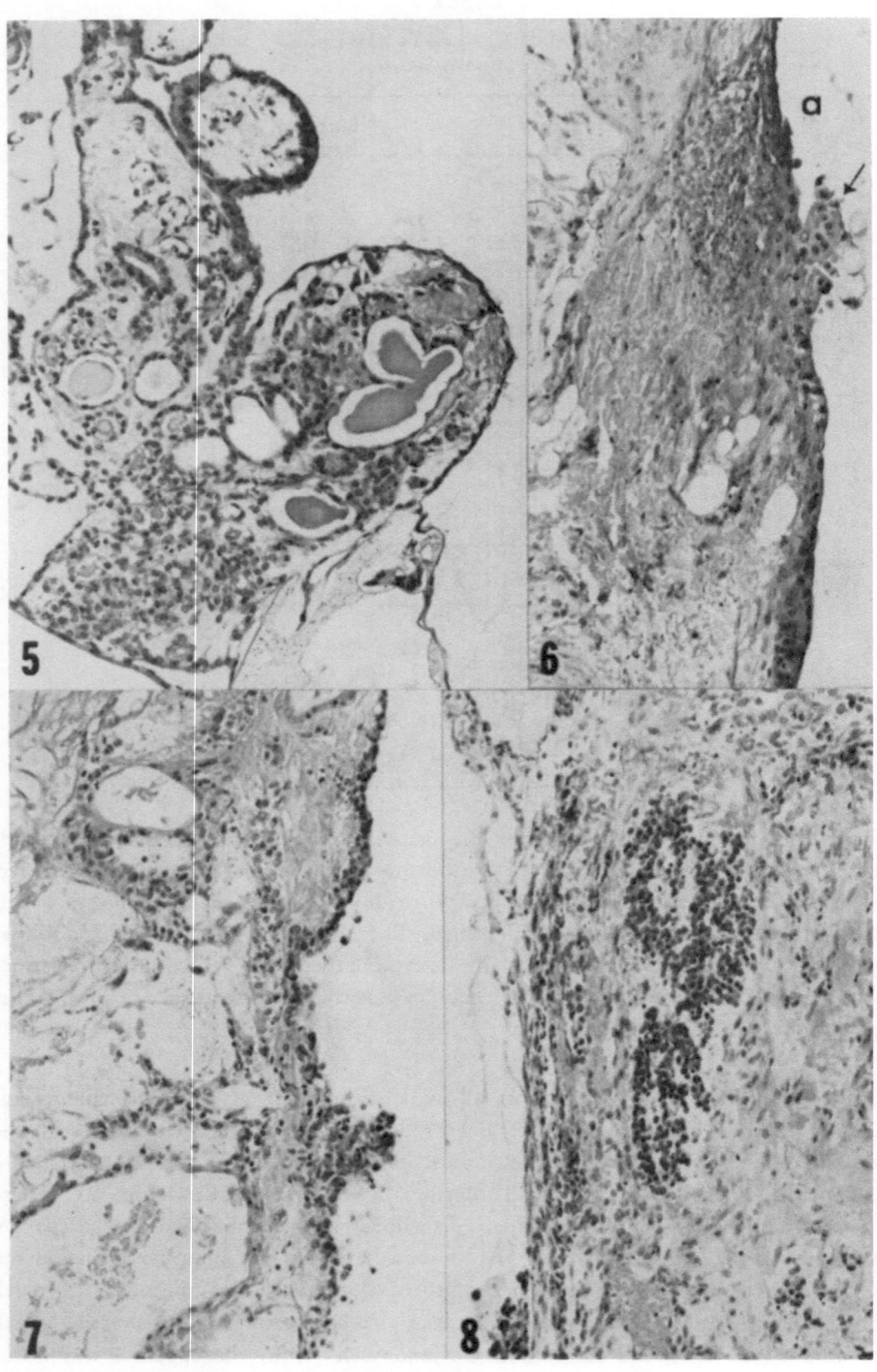

(PLATE 1, Fig. 3 and PLATE 2, Fig. 7). The pleural mesothelioma, cultured without accompanying normal tissue, gave rise to an extensive migration of spindle shaped cells into the interstices of the sponge (PLATE 1, Fig. 4).

A varied picture of viability was seen among cultured explants from all cases of carcinoma of the breast and from the melanotic progonoma. Some explants contained many viable groups of tumor cells, others from the same specimen consisted of dense acellular fibrous tissue or necrotic tissue. This variation was probably a reflection of the heterogeneous composition of the original explants, since a similar variation was seen in histologic preparations of samples of the donor fragments. Outgrowth of tumor cells from the mammary cancer was minimal, even for explants with large numbers of viable tumor cells (PLATE 3, Fig. 9). The presence of normal tissues of the chick embryo, and in one case of normal ovary from the same patient, did not enhance the outgrowth of tumor cells (PLATE 3, Fig. 12). However, the tumor in contact with the autologous ovary had a larger population of viable tumor cells than did explants of tumor only.

A very low level of viability was evident in the cultures of a Wilms' tumor, a renal cell carcinoma, and a carcinoma of the lung. Only a few small foci of tumor were seen in the cultures of carcinoma of the lung (PLATE 2, Fig. 6). In the case of the lung, the poor result may be explained by the fact that the donor tissue consisted primarily of necrotic lung cancer. The same explanation cannot apply to the Wilms' tumor or the renal cell carcinoma. In both of these cases the donor tissue was cellular and apparently viable.

Mince of Solid Tumors. The consistency of carcinoma of the colon may vary within a small piece of tissue from a firm fibrous texture to a soft mushy one. Our inocula from three of these tumors consisted of fragments of varying size, ranging from discrete explants to small clumps of cells. In all cases, the morphologic identity

---

PLATE 2

Fig. 5. Seven-day-old culture of metastatic papillary adenocarcinoma of the thyroid. The tissue explant retains the architecture of the original tumor, including the presence of follicles of different sizes. Flattened sheets of epithelium extend onto the adjacent trabecular surfaces. Hematoxylin and Eosin, ×150.

Fig. 6. Six-day-old culture of carcinoma of the lung growing in association with chick embryonic intestine. A thin layer of tumor cells is seen on the surface of the combined tissue. One group of tumor cells projects from the free surface (arrow). Deep to the layer of tumor cells is a broad zone of sparsely cellular collagenous tissue. Embryonic tissue is in the upper part of the figure (a). Hematoxylin and Eosin, ×150.

Fig. 7. Seven-day-old culture of carcinoma of the larynx growing in combination with fragments of chick embryonic lung. The cells in this figure are almost entirely from the tumor and its outgrowth. Part of the tumor explant is in the upper part of the field. Tumor cells have migrated from the explant onto the contiguous collagen-coated sponge surfaces. Hematoxylin and Eosin, ×150.

Fig. 8. Six-day-old culture of a fine mince of neuroblastoma growing in association with a mince of chick embryonic lung. Characteristic tumor cells with prominent nuclei and scant cytoplasm appear as groups in the substance of the chick embryonic connective tissue. A small group of tumor cells is seen in the lower left, on the medium bathed surface of the embryonic connective tissue. Hematoxylin and Eosin, ×150.

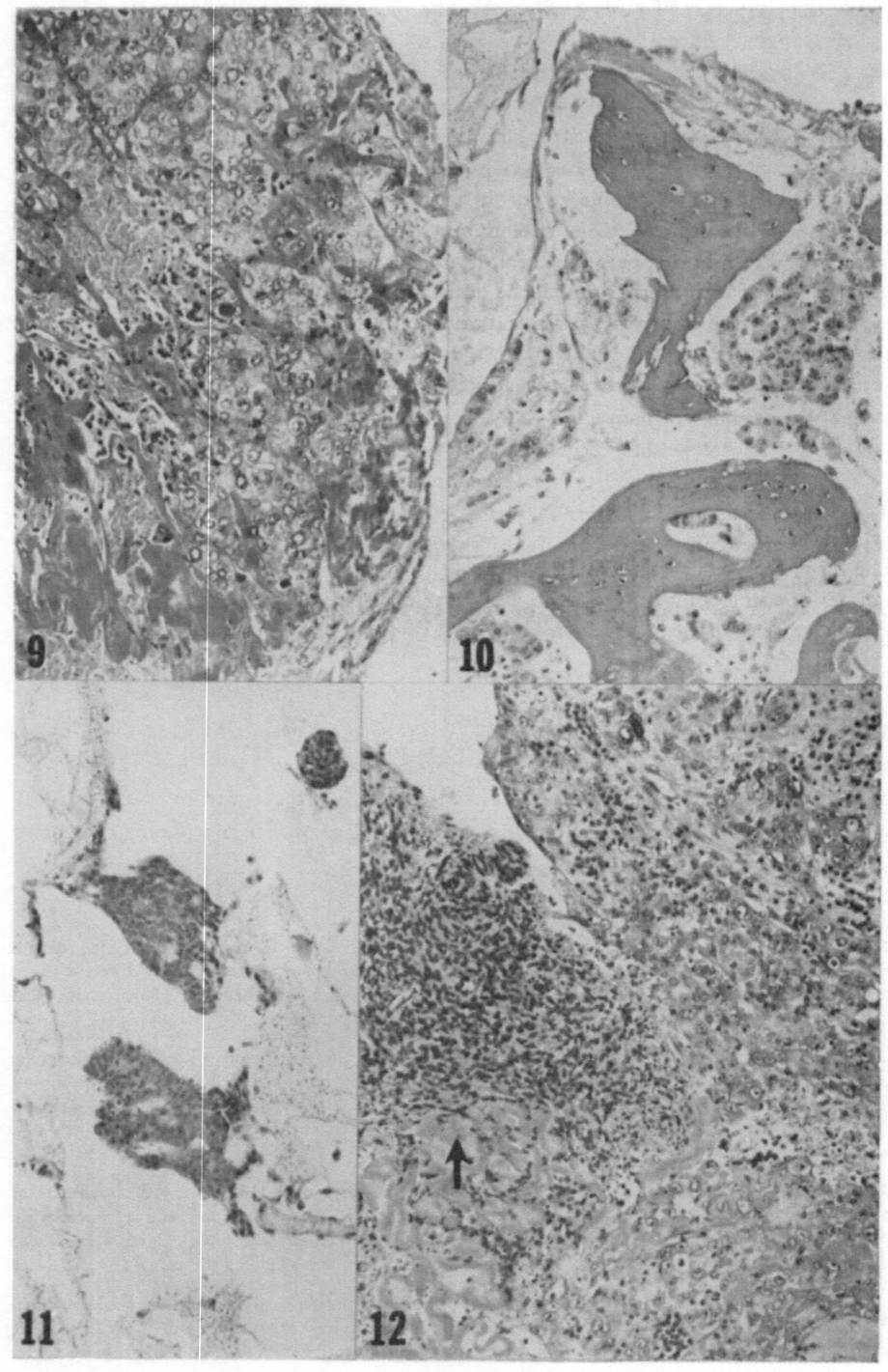

of the tumor was maintained (PLATE 4, Figs. 13, 14, 15, and 16). The last two figures, from a case in which the explants were all small clumps, suggest that such fragments may be the most interesting inocula since they can be intimately combined with equally small pieces of embryonic tissues. The interaction between small populations of normal and tumor cells may be studied in a few serial sections without any concurrent central necrosis of either micro-explant (PLATE 4, Fig. 16).

The neuroblastoma, a soft friable tumor, was prepared as a very fine mince and in all the cultures was combined with a mince of embryonic lung. This tumor thrived in the substance of the proliferating embryonic tissue, as seen in PLATE 2, Fig. 8.

Effusion Tumors. The growth of the effusion tumors varied with two factors, the density of tumor cells in the centrifuge sediment, and whether or not normal tissue was added to the culture.

In general, the sediment from effusions of carcinoma of the breast contained mainly erythrocytes and mesothelial cells, with only rare tumor cells. These inocula showed persistent viability of mesothelial cells, which adhered to the trabeculae of the sponge and in 3 or 4 days gave rise to numerous multinucleated foreign body giant cell forms. The rare tumor cells found in the initial sediment disappeared after a few days in culture. The effusion tumors that gave rise to distinct growth of carcinoma cells in matrix culture were those having large numbers of tumor cells in the original sediment. Four cases were in this category. They were carcinomas of the breast, stomach, ovary, and one whose primary site was unknown. The growth of these populations was more luxuriant and histologically complex in association with a mince of embryonic tissue than when cultured alone (PLATE 5, Figs. 17, 18, 19, and 20). The best growth among the effusion tumors was produced by the sediment of the carcinoma of the ovary, illustrated in PLATE 5, Fig. 20.

PLATE 3

Fig. 9. Five-day-old culture of carcinoma of the breast growing in association with chick embryonic mesonephros. This field shows only a part of the outer surface of the tumor explant. Visable carcinoma cells are in abundance and cells in mitosis are also seen. In adjacent fields, not in the figure, both tissues were in contact. There was some migration of mesonephric stroma around the tumor, but no indication of migratory growth of tumor cells. Hematoxylin and Eosin, ×150.

Fig. 10. Five-day-old culture of carcinoma of the breast metastatic to bone. Nests of tumor cells are seen in the stroma of the bony fragment. Although there has been no migration of tumor cells into the spongy matrix (upper left), migration of cells to the surface of the explant has occurred. Hematoxylin and Eosin, ×150.

Fig. 11. Eight-day-old culture of mucinous carcinoma of the breast. Only scanty collections of viable tumor cells are found; these are irregularly adherent to the collagen-coated sponge surfaces. Hematoxylin and Eosin, ×150.

Fig. 12. Four-day-old culture of carcinoma of the breast growing in association with autologous ovarian tissue. This field contains three explants in contact, one of ovarian tissue and two of carcinoma. The ovarian stroma, seen on the left, has small, dark, elongated nuclei (arrow). The two tumor fragments occupy the right half of the field. Tumor fragments grown with ovary were more cellular than tumor cultivated alone. Hematoxylin and Eosin, ×150.

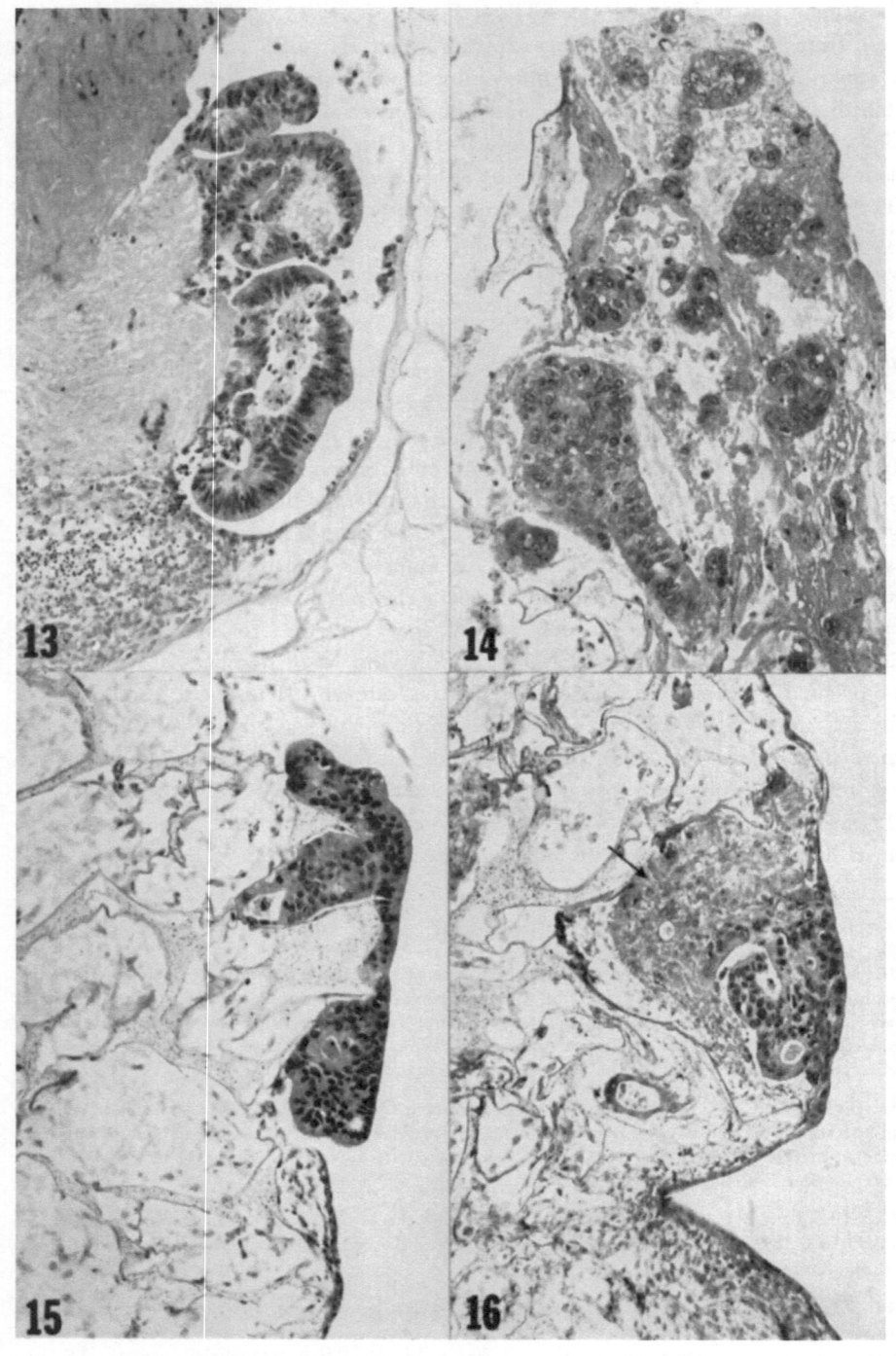

Effect of Normal Tissue. Migratory outgrowth from discrete explants was generally unimpressive when tumor tissue was cultured alone. In contrast, extensive migration of tumor epithelium was seen in the carcinoma of the larynx when tumor and embryonic lung were combined (PLATE 2, Fig. 7). Where the inoculum consisted of a fine mince of tumor in combination with embryonic tissue, a broad zone of growth developed along the diagonal line of inoculation and on the edges of the sponge at the ends of the diagonal band (Fig. 1). Dense growth, consisting predominantly of embryonic tissue sometimes accompanied by scattered foci of tumor, extended into the sponge to a depth of 100 to 300 microns. The growth of effusion tumors was consistently more abundant in association with a stroma of chick embryonic tissue than where the sediment was cultured alone (PLATE 5, Figs. 17 through 20). The supplementary stroma also enhanced the architectural complexity of the groups of cancer cells.

The mechanism of this supportive effect is not evident. In some cases the sticky quality of embryonic tissue was imparted to the tumor, aiding tumor fragments in establishing adherence to the matrix. Other mechanisms may be operating as well. This was suggested by our observations in a case where mammary carcinoma was cultivated alone and in contact with autologous ovary. Although living tumor was seen in both series, the extent of tumor viability was obviously greater where tumor and ovary were cultivated together.

Discussion

Our survey of a small sample of different human tumors parrallels our earlier experience with rodent tumors (5). A variety of neoplasms can be cultivated for at least a few days on a matrix of collagen coated cellulose sponge. From the point of view of bioassay and clinical correlation, attention must now be concentrated on

---

PLATE 4

Fig. 13. Seven-day-old culture of carcinoma of the colon growing in combination with chick embryonic intestine. Tumor cells form several papillary glandular structures on the residual fibrous core of the tumor explant. The connective tissue in the lower left is of embryonic origin. Hematoxylin and Eosin, ×150.

Fig. 14. Five-day-old culture of a mucinous carcinoma of the colon grown in combination with chick embryonic intestine. This field is limited to an ill-defined explant of tumor. The clusters of tumor cells remain within their matrix of mucin. The sponge matrix is seen on the left side of the figure. Hematoxylin and Eosin, ×150.

Fig. 15 and Fig. 16. Two fields from the same culture of carcinoma of the colon grown with chick embryonic tissue, five days after preparation. In Fig. 15, a fragment of glandular neoplastic epithelium has insinuated itself into the contours of the collagen-coated sponge. In Fig. 16, tumor tissue and chick embryonic are in intimate association. At the fluid bathed surface of the combination (on the right) tumor tissue with dark staining nuclei appears to be progressively covering the fragment of liver parenchyma (arrow). Hematoxylin and Eosin, ×150.

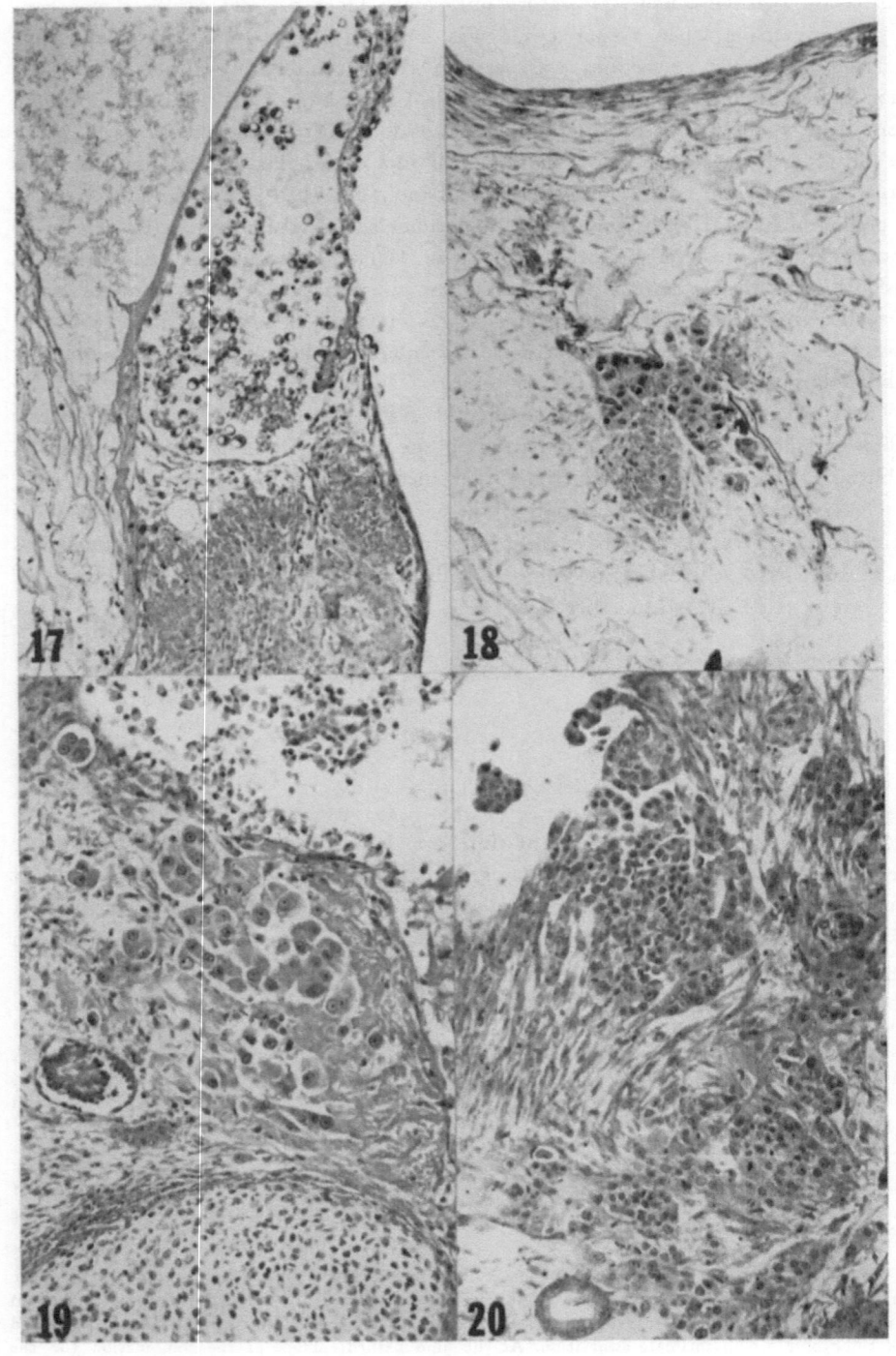

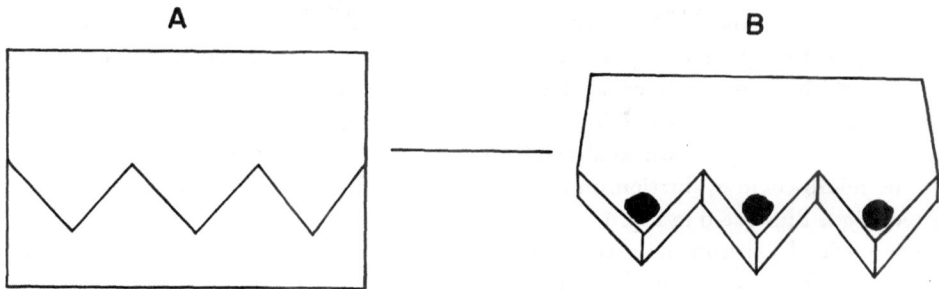

Fig. 2

a limited group of tumors. We have chosen to study, in the immediate future, carcinoma of the colon, a common type of cancer that displays excellent histotypic architecture when cultured on collagen coated sponge (PLATE 4, Figs. 13, 14, 15 and 16). Furthermore, earlier studies in our laboratory with our *in-vivo* model, the chick embryo, demonstrated that this type of tumor transplants readily to the chorioallantois with excellent persistence of histologic organization (1).

A consideration of Fig. 1 indicates that an effort might be made to reduce the expense of histologic evaluation of matrix cultures. Growth was seen on the surface of the sponge and was especially good on the two edges of the sponge section. We have, therefore, been exploring means of increasing the number of edges examined per microscopic section. Cutting the sponges with pinking shears (Fig. 2A) has provided a ready means of increasing the number of edges available for each microscopic section. The sequence of events in this procedure is illustrated by Fig. 2 In a typical piece of sponge there are three points. The upper surface of each point is inoculated with an explant of tissue (Fig. 2B). Each of the clefts between the points may also be the site of inoculation, providing five inoculation sites in all. The tissues used in developing this procedure have been those of the chick embryo, experimental tumors of mice, and tissue culture cell lines. On embedding, the sponge

---

PLATE 5

Fig. 17. Two-day-old culture of ascites sediment from a patient with carcinoma of the stomach, linitis plastica type, combined with chick embryonic heart. A number of isolated signet ring cells are seen in the center of the field. Hematoxylin and Eosin, $\times 150$.

Fig. 18. Four-day-old culture of ascites sediment from a patient with disseminated carcinoma of the breast, combined with a mince of embryonic tissues. Groups of tumor cells are seen in a stroma of embryonic connective tissues. Hematoxylin and Eosin, $\times 150$.

Fig. 19. Three-day-old culture of pleural fluid sediment, primary site unknown, combined with a mince of entire six-day-old chick embryos. In addition to the large anaplastic tumor cells, several other cell types can be identified. The loose small cells in the upper part of the field are mainly of pleural mesothelial origin. A glomerulus (probably chick mesonephros) is seen to the left of center, and a mass of embryonic cartilage occupies the lower part of the field. Hematoxylin and Eosin, $\times 150$.

Fig. 20. Four-day-old culture of ascitic fluid from patient with carcinoma of the ovary combined with a mince of the mesonephric region of an eight-day-old embryo. The tumor appears as many nests of cells, some in papillary patterns, in the embryonic stroma. The tubule in the lower left of the field is of mesonephric origin. Hematoxylin and Eosin, $\times 150$.

is oriented so that the points are down, that is the microtome knife makes its first contact with the apices of the three points. Sections are cut to the extent of 10 to 15 slides. Within this range of sections the entire area of the protruding triangles is displayed on the microscope slides. The available edge area has been increased three-fold over the technique illustrated in PLATE 1, Fig. 1. The amount of growth available for microscopic evaluation on a few slides exceeds by far the growth seen with the technique illustrated in Fig. 1.

For optimal experimental study of tumor tissue we need repeated opportunities to examine the same specimen of tumor. This is an outstanding attraction of the many transplantable tumors of rodents. The closest clinical parallel to this situation occurs in the case of effusion tumors. Patients with carcinomatous effusions are usually subject to several paracenteses during the terminal part of their illness, and one can therefore obtain specimens on more than a single occasion. However, the matter is complicated by the fact that the clinician usually introduces chemothera-peutic agents with the first or second tap. One cannot be sure that a cell population obtained at a subsequent tap has not been modified by the chemotherapy. There are other difficulties as well. Scheduling follow-up taps at the mutual convenience of the patient, the clinician, and the tissue culture laboratory presents its own problems.

We are now examining the possibility that freezing preservation techniques will permit us to examine uniform aliquots of tumor tissue at time intervals of our choice after operation. To study the feasibility of this idea, we are now attempting to culture frozen human tumors from the tissue bank at the Roswell Park Memorial Institute. We are also preparing to use a freezing technique in studying carcinoma of the colon from our own hospital, the Presbyterian-University Hospital of Pittsburgh. In this case, our procedure is to cut a tumor into many fragments of explant size, cultivate some at once, inoculate others on the chorioallantois of the chick, and im-mediately freeze the remainder in 9 or 18 aliquots over liquid nitrogen, according to established procedures. When tumors grow from the primary cultivation, one or two aliquots from the freezer will be thawed and prepared for study in the same manner as that of the primary series. For tumors in which both primary study and freezing recovery results are satisfactory, we plan a variety of follow-up studies.

Our data suggest that several qualities of neoplastic behavior may be studied in matrix culture. Recognition and interaction between tumor cells may be expressed by a number of morphologic patterns, i.e., the formation, shape, and size of glands, papillary structures, cords, or cell aggregates. Cells that migrate from explants ap-pear in monolayers or stratified multilayers. In combinations of tumor and normal tissues these organoid characteristics of neoplastic growth may be modified. In ad-dition some tumors may envelop normal tissue, others invade and replace it. The histologic localization of synthetic biochemical events in the cultures should be pos-sible using appropriately labeled precursors and autoradiography.

We are now in a position to examine selected types of clinical cancer, such as carcinoma of the colon, with the real possibility that behavioral expression by tumors in the laboratory can eventually be correlated with the clinical course of individual patients.

References

1. LEIGHTON, J.: The Spread of Cancer. Academic Press, New York, 131, 1967.
2. LEIGHTON, J.: A sponge matrix method for tissue culture. Formation of organized aggregates of cells *in vitro*. J. Nat. Cancer Inst. 12, 545 (1951).
3. LEIGHTON, J.: Invasive growth and metastasis in tissue culture systems. *In:* Methods in Cancer Research IV. H. Busch (ed.), Academic Press, New York, 86 (1967).
4. LEIGHTON, J., JUSTH, G., ESPER, M., and KRONENTHAL, R. L.: Collagen coated cellulose sponge: Three-dimensional matrix for tissue culture of Walker tumor 256. Science 155, 1259 (1967).
5. LEIGHTON, J., MARK, R., and JUSTH, G.: Patterns of three-dimensional growth *in vitro* in collagen coated cellulose sponge: Carcinomas and embryonic tissues. Cancer Research, in press.
6. LEIGHTON, J.: Bioassay of cancer in matrix tissue culture systems. Presented at the 21st Annual Symposium of the M. D. Anderson Hospital, Houston, Texas. Texas U. Press, in press (1967).
7. LEIGHTON, J., and ESPER, M.: Culture tube and pipette for cultivation of tissues on standard microscope slide. Public Health Reports, 79, 642 (1964).

Discussion

The Use of Three-Dimensional Matrix Tissue Culture for Bioassay of Cancer

KATHERINE SANFORD

National Cancer Institute, Bethesda, Maryland

Dr. Leighton has developed a technique that appears to be particularly useful for studying the behavior of tumor cells in forming organized patterns and for examining interactions between tumor cells and normal tissues *in vitro*. With such three-dimensional preparations, the usual histologic techniques and interpretations can be applied more readily than with two-dimensional substrate cultures. Since the sponge is providing a three-dimensional support for cell outgrowth, the conformation of the sponge surfaces might influence the architecture of the culture. However, it appears that the cells fill the interstices and in these lacunae organize into acini, cords, glands, and other structures. For this reason, I wonder if the size and arrangement of pores is not critical. It would seem that they must be relatively small and yet large enough to permit moderate flow of nutrients and development of organoid structures.

This type of culture as well as the organ cultures used by Wolff and Wolff (13—14) for maintaining human and animal tumors in embryonic chick mesonephros are useful in studying the invasion of normal tissues by neoplastic cells. Dr. Leighton's results suggest that the culture medium for certain of the human tumor tissues may have been deficient and that the added chick embryonic tissues provided substances needed for survival and growth as has been shown by Wolff and Wolff (13). The slow diffusion of the medium through the interstices of the sponge probably prevents the washing out of cellular products possibly necessary for continued maintenance of differentiated structure.

Our earliest experience in culturing tissue was with the three-dimensional plasma clot, which unlike gels such as agar or gelatin, consists of 1. a dense network of fibrin filaments along which the cells migrate and divide, and 2. a continuous fluid phase. In the plasma matrix cultures, cells tend to migrate out from the explant surface through the matrix and collect at the glass/plasma interface of the culture and in the plasma at the fluid interface (2). The morphology of cells at these two interfaces, even in the same culture, may be radically different as was shown by Earle in studies on strain L and related cell lines treated with the carcinogen 3-methylcholanthrene (3, 4). However, in the plasma matrix, histotypic characters of individual neoplasms or normal tissues may be maintained near the explanted tissue. As the cells migrate outward and are serially subcultured and dispersed, greater disorganization occurs. Even with cellular dispersion and continuous culture on glass, the potential for organized structure may frequently persist. We cultured one strain of C3H mouse mammary carcinoma cells in a serum supplemented, chemically defined medium that continued to reproduce when implanted in mice the epithelial glandular architecture of the original tumor after 1½ years and 35 transplant generations of growth *in vitro*. The high arginase activity characteristic of C3H mammary carcinomas was also maintained (10). Other examples of retention of differentiated function or structure during long term culture of dispersed cell populations have been reported (8, review). In general, however, many differentiated characters tend to be lost.

Another phenomenon that occurs repeatedly during the continuous subculturing of dispersed normal tissue cells is their neoplastic conversion as evidenced by their capacity to grow as malignant neoplasmas when implanted in animals of the strain of origin. This phenomenon has now been observed in cell lines derived from a wide variety of tissues from different strains of several different species of animals including the mouse, rat, hamster, and man (7, review). Since no known carcinogenic chemical or virus was deliberately added to the cultures, these conversions of unknown cause have been referred to as "spontaneous" which means proceeding without external stimulus. However, several recent observations strongly suggest that these conversions are not spontaneous but may be induced by specific extrinsic factors. Evans and Andresen (5) have found that the type of serum used to supplement chemically defined medium NCTC 135 can delay or prevent the conversion of C3H mouse embryo cells. Neoplastic conversion in these cells usually occurs at 90 to 180 days of culture in horse or calf serum medium but may be prevented or delayed significantly if cells from the same original pool are cultured in fetal calf serum. Studies are currently in progress to detect what fractions of horse serum may be carcinogenic or what moiety of the fetal calf serum may prevent neoplastic conversion. High multiplicities of tumor viruses may also induce neoplastic conversion of cells *in vitro*.

Since this is a symposium on normal and neoplastic cell growth, I would like to comment briefly on some growth responses of cells during neoplastic conversion *in vitro*. A distinguishing feature of neoplastic cells is their uncontrolled growth in the organism. The growth controlling mechanism from which the cells have escaped is unknown and may be intracellular, intercellular, or systemic. If intracellular, some differences in the growth potential of neoplastic and normal cells *in vitro* might be expected under certain culture conditions. One such difference has been noted. When dispersed embryonic cells are first explanted *in vitro*, they may proliferate rapidly. With certain species such as the Syrian hamster, the cells may then show a decline in proliferation. If at this time the cultures have been treated with a high multiplicity of tumor virus such as polyoma, the cells may proliferate more rapidly, loosen from the floor of the flask, pile up into "criss-cross" networks and continue to grow to a higher cell density per culture than control, untreated cells (9, review). These altered cells, if implanted *in vivo*, usually grow as sarcomas. The alteration in growth pattern has been interpreted as resulting from a loss of "contact inhibition" by the cells, either contact inhibition of locomotion or of mitosis. The term "contact inhibition of locomotion" was applied by Abercrombie and associates (1) to the behavior of freshly isolated chick embryo heart fibroblasts. "Contact inhibition" was defined as the stopping of locomotion of a cell in a particular direction by contact with another cell. Cells exhibiting contact inhibition formed a monolayer with little or no overlap. Since this phenomenon was observed in freshly isolated chick and mouse fibroblasts but not in mouse sarcoma cells, Abercrombie and associates proposed the hypothesis that malignancy involves the loss or diminution of contact inhibition. Subsequently, many workers have assumed that if cells form a monolayer, the cells exhibit contact inhibition of locomotion. It appears, however, that monolayer growth may result from other conditions such as tight adhesion of cells to substrate. The term "contact inhibition of mitosis" has been applied to the inhibition of mitosis or reduced growth rate observed in certain cultures when the cells have grown into a confluent monolayer (11). Cells transformed by polyoma virus and made neoplastic are no longer considered susceptible to contact inhibition of mitosis since they can grow in multilayers to a higher cell density or "saturation density" than normal or non-neoplastic cells. However, control cultures if carefully handled may also survive and ultimately show similar proliferation rates. Some of these may become neoplastic; others may grow as rapidly *in vitro* but test as non-neoplastic (9). Non-neoplastic cells under favorable culture conditions can also grow in multilayers (6). Cells that have undergone spontaneous neoplastic conversion or cells derived from tumors *in vivo*, on the other hand, may tend to grow as monolayers (10, 9). The degree or extent of monolayering or multilayering thus appears to depend more on the cell type and culture conditions than on the neoplastic or non-neoplastic state of the cells. Furthermore, the phenomenon of inhibition of mitosis by cell contact has not been clearly demonstrated. In fact, cell mitosis in lightly seeded cultures is enhanced by cell contacts. In a confluent culture, mitosis may be inhibited as a result of cell crowding and the consequent poor exchange of nutrients and waste products in the microenvironment of each cell. Furthermore, some cells require a solid substrate which seems to act as a stimulus for migration and division. Thus, cell crowding with inadequate perfusion of nutrients and wastes and lack of surface substrate may lead to reduced mitosis and the stationary phase of growth. Such stationary growth phases also occur in suspension culture where cell contact may be minimal.

It is interesting that a tumor virus induces a proliferative response apparent when the cultures are in a decline or stationary phase during their early adaptation to culture and that such altered cells are neoplastic. Since polyoma virus has been reported to induce synthesis of cellular DNA and associated enzymes, which, of course, would be requisite for the proliferative response, it appears that the cells during this phase of adaptation to culture have become more biosynthetically active and can survive and grow better than untreated control cells. The mechanism of this effect, whether resulting from activation or derepression of genetic material, alterations in membrane permeability and transport, or synthesis of growth stimulants or other regulatory substances, needs further clarification.

In summation, we have referred to two types of culture, the short term 3-dimensional matrix culture in which differentiated structure and function may be retained for short intervals and in which cell interactions may more closely resemble those occurring *in vivo*, and the long term dispersed cell culture in which after repeated subcultures differentiated structures and functions may disappear in both neoplastic and normal tissue cells. Also, in populations of normal tissue cells, neoplastic conversion may occur presumably through some influence of the type of serum in the medium. Finally, one difference in growth response of normal and virus induced neoplastic cells has been described.

References

1. ABERCROMBIE, M., HEAYSMAN, J. E. M., and KARTHAUSER, H. M.: Social behavior of cells in tissue culture. III. Mutual influences of sarcoma cells and fibroblasts. Exp. Cell, Res. **13**, 276 (1957).

2. EARLE, W. R.: Some morphologic variations of certain cells under controlled experimental conditions. Nat. Cancer Inst. **7**, 213 (1962).

3. EARLE, W. R., SCHILLING, E. L., and SHELTON, E.: Production of malignancy *in vitro*. IX. Description of cells at the fluid interface of the culture. J. Nat. Cancer Inst. **10**, 865 (1950).

4. EARLE, W. R., SCHILLING, E., and SHELTON, E.: Production of malignancy *in vitro*. X. Continued description of cells at the glass interface of the cultures. J. Nat. Cancer Inst. **10**, 1067 (1950).

5. EVANS, V. J., and ANDRESEN, W. F.: Effect of serum on spontaneous neoplastic transformation *in vitro*. J. Nat. Cancer Inst. **37**, 247 (1966).

6. KRUSE, P. F., JR., and MIEDEMA, E.: Production and characterization of multiple-layered populations of animal cells. J. Cell. Biol. **27**, 273 (1965).

7. SANFORD, K. K.: "Spontaneous" neoplastic transformation of cells *in vitro*: Some facts and theories. Nat. Cancer Inst. **26**, 387 (1967).

8. SANFORD, K. K.: Malignant transformation of cells *in vitro*. Intl. Rev. Cytol. **18**, 249 (1965).

9. SANFORD, K. K., BARKER, B. E., WOODS, M. W., PARSHAD, R., and LAW, L. W.: Search for "indicators" of neoplastic conversion *in vitro*. J. Nat. Cancer Inst. **39**, 705 (1967).

10. SANFORD, K. K., DUNN, T. B., WESTFALL, B. B., COVALESKY, A. B., DUPREE, L. T., and EARLE, W. R.: Sarcomatous change and maintenance of differentiation in long term cultures of mouse mammary carcinoma. J. Nat. Cancer Inst. 26, 1139 (1961).

11. TODARO, G. J., LAZAR, G. K., and GREEN, H.: The initiation of cell division in a contact inhibited mammalian cell line. J. Cell. Comp. Physiol. 66, 325 (1965).

12. WOLFF, E., BARSKI, G., and WOLFF, E.: Mise en evidence de differents degres de malignité de souches cellulaires de Souris en culture d'organes embryonnaires de Poulet. Compt. Rend. Acad. Sci. [Paris] 251, 479 (1960).

13. WOLFF, E., and WOLFF, E.: Cultures organotypiques de longue durée de deux tumeurs humaines du tube digestif. Europ. J. Cancer 2, 93 (1966).

14. WOLFF, E., and WOLFF, E.: Les résultats d'une nouvelle méthode de culture de cellules cancéreuses "in vitro." Rev. Franc d'etudes Clin. et Biol. 3, 945 (1958).

Importance of the Non-Dividing Leukemic Cell *

Alvin M. Mauer, E. F. Saunders and Beatrice C. Lampkin

Children's Hospital Research Foundation and Department of Pediatrics
University of Cincinnati
Cincinnati, Ohio

A study of the characteristics of cell proliferation in acute leukemia has potentially three things to offer. First, we may learn the mechanism by which leukemic cells have an advantageous growth differential with respect to the normal marrow cell population. Second, information may be derived concerning the origin of the leukemic cells with particular reference to the need for continued transformation of a normal cell population. Finally, therapy for acute leukemia has been primarily directed against the parts of the cell cycle related to division, that is the synthesis of DNA and mitosis. Further information concerning the nature of the leukemic cell population may give us better methods of using current therapeutic measures and point the way toward new approaches for therapy.

It will be the purpose of this paper to review briefly the studies available so far about the characteristics of leukemic cell proliferation and then to present the results of a recent study which has had some implications for therapy.

Methodology

The earliest attempts to measure proliferative activity in the leukemic cell population were those of Astaldi and Mauri in 1953 (1). It was interesting that their measurement of the numbers of mitotic figures among the cells gave low values in contrast to the concepts then current of the leukemic cells being a wildly proliferating group. These cells in mitosis can be identified because of the morphological alteration occurring during the time of mitotic division. A modification of the method described by Japa (13) provides a simple technique for determining the mitotic index.

A major advance in the study of leukemic cell proliferation came from the development of tritiated thymidine as a cell label for use in humans by means of autoradiographic techniques (7, 6). This material is only incorporated into cells during the DNA synthesizing phase of the mitotic cycle. After intravenous in-

* This investigation was supported by Public Health Service Research Grants CA 04826 and FR 00123. Dr. Mauer was a recipient of a research career development award from the National Institutes of Health. Dr. Saunders is supported by The Leukemia Society, Inc. Dr. Lampkin is an Advanced Clinical Fellow of the American Cancer Society, Inc.

jection it is available briefly for incorporation (26), although a variable degree of label reutilization may occur later. Some of the assumptions and general considerations concerning the label and autoradiography have been discussed by Cronkite and his coworkers (6, 15).

Several special considerations needed study before the label could be accepted for application to patients with acute leukemia. The label was incorporated by all dividing leukemic cells (17, 18). Although the proliferative activity of blood and bone marrow leukemic cells were different as measured by percent of cells in DNA synthesis (19), measurement of the percent of labeled cells and the concentration of label per cell at different marrow sites gave similar results (18). Thus determination of proliferative activity at a single marrow site reflected the whole marrow population. The results of *in vivo* and *in vitro* labeling studies of marrow cells were similar and both labeling and mitotic indices in the same patient gave parallel indications of proliferation rates (27). From these studies, then, the label can be used as a valid method of studying cell kinetics in patients with acute leukemia.

Generation Time

One of the earliest areas of interest was the measurement of generation time for the leukemic cell. The anticipated result was a shortened cycle in keeping with the apparently accelerated growth rate for these cells. An early attempt to define an aspect of the proliferative cycle was the determination of the labeling index for blood leukemic cells (5). By assuming a homogeneous cell population with respect to proliferative activity, the authors concluded that a long generation cycle was present because of the low labeling index. Subsequently it has been learned that the blood is not a proliferative compartment and the cell population is not homogeneous. The labeling index by itself does not therefore yield information concerning the generation time.

The attempt to measure generation time by the decreasing mean grain count in serial samples of the cell population (16) is based on the division of label equally between daughter cells after mitosis. Thus a decrease in mean grain count by one-half should mark the conclusion of one division. Too many technical problems involving autoradiography, the non-uniform nature of the cell population and label reutilization make this method an invalid one.

Changes in the time course for labeled cells determined from serial marrow samples after a single injection of label and study of changes in cell label after serial injections of tritiated thymidine have been used to measure the generation time of dividing cells (18). These results have been in keeping with a mitotic cycle for dividing cells of about 20 hours. Another group of three patients studied by means of the "mitotic window" technique have had generation times that are somewhat longer, about 60 hours (27).

Generation times for these malignant cell populations, ranging from 20 to 60 hours, would be similar to the results of some studies comparing normal and malignant animal (23, 2) and human (12) tissues of the same derivation wherein generation times for the malignant cells are the same as or longer than the normal cell. No information concerning generation times for normal lymphocytes is available but 20 hours would be in the usual range for normal marrow precursor cells.

A further complication in measuring generation times for leukemic cells comes from the observation that the cell cycles may not be uniform in this respect. In one patient we have studied, the generation time has varied from a minimal figure of 60 hours to a maximal demonstrated time of 210 hours (20).

The results of generation time studies have indicated that the differential growth rate for the leukemic cell population does not arise from a more rapid rate of division. Other aspects of the leukemic cell characteristics must therefore be important in this regard.

Leukemic Cell Life Cycle

Several studies have now yielded information regarding the cell cycle. The marrow cell population is not uniform but is comprised of dividing and non-dividing elements (18, 10, 14). The two compartments are interrelated in that the dividing compartment feeds cells into the non-dividing compartment in much the same manner as myelocytes become metamyelocytes (18, 10). Some cells leave the marrow and enter the blood (18). The dividing cells can be distinguished morphologically in that they are larger and have finer nuclear chromatin patterns.

The proportion of dividing to non-dividing cells is constant but varies from patient to patient and in the same patient during different stages of his disease (27). The labeling index and proportion of dividing leukemic cells in the marrow are generally least at the time of diagnosis and greatest when studied during subsequent relapses (27, 25, 8).

The patient at the time of diagnosis has generally had symptoms for several weeks and presumably has had growth of his leukemic cell population for at least that time. Just before a subsequent relapse, the patient is followed closely in clinic and studies are usually done at the earliest time after onset of symptoms or changes in blood counts. In this instance, the leukemic cell population might be presumed to have had a shorter period of growth before study. If these assumptions are true, then the accumulation of non-dividing cells seems to be a progressive function of a growing population.

Similar accumulation of non-dividing cells occurs in some animal tumors as well (21, 22, 3, 9). As these tumors start to grow, all cells participate in cell division. Consequently, as the population grows, progressive accumulation of non-proliferating cells occurs. Accumulation of these cells could indeed account for the observed replacement of normal tissues. Thus, leukemia may be primarily a disease of accumulation rather than proliferation.

The observed variability of proliferative activity found in marrow samples from leukemic patients could not be correlated with age of the patient, sex, type of leukemia, degree of marrow replacement, blood leukemic cell concentration or response to chemotherapy (27). There has not been found a significant variation of labeling indices as a function of the time of day (27). This feature of cell kinetics indicates that there is no particularly advantageous time of day during which to give chemotherapeutic agents which inhibit DNA synthesis. An interesting observation has been that some patients maintain a normal diurnal variation of mitotic indices in the marrow even when complete replacement by leukemic cells has occurred (27). These cells may respond at least in part to some normal control mechanisms for cellular proliferation.

A summary of our knowledge of leukemic cell kinetics is schematically presented in simplified form in Fig. 1. A proliferating population of cells, morphologically distinguishable, is dividing with a generation time from 20 to 60 hours. The minimal generation time for the dividing cells is consistent within the individual patient although a variable portion of the cells may have longer generation times related to a prolongation of the G_1 interphase. After one or more mitotic divisions, the cells become smaller and stop dividing. This non-dividing segment accumulates progressively with growth of the cell population.

Several important questions remain. The blood leukemic cell is not a proliferative one but what is its role? The blood leukemic cell population turns over but do the cells leaving the compartment return to tissues to recycle as does the lymphocyte? Or does the turnover indicate a cell death function as in the case of the neutrophil? Clearly no kinetic measurements based on blood cell turnover rate can be made until this information is available.

Gavosto and his coworkers (11) have recently indicated that the proliferating cell compartment is not a self-maintaining stem cell population. That is, based on observations of rates of cell production and rates of flux out of the compartment, an influx of cells is required to prevent depletion of the dividing cells. The question marks over the two arrows into the compartment indicate the need for information concerning this point.

If replacement for the proliferating compartment comes from the left-hand arrow by means of continuing leukemic transformation of normal cells, then there would be indication that the transforming agent would still be active. Therapy directed toward cure of the disease would then have to take the continued presence of the leukemogenic agent into account.

If, on the other hand, replacement comes from the right-hand direction, that is recycling of non-dividing cells through a phase of cell proliferation, then an entirely different approach might be indicated. Such a re-entry of non-dividing ascites

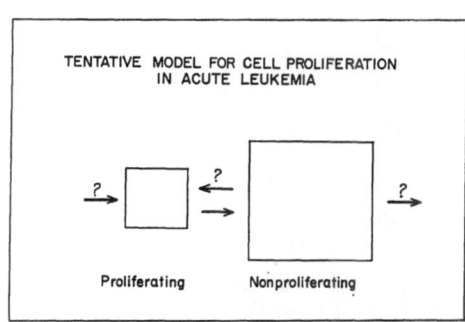

Fig. 1. A schematic model for cell kinetics in acute leukemia.

tumor cells into a proliferative phase has been demonstrated by Baserga and Gold (4). Certainly normal resting lymphocytes can re-enter proliferation under such non-specific stimulus as phytohemagglutinin or the specific stimulus of antigen re-exposure in the sensitized cell.

The capacity for the resting leukemic cell to re-enter division has potential therapeutic significance. Miller and Cole (24) have recently reported on the relative resistance of resting small lymphocytes to such chemotherapeutic agents as prednisone, cyclophosphamide, 6-mercaptopurine, and actinomycin D. These cells are capable of subsequent cell division. If resting leukemic cells were, in a similar fashion, resistant to chemotherapy, capable of surviving therapy into disease remission and then, having achieved drug resistance if the cells could re-enter the proliferative phase to mark the onset of disease relapse, then the small resting cell holds the key to successful and permanent treatment for the disease.

Re-entry of Resting Leukemic Cells into a Proliferative Phase

The following *in vivo* experiment was designed to explore the possibility of re-entry of small, non-proliferative leukemic cells back into cell division. An untreated patient with acute lymphoblastic leukemia was given three injections of tritiated thymidine at twelve hour intervals as shown in Fig. 2. At the end of that time, most of the proliferating cells were labeled. The rate with which the proliferating cells left that compartment to become small, non-proliferating cells was then determined by serial marrow samples over the next 48 hours. As the cells left, they were replaced by unlabeled cells and the compartment was maintained in this manner.

Then nine injections of tritiated thymidine were given at twelve hour intervals.

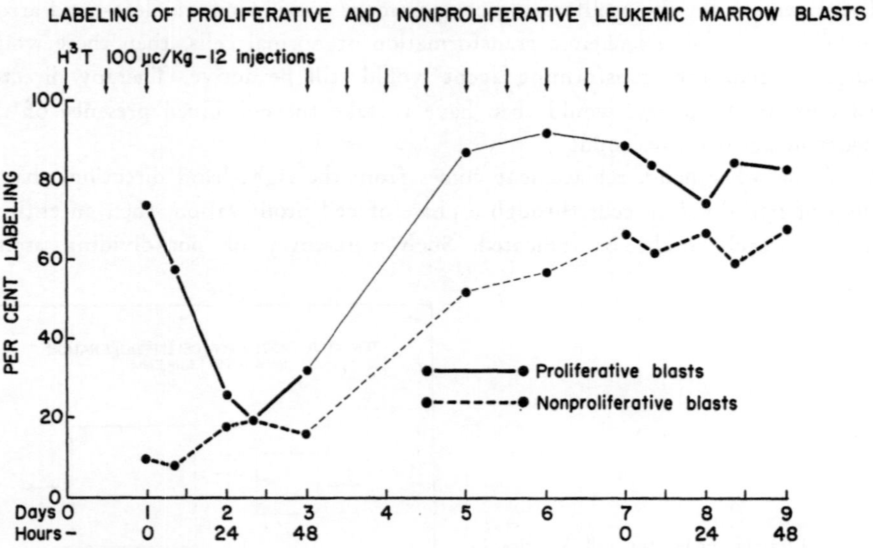

Fig. 2. The time course for labeled leukemic cells in bone marrow after serial injection of tritiated thymidine.

At the end of this time, again, most of the proliferative cells were labeled but now two-thirds of the non-proliferative cells were also labeled. This compartment became labeled by an influx of cells from the proliferative compartment. The time course for labeled cells was then followed by serial marrow samples during the following 48 hours. The percent of labeled proliferative cells did not significantly change, indicating that as cells left the compartment they were replaced by labeled cells which must have come from the labeled small, non-proliferative cell population.

Summary

Thus the non-proliferative leukemic cell is a resting cell capable of re-entering a phase of cell division. Also the leukemic cell population is most probably a closed, self-maintaining population which does not require continued leukemic transformation of normal cells for replacement. The leukemic cell may be a long-lived cell, explaining the accumulation phenomenon. Finally, the relatively resistant non-proliferative cell may survive therapy into the period of remission and serve as the focus for eventual regrowth of drug-resistant cells to bring about relapse.

References

1. ASTALDI, G., and MAURI, C.: Recherches sur l'activité proliférative de l'hemocytoblaste de la leucémie aiguë. Revue. Belge. Path. Méd. Exp. **23**, 69 (1953).
2. BANERJEE, M. R., and WALKER, R. J.: Duration of DNA synthesis in hyperplastic alveolar nodules of C3H/He mouse mammary gland. J. Natl. Cancer Inst. **39**, 551 (1967).
3. BASERGA, R.: Mitotic cycle of ascites tumor cells. Arch. Path. **75**, 156 (1963).
4. BASERGA, R., and GOLD, R.: The uptake of tritiated thymidine by newly transplanted Ehrlich ascites tumor cells. Exp. Cell Res. **31**, 576 (1963).
5. CRADDOCK, C. G., and NAKAI, G. S.: Leukemic cell proliferation as determined by *in vitro* deoxyribonucleic acid synthesis. J. Clin. Invest. **41**, 360 (1962).
6. CRONKITE, E. P., BOND, V. P., FLIEDNER, T. M., and RUBINI, J. R.: The use of tritiated thymidine in the study of DNA synthesis and cell turnover in hemopoietic tissues. Lab. Invest. **8**, 263 (1959).
7. CRONKITE, E. P., FLIEDNER, T. M., BOND, V. P., and RUBINI, J. R.: Dynamics of hematopoietic proliferation in man and mice studied by H^3-thymidine incorporation into DNA. Ann. N.Y. Acad. Sci. **77**, 803 (1959).
8. FOADI, M. D., COOPER, E. H., and HARDISTY, R. M.: DNA synthesis and DNA content of leukocytes in acute leukemia. Nature (London) **216**, 134 (1967).
9. FRINDEL, E., MALAISE, E. P., ALPEN, E., and TUBIANA, M.: Kinetics of cell proliferation of an experimental tumor. Cancer Res. **27**, 1122 (1967).
10. GAVOSTO, F., PILERI, A., BACHI, C., and PEGORARO, L.: Proliferation and maturation defect in acute leukaemia cells. Nature (London) **203**, 92 (1964).
11. GAVOSTO, F., PILERI, A., GABUTTI, V., and MASERA, P.: Non-self-maintaining kinetics of proliferating blasts in human acute leukaemia. Nature (London) **216**, 188 (1967).
12. HOFFMAN, J., and POST, J.: *In vivo* studies of DNA synthesis in human normal and tumor cells. Cancer Res. **27**, 898 (1967).

13. JAPA, J.: A study of the mitotic activity of normal human bone marrow. Brit. J. Exp. Path. 23, 272 (1942).

14. KILLMAN, S. A.: Proliferative activity of blast cells in leukemia and myelofibrosis. Morphological differences between proliferating and non-proliferating blast cells. Acta Med. Scand. 178, 263 (1965).

15. KILLMAN, S. A., CRONKITE, E. P., FLIEDNER, T. M., and BOND, V. P.: Cell proliferation in multiple myeloma studied with tritiated thymidine in vivo. Lab. Invest. 11, 845 (1962).

16. KILLMAN, S. A., CRONKITE, E. P., ROBERTSON, J. S., FLIEDNER, T. M., and BOND, V. P.: Estimation of phases of the life cycle of leukemic cells from labeling in human beings in vivo with tritiated thymidine. Lab. Invest. 12, 671 (1963).

17. MAUER, A. M.: Characteristics of cell proliferation in a patient with acute leukemia. Lancet 2, 675 (1964).

18. MAUER, A. M., and FISHER, V.: Characteristics of cell proliferation in four patients with untreated acute leukemia. Blood 28, 428 (1966).

19. MAUER, A. M., and FISHER, V.: Comparison of the proliferative capacity of acute leukaemia cells in bone marrow and blood. Nature (London) 193, 1085 (1962).

20. MAUER, A. M., SAUNDERS, E. F., and LAMPKIN, B. C.: The nature and causes of the variability of proliferative activity in marrow cell populations in human acute leukemia. Proceedings of the Twenty-first Annual Symposium on Fundamental Cancer Research. The University of Texas. (In press.)

21. MENDELSOHN, M. L.: Chronic infusion of tritiated thymidine into mice with tumors. Science 135, 213 (1962).

22. MENDELSOHN, M. L.: Autoradiographic analysis of cell proliferation in spontaneous breast cancer of the C3H mouse. III. The growth fraction. J. Natl. Cancer Inst. 28, 1015 (1962).

23. METCALF, D., and WIADROWSKI, M.: Autoradiographic analysis of lymphocyte proliferation in the thymus and in thymic lymphoma tissue. Cancer Res. 26, 483 (1966).

24. MILLER, J. J., and COLE, L. J.: Resistance of long-lived lymphocytes and plasma cells in rat lymph nodes to treatment with prednisone, cyclophosphamide, 6-mercaptopurine and actinomycin D. J. Exp. Med. 126, 109 (1967).

25. PILERI, A., GABUTTI, V., MASERA, P., and GAVOSTO, F.: Proliferative activity of the cells of acute leukemia in relapse and in steady state. Acta Haemat. 38, 193 (1967).

26. RUBINI, J. R., CRONKITE, E. P., BOND, V. P., and FLIEDNER, T. M.: Metabolism and fate of tritiated thymidine in man. J. Clin. Invest. 39, 909 (1960).

27. SAUNDERS, E. F., LAMPKIN, B. C., and MAUER, A. M.: Variation of proliferative activity in leukemic cell populations of patients with acute leukemia. J. Clin. Invest. 46, 1356 (1967).

Discussion

Magnitude of Proliferating Fraction and Rate of Proliferation of Populations of Leukemic Cells in Man [*]

B. D. CLARKSON, J. FRIED, and M. OGAWA

Divisions of Chemotherapy Research and Biophysics,
Sloan Kittering Institute for Cancer Research, and
Department of Medicine, Memorial and James Ewing
Hospitals for Cancer and Allied Diseases, and
Cornell University Medical College, New York, New York

In the past our findings in regard to the proliferation kinetics of acute leukemia have differed from those of Dr. Mauer and his colleagues in two major respects. The first concerns the size of the proliferating fraction. Drs. Mauer and Fisher have reported the actively dividing fraction to be as small as 12 percent in some patients (12) while our estimates have been much larger (3, 2). The second point of disagreement concerns the generation times of the proliferating fractions. Dr. Mauer has previously reported generation times as short as 15–20 hours (2) whereas we have never found the mean generation time to be less than about 2 days and in most patients it was appreciably longer. We have also found considerable variability in the generation time within any one population of leukemic cells (3, 2, 7, 8). Since our studies were in adults while Dr. Mauer's were in children, it is important to know if a real difference exists between adult and childhood leukemia. The more recent studies of Dr. Mauer and his colleagues are much more in accord with our own; that is, mean generation times of the order of 60 hours (16); recognition that there may be wide variability of generation times within one population; and redefinition of the so-called "non-proliferative" cells to include resting cells which are capable of resuming active proliferation.

We would like to illustrate our methods and show representative results by presenting a recent study in one patient, a young girl with acute myeloblastic leukemia. Her course is shown in Fig. 1; it can be seen that her disease progressed clinically in a rather indolent fashion. She had had two remissions induced by cytosine arabinoside prior to the kinetic study in June, 1967. Although almost no maintenance therapy was given, the first remission lasted almost a year and the second about 5 months.

The most reliable method for determining the size of the proliferating fraction of

[*] This investigation was supported in part by research grants CA-05826 and CA-08748 from the National Cancer Institute, United States Public Health Service and #P-494 from the American Cancer Society.

G.S. 18 YR ♀ ACUTE MYELOBLASTIC LEUKEMIA

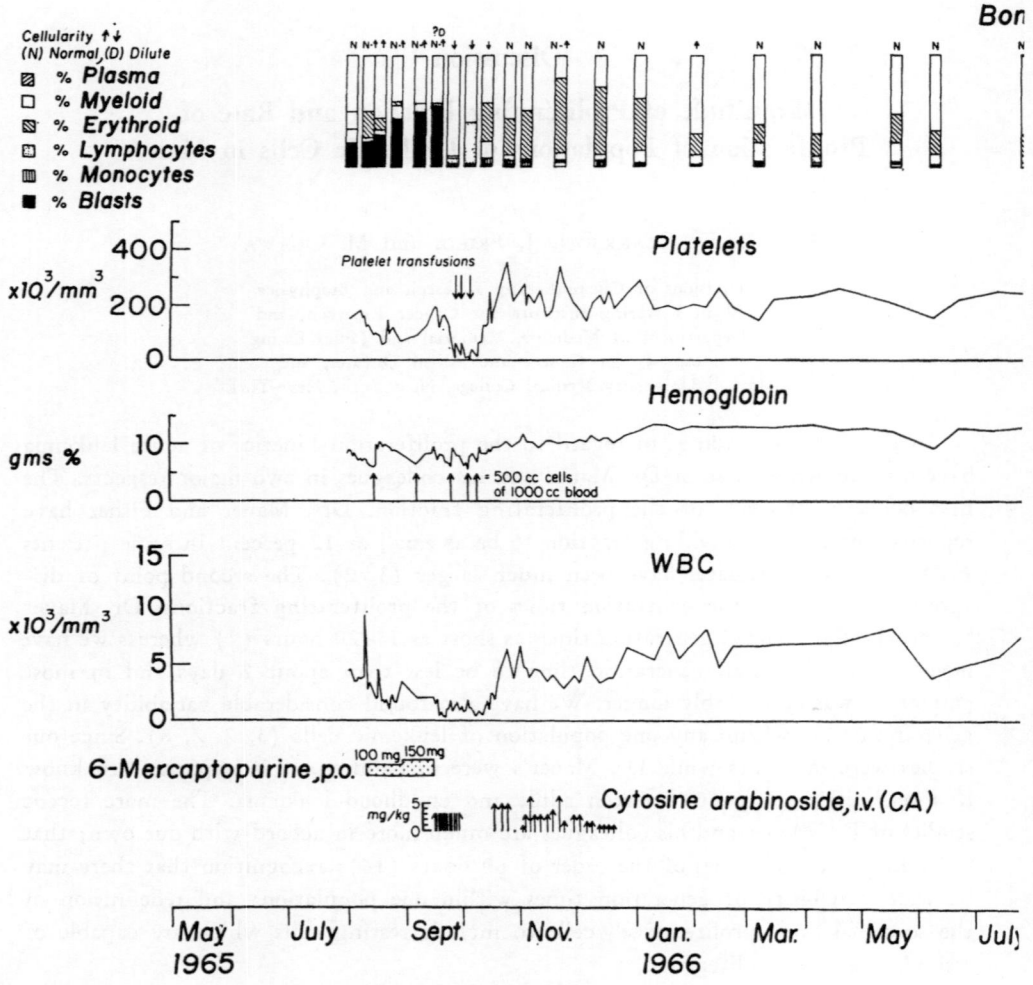

Fig. 1. Clinical course of G.S.

any population of cells is to expose them continuously to an isotope such as ^{3}H-thymidine which, under appropriate experimental conditions, is incorporated only by actively proliferating cells. Autoradiographic methods can then be used to determine both the fraction of cells labeled and their generation time; the latter can be derived from analysis of the grain count data by methods described in detail elsewhere (2, 7, 8). In the present investigation, ^{3}H-thymidine was infused continuously for 20 days. This rather long duration was chosen because at the end of previous continuous infusions for 8–10 days in 4 other patients with acute leukemia, 7–12 percent of the leukemic cells were still unlabeled and were therefore presumably resting cells (3, 8, 1), and because we anticipated that a greater pro-

Marrows

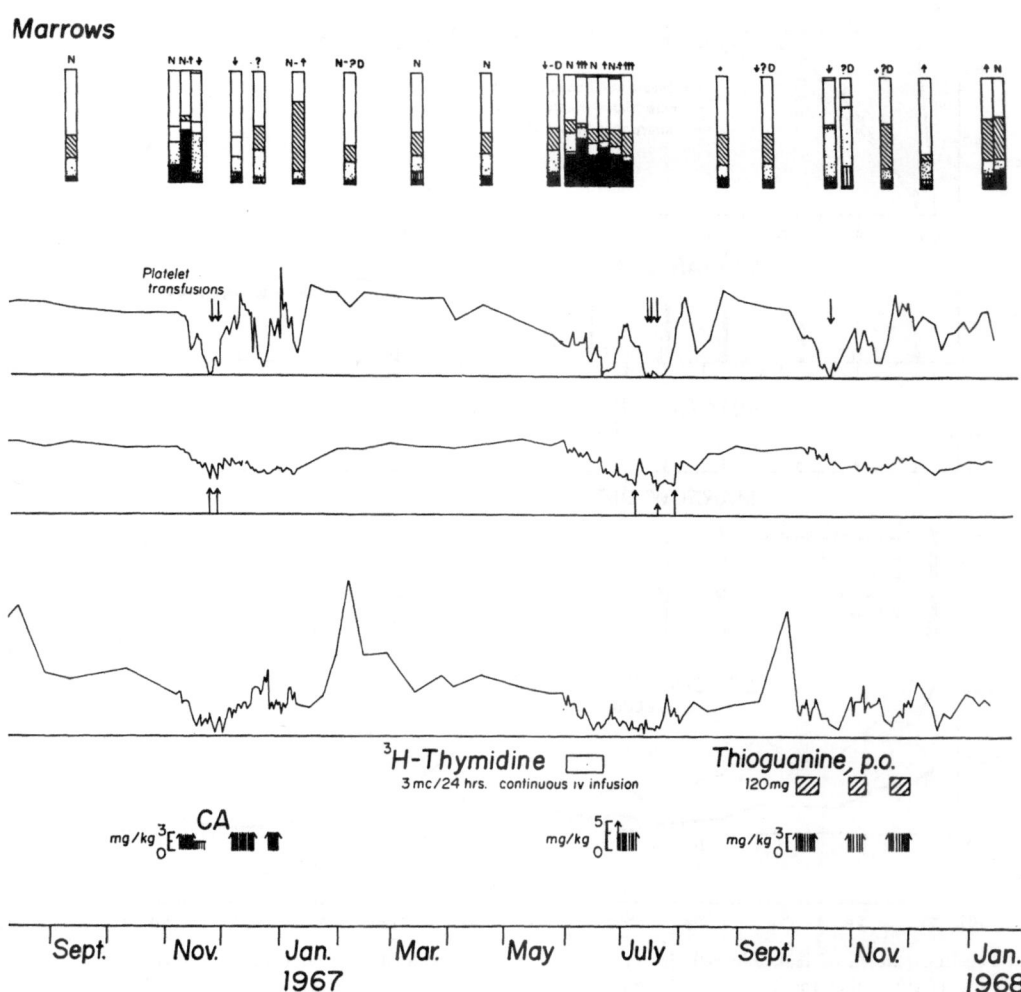

^{3}H-Thymidine ☐
3 mc/24 hrs. continuous iv infusion

Thioguanine, p.o.
120mg ▨ ▨ ▨

CA

Sept.   Nov.   Jan.   Mar.   May   July   Sept.   Nov.   Jan.
                 1967   1968

portion of the leukemic cells in the present patient might be dormant in view of
the slow clinical progression of her disease.

The results of the present study are shown in Fig. 2. The initial labeling index
(LI) of the leukemic cells in the marrow was 6.3 percent and in the blood, 0.5 percent as determined by *in vitro* incubation of the cells with ^{3}H-thymidine for 1 hour.
After continuous infusion for 20 days, 99 percent of leukemic cells were labeled in
the marrow and 99.8 percent in the blood. If one defines the proliferative fraction
as that fraction of cells which will pass through the division cycle within a given
period of observation, then, discounting cells which may have died, the proliferative
fraction in this patient was close to 100 percent. We have recently given a 21-day
continuous infusion of ^{3}H-thymidine to another adult with slowly progressive acute

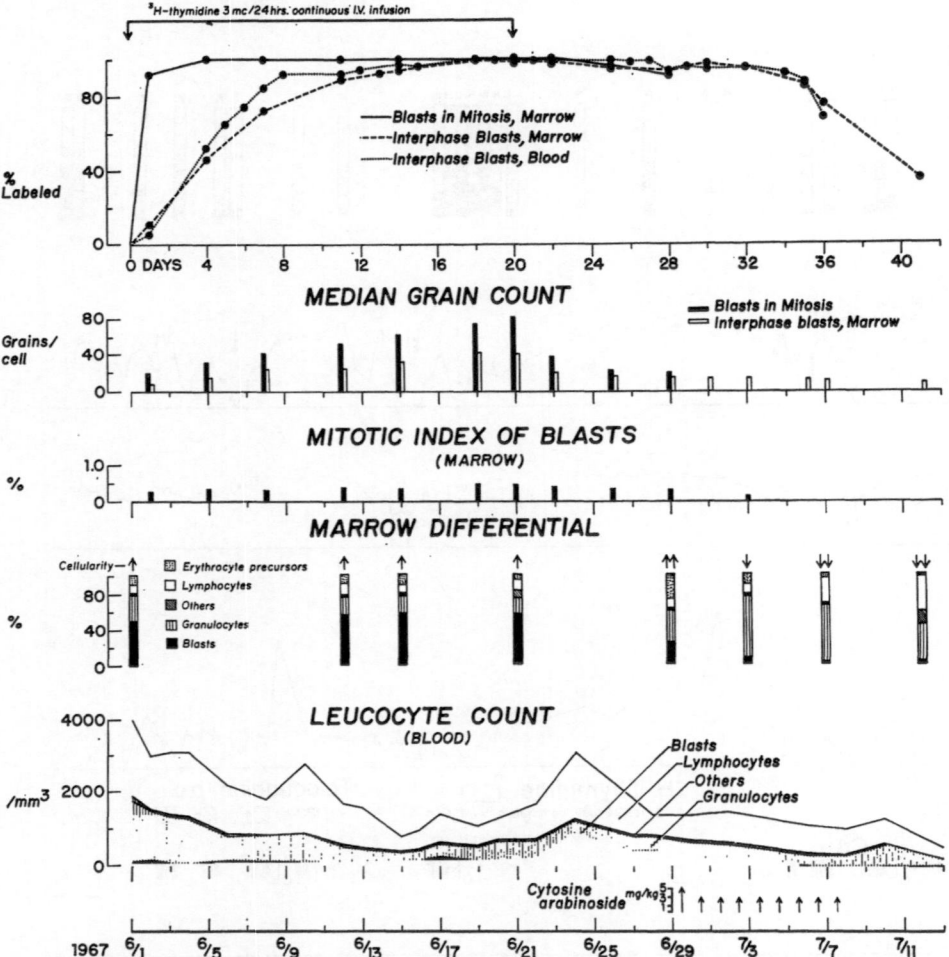

Fig. 2. Labeling pattern of leukemic cells in marrow and blood of G.S. during continuous intravenous infusion of ³H-thymidine for 20 days. The median grain counts of the leukemic cells in the blood were very similar to those in the marrow.

leukemia and have similarly found that almost all of the leukemic cells were labeled.

Two independent methods were used to estimate the generation time of the proliferating cells, as shown in Fig. 3. All determinations were performed with the aid of an IBM 1800 computer as previously described (7, 8). Only the marrow leukemic cells in mitosis are considered in this illustration. In the first method, the time taken for the median grain count of the labeled mitoses to halve after the end of the ³H-thymidine infusion reflects the mean generation time. The observed values for the median are adjusted to compensate for the changes due to lightly labeled cells falling below the grain counting threshold after division. For reasons

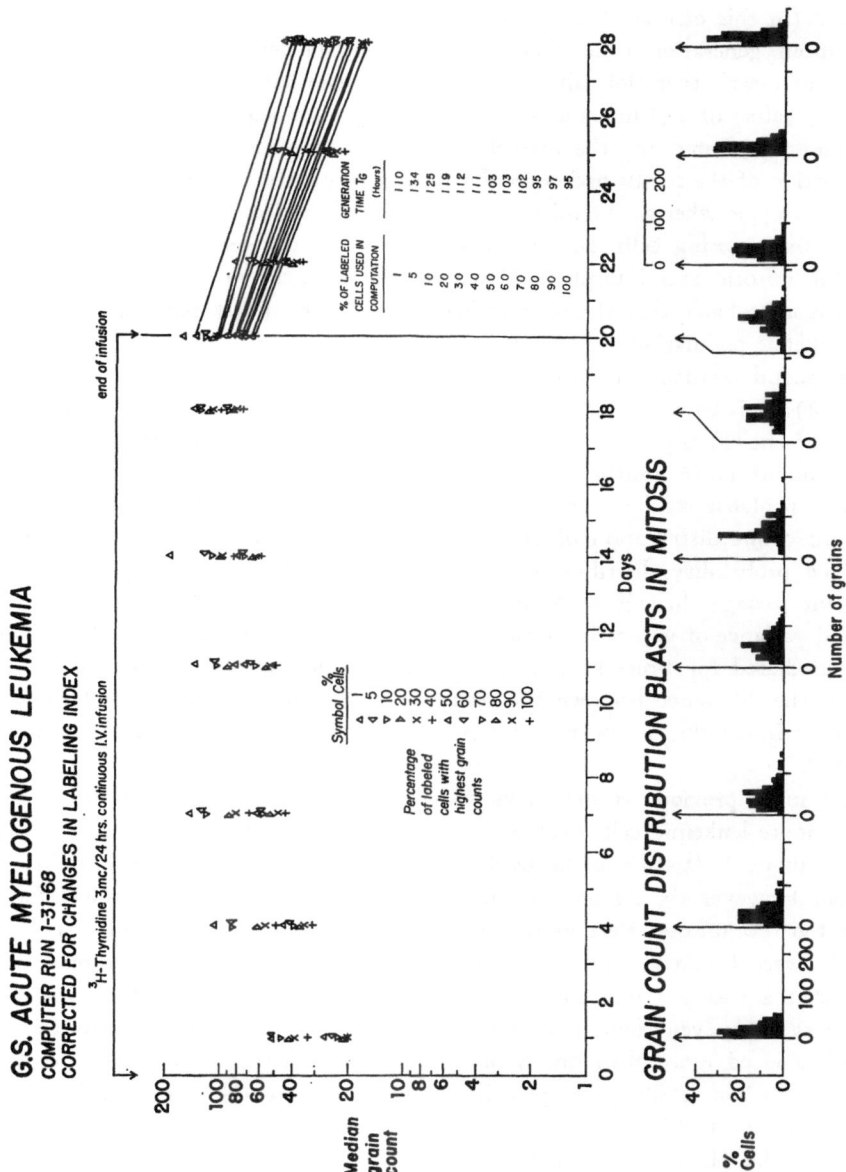

Fig. 3. Computer curves of median grain counts (MGCs) of labeled blasts in mitosis in the marrow of G.S. to illustrate methods used in determining their generation time after stopping the ^{3}H-thymidine infusion (Method 1) and during the infusion (Method 2). No therapy was given until the 8th day after the end of the infusion.

presented elsewhere (8), the generation time estimate generally tends to decrease as
the percentage of labeled cells included in the computation increases until a plateau
is reached (in this case at about 95 hours); this value is taken as the best estimate
of the mean generation time. The same method was employed (not shown) to
estimate the mean generation time using the interphase leukemic cells in the marrow
and blood; values of 130 hours and 138 hours were obtained respectively. The longer
generation time found for the interphase blasts in this instance probably indicates
that a portion of these cells had entered a resting phase after passing through at least
one division cycle whereas the mitotic blasts were selected cells in that they included
few long term resting cells. In certain other patients, the generation time estimates
found for mitotic and interphase blasts were almost the same (8), and in these
patients it is probable that the mitotic blasts were more nearly representative of the
whole leukemic population.

The second method for estimating the generation time has been described previously (8). It is based, in part, on the assumption that at a suitable time following
the start of the ³H-thymidine infusion, the mitotic cells have all traversed one complete period of DNA synthesis (S phase) subsequent to the time when the body
thymidine pool has reached a steady state with respect to specific activity of label.
The grain count distribution of this sample of mitotic cells is then taken to represent the probability distribution for grains "taken up" by any cell during its
subsequent passage through S during the infusion. By means of an assumed "trial"
mean and variance of generation times, the grain count distribution of cells in mitosis
can be predicted for times between the initial sample and the end of the infusion.
Based on the difference between the resulting predicted distributions and those observed experimentally, a new trial mean and variance is postulated and the process
is repeated.

Since most previous studies have shown that the average duration of the S
phase in acute leukemic cells is about 20 hours (3, 2, 16, 14, 19), ideally a sample
taken at about 1 day should be used to establish the grain count probability distribution. However the 24 hour sample in the present study proved unsatisfactory
because too few mitoses were present to establish a reliable grain count distribution
(only 56 were found on the entire slide) and because their labeling intensity was
so low that a steady state could not yet have been reached. Therefore, the 4-day
sample was used, even though it undoubtedly included a number of cells that had
already traversed more than one S phase during the infusion. The observed grain
count distribution is shown graphically in Fig. 3 where the mitotic cells in each
sample were classified into 20 groups of 10 grains each: 0–10, 11–20, and so forth.
In Fig. 4, the observed and best predicted grain distributions are compared in
tabular form. In this case the mean generation time was 95 hours; 67 percent of
cells had generation times between 50 and 185 hours, and 95 percent between 25
and 360 hours.

Numerous patients with acute leukemia have now been studied by us (2–5, 10)
using one or both of these methods and by others (14, 19, 11) using techniques
similar to the first method described above. In untreated patients or in those not
receiving treatment during the study, mean generation times of 2–8 days have been

COMPARISON OF OBSERVED AND PREDICTED DISTRIBUTION OF GRAINS IN MITOTIC LEUKEMIC CELLS

Grain level	Range of grain counts	TIME AFTER START OF ^{3}H-THYMIDINE INFUSION (DAYS)											
		1	4*	7		11		14		18		20	
		Observed %	Observed %	Predicted %	Observed %	Predicted %	Observed %	Predicted %	Observed %	Predicted %	Observed %	Predicted %	Observed %
1	0- 10	27	8	3	2	1	0	0.4	0	0	0	0	1
2	11- 20	30	19	9	12	5	8	2	2	1	0	0.7	1
3	21- 30	20	20	14	15	10	12	7	2	5	5	4	3
4	31- 40	11	20	18	16	15	10	12	3	10	4	10	1
5	41- 50	9	12	16	12	17	14	16	9	15	9	15	7
6	51- 60	4	10	14	17	16	19	17	30	17	19	17	11
7	61- 70	0	2	9	9	12	7	14	14	16	15	16	8
8	71- 80	0	3	6	4	8	8	11	10	12	9	13	16
9	81- 90	0	3	4	5	5	10	7	10	8	15	9	21
10	91-100	0	0	2	3	4	5	5	4	5	9	6	13
11	101-110	0	2	2	0	3	4	3	8	4	6	4	8
12	111-120	0	0	1	2	2	0	2	3	2	4	3	5
13	121-130	0	0	0.6	2	1	1	1	1	2	3	2	1
14	131-140	0	0	0.2	0	0.5	0	0.8	1	1	2	1	1
15	141-150	0	1	0.4	0.9	0.3	2	0.4	0	0.5	0.7	0.5	0
16	151-160	0	0	0.3	0.9	0.3	0	0.3	0	0.3	0.7	0.3	0
17	161-170	0	0	0.2	0	0.3	0	0.3	0	0.3	0.7	0.3	1
18	171-180	0	0	0.1	0	0.1	0	0.2	0	0.3	0	0.3	0
19	181-190	0	0	0	0	0	0	0.1	0	0.1	0	0.1	0
20	191-200	0	0	0	0	0	0	0	1	0	0	0	0
Number labeled mitoses counted		56	156		101		100		96		151		75

* 4 Days sample was used to define probability distribution of grains taken up by cell in passing through subsequent S phases during remainder of infusion.

Predicted values based on assumed mean generation time of 95 hours with 95 % of cells having generation times between 25 and 360 hours (log normal distribution)

Fig. 4. Comparison of observed and predicted distribution of grains in blasts in mitosis during ^{3}H-thymidine infusion. Since in this case the cells had incorporated insufficient label after only 24 hours' exposure to give representative initial values, the 4-day sample was used to define the probability distribution of grain counts taken up by cells in passing through S again during the remainder of the infusion. Percentage totals do not necessarily add up to 100 due to rounding off of values above 1%.

found in different patients. Moreover, there has been considerable variability in the generation time of the leukemic cells in any one patient (2, 7, 8).

Treatment with cytotoxic drugs can prolong the generation time, presumably either by selectively killing the more rapidly dividing cells or else by sublethally damaging other cells and slowing their passage through the mitotic cycle (7, 8). In patients in whom we have estimated generation times by the median grain count halving method before and during treatment, we have almost always found it to be prolonged by chemotherapy. However, these studies lacked precision because the grain counts were usually too low by the time treatment was started to obtain reliable estimates during therapy and more accurate measurements of the effects of treatment with different drugs are needed. Even after therapy has been discontinued, some drugs may exert a delayed effect in prolonging the generation time. We have studied one patient who had previously been treated with multiple drugs (7). Although he had received no treatment for 2 weeks prior to study, the generation time of the most immature leukemic cells was greater than 8 days and about 60 percent of those cells remained dormant for at least 10 days.

Gavosto et al. (12) first noted that large leukemic cells have a higher initial ^{3}H-thymidine LI than small ones and this observation has now been confirmed repeatedly (12, 7, 8, 16, 14). Most of the larger cells are labeled following a single rapid injection of ^{3}H-thymidine, and it can be shown by serial sampling that the smaller cells later become labeled as a consequence of the larger ones halving their volumes by division (7). The small leukemic cells have four possible alternatives:

1. They can die, either in situ in the marrow or else after passing into the circulation. We have no information regarding their death rate in the marrow. However we have carried out several experiments in which circulating leukemic cells were labeled for short periods in vitro with ^{3}H-uridine and then reinjected into the same patient (2, 4). The labeled cells disappeared with half-times of about 1–1.5 days and there was no evidence that any significant number returned to the marrow to resume proliferation. Based on these experiments and other considerations previously presented (2, 8, 11), it would appear that most leukemic cells which enter the blood are destined to die, although it is obvious that all of them do not invariably do so since they may sometimes infiltrate and grow in extramedullary sites.

2. The second alternative is that some leukemic cells may partially mature, sometimes to the extent of losing their capacity to divide; such maturation has been demonstrated in several patients with acute myelomonocytic leukemia (3, 7). We believe it is a common occurrence in such patients, and that at least in this type of leukemia, it is a process which must be considered separately from that of differences in cell size in relation to proliferative activity. In other patients the leukemic cells are homogeneous and show no morphological evidence of maturation.

3. A third possibility is that the small cells can grow and divide again (7, 8). It is apparently necessary for them to attain a certain sufficient mass before they are again able to begin DNA synthesis.

4. Finally, they can remain in the marrow as dormant small cells (i.e., in G_0).

The factors determining which pathway is followed by a given cell are unknown.

In previous continuous ^{3}H-thymidine infusion studies of 8–10 days' duration, almost all large cells were labeled by the end of the infusions but some of the small ones remained unlabeled (8). Thus some small cells may remain dormant in the marrow for more than 10 days. In the patient described above who was given a continuous infusion for 20 days, almost all leukemic cells were labeled regardless of size (Fig. 5); however the few cells remaining unlabeled were generally small ones. The size distribution of the leukemic cells did not change significantly during the infusion. As in previous studies (8), the large cells had higher labeling intensities at the end of the infusion, indicating that they had passed through more division cycles during the 20-day period than the small ones. This supports the previous conclusion that the rate of division is usually variable among a population of leukemic cells. Further prolonged ^{3}H-thymidine infusions in other patients will be necessary to confirm these observations, but it appears that while some of the small

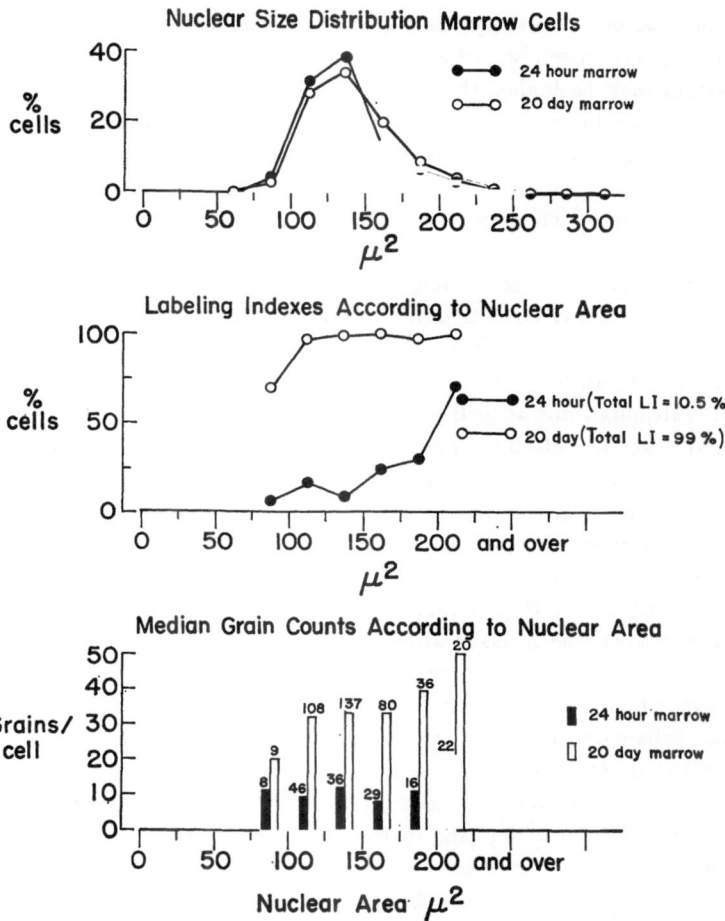

Fig. 5. Relation of nuclear size of leukemic cells in marrow of G.S. to ^{3}H-thymidine labeling index and labeling intensity after 24 hours and after 20 days' infusion of ^{3}H-thymidine *in vivo*. The areas of 500 cells were measured in each sample (5); the number of labeled cells in each size category which were counted to determine the median grain counts are indicated above each column of grains/cell.

leukemic cells may remain dormant in the marrow for longer than 10 days, very few of them do so indefinitely and they either resume proliferating or die.

There are several reports indicating that the ^{3}H-thymidine LI of leukemic cells in any one patient frequently increases significantly above the pretreatment value during antileukemic therapy or when the disease relapses (16, 17, 18, 9, 15), and we have also observed several such cases (7, 8). Insufficient details regarding exact relation to treatment were given in many of the reported cases to allow proper interpretation, but we believe several factors may be operative depending on the situation.

1. Some drugs by causing sublethal damage may either prolong the S phase during treatment, or, shortly after stopping therapy, partial synchronization of the cells may occur temporarily. Either effect might alter the LI (7, 8).

2. Since one cannot ordinarily distinguish between leukemic and normal blasts, when the former are severely reduced by chemotherapy, the average LI of the mixed population may be higher than prior to treatment because generally a higher percentage of normal blasts are synthesizing DNA than leukemic blasts (2). This effect is probably significant only when the marrow is nearly in complete remission (8).

3. A third factor which may affect the LI is cellular concentration. It is well established that bacteria and mammalian cells will only grow *in vitro* up to a certain maximum concentration after which growth ceases although viability remains good for a time (7, 6, 5). Growth inhibition cannot be explained by exhaustion of essential components in the medium since if the concentration of cells is simply reduced by removing some of them, the remaining cells will resume growth in the same medium (although not as well as in fresh medium). Under such circumstances we have found that the ^{3}H-thymidine LI of human hematopoietic cells (6) in suspension cultures may change from about 50–60% during exponential growth to around 10–20% during the stationary phase (5). It seems probable that a similar effect may occur *in vivo*; that is when the marrow is densely crowded with leukemic cells, their rate of proliferation may be less (and the LI lower) than when many cells have been killed and their concentration reduced by therapy. We think this effect is most probably due to elaboration by the cells of an inhibitory factor which reaches an effective concentration when they exist under crowded conditions; not only is the growth of the leukemic cells inhibited but that of the normal hematopoietic stem cells even more so. The evidence for such an effect *in vivo* is as yet only circumstantial (2, 8). However, we have recently found that suspension cultures of human hematopoietic cells in high concentration (stationary phase) will, when separated by a cellophane membrane, inhibit the growth of cells of the same or other lines present at lower cellular concentrations (at which they would ordinarily grow exponentially) (5). We believe this effect is due to production by the concentrated cells of a dialyzable labile inhibitory factor and that its influence is distinct from that of other factors which may inhibit growth (*e.g.*, pH change, exhaustion of critical nutrients, *etc.*). Further experiments are currently being done to try to prove the existence of such a factor and to characterize its properties.

References

1. Clarkson, B. D., Kimura, T. and Fried, J.: Studies of cellular proliferation in human leukemia. IV. Kinetics of cellular proliferation in an adult with acute lymphoblastic leukemia who had a spontaneous remission. (In preparation.)
2. Clarkson, B. D., Ohkita, T., Ota, K. and Fried, J.: Studies of cellular proliferation in human leukemia. I. Estimation of growth rates of leukemic and normal hematopoietic cells in two adults with acute leukemia given single injections of tritiated thymidine. J. Clin. Invest. **46**, 506 (1967).
3. Clarkson, B. D., Ohkita, T., Ota, K. and O'Connor, A.: Studies of cellular proliferation in acute leukemia. J. Clin. Invest. **44**, 1035 (1965).
4. Clarkson, B. D., Ohkita, K., Sakai, Y. and Todo, A.: Unpublished observations (1968).

5. CLARKSON, B. D. and STRIFE, A.: Unpublished observations (1968).

6. CLARKSON, B. D., STRIFE, A. and DE HARVEN, E.: Continuous culture of seven new cell lines (SK-L1 to 7) from patients with acute leukemia. Cancer 20, 926 (1967).

7. CLARKSON, B. D., SAKAI, Y., KIMURA, T., OHKITA, T. and FRIED, J.: Studies of cellular proliferation in human leukemia. II. Variability in rates of growth and cellular differentiation in acute myelomonoblastic leukemia and effects of treatment. Twenty-first Annual Symposium on Fundamental Cancer Research, The Proliferation and Spread of Neoplastic Cells. The University of Texas, M. D. Anderson Hospital and Tumor Institute, Houston, Texas. (In press.)

8. CLARKSON, B. D., SAKAI, Y., STRIFE, A., OTA, K., OHKITA, T. and FRIED, J.: Studies of cellular proliferation in human leukemia. III. Continuous infusion of ^{3}H-thymidine in three adults with acute leukemia. J. Clin. Invest. (In press.)

9. FOADI, M. D., COOPER, E. H. and HARDISTY, R. M.: DNA synthesis and DNA content of leucocytes in acute leukemia. Nature 216, 134 (1967).

10. GAVOSTO, F., PELERI, A., BACHI, C. and PEGORARO, L.: Proliferation and maturation defect in acute leukemia cells. Nature 203, 92 (1964).

11. KILLMANN, S. A., CRONKITE, E. P., ROBERTSON, J. S., FLIEDNER, T. M. and BOND, V. P.: Estimation of phases of the life cycle of leukemic cells from labeling in humans in vivo with tritiated thymidine. Lab. Invest. 12, 671 (1963).

12. MAUER, A. M. and FISHER, V.: Characteristics of cell proliferation in four patients with untreated acute leukemia. Blood 28, 428 (1966).

13. OGAWA, M.: Studies of cellular proliferation in acute leukemia using H^3-thymidine. Nagoya Medical Association Journal 90, 91 (1967).

14. OTA, K.: Kinetics of cellular proliferation in leukemia and cancer. Acta Haemat. Jap. 27, 693 (1964).

15. PILERI, A., GABUTTI, V., MASERA, P. and GAVOSTO, F.: Proliferation activity of the cells of acute leukemia in relapse and in steady state. Acta Haemat. 38, 193 (1967).

16. SAUNDERS, E. F., LAMPKIN, B. C. and MAUER, A. M.: Variation of proliferative activity in leukemic cell populations of patients with acute leukemia. J. Clin. Invest. 46, 1356 (1967).

17. SCHMID, J. R., KIELY, J. M., TAUXE, W. N. and OWEN, C. A., JR.: Cell proliferation in leukemia during relapse and remission. I. DNA and RNA synthesis of leukemic cells in the bone marrow in vitro. Acta Haemat. 36, 313 (1966).

18. SCHMID, J. R., OECHSLIN, R. J., FRICK, P. G. and MOESCHLIN, S.: Cell proliferation in leukemia during relapse and remission. II. DNA synthesis of leukemic cells in the peripheral blood in vitro. Acta Haemat. 37, 16 (1967).

19. TODO, A.: Proliferation and differentiation of hematopoietic cells in hematologic disorders. III. In vivo radioautographic study of leukemia including erythroleukemia. Acta Haemat. Jap. (In press.)

Incorporation of [125]Iodine-Labeled 5-Iodo-2'-Deoxyuridine into the DNA of Mouse Mammary Tumors *

LYLE A. DETHLEFSEN

Department of Radiology
University of Pennsylvania
Philadelphia, Pennsylvania

Introduction

The symposium papers of the past two days attest to the successful use of labeled DNA precursors in the autoradiographic analysis of normal and malignant cell proliferation. The advances in the analysis of cell cycle kinetics over the last decade have been both broad and profound. Unfortunately, autoradiographic analysis is not without its disadvantages and limitations. For example, the long exposure times often needed for autoradiography make experimental "turn-around" times burdensome, and the frequent inability to obtain reliable, unperturbed serial samples *in vivo* is a major frustration. In tumor biology, one can combine studies on volumetric growth with autoradiographic analysis of the cell cycle for added insight (17, 35, 26), but such studies still do not permit one to get sequential measurements on the interactions between tumor cell proliferation and volumetric growth in the same intact host. Experiments, *in situ*, may also permit one to measure concomitant chemotherapeutic effects on cellular proliferation and volumetric growth in the same tumor.

The synthesis of radioactive labeled 5-iodo-2'-deoxyuridine (IUdR) by Prusoff (30, 31) opened the possibility for studying certain aspects of tumor cell proliferation *in situ* (8, 9, 10). IUdR is an analogue of thymidine, and the photons from both [131]Iodine (energy of principal photon = 364 KeV) and [125]Iodine (energy of principal photon = 27.4 KeV) are energetic enough to traverse several centimeters of soft tissue. IUdR is incorporated into the DNA of proliferating cells in a variety of

* This work was supported in part by USPHS Grants 5T1-CA5097, 5T1 GM-694, and 5 R01 CA03896; by an American Cancer Society Institutional Grant (IN 30-H, Subproject #8); and by the Atomic Energy Commission (NYO-3924-1).

Some of these data were included in a dissertation submitted in 1966 to the Graduate School of Arts and Sciences, University of Pennsylvania, in partial fulfillment of the requirements for the Doctor of Philosophy degree.

The author thanks Dr. Mortimer L. Mendelsohn for his generous support and constructive criticisms of this work and manuscript; also Virginia Lieblein and Elsie deLong for their competent technical assistance.

in vitro and *in vivo* systems (for example see 4, 7, 12, 25, 28, and 32). Also its potential as a chemotherapeutic agent (3, 5, 23) and radiosensitizing agent (2, 13) has been evaluated. In 1960, Kreuger *et al.* (24) reported on IUdR as a tracer of DNA metabolism *in vivo,* and in 1961, Gitlin *et al.* (18) demonstrated that x-irradiation affected the *in vivo* incorporation of IUdR into DNA. Dethlefsen and Mendelsohn (10) and Dethlefsen (8, 9) discussed the possible *in situ* use of ^{125}I-IUdR for studies involving the mouse mammary tumor, while Hughes *et al.* (22) discussed the use of IUdR for studying normal murine cell proliferation and cell death *in vivo*. Hughes *et al.* (22) and Feinendegen *et al.* (15) reported on the apparent nonreutilization of this DNA precursor, and Commerford (6) discussed the long-term stability of the ^{125}I-label in DNA containing ^{125}I-IUdR.

This report will be concerned with studies evaluating ^{125}I-IUdR as a tracer for DNA metabolism in the C3H mouse mammary tumor, with special emphasis on the feasibility of using *in situ*, externally counted, tumor radioactivity as an index of DNA accumulation in the intact tumor.

Materials and Methods

The experimental design is briefly summarized in Fig. 1. The techniques for tumor implantation, tumor mensuration, and computer analysis of the data have been published previously (9, 11) so they will not be repeated here. The mice were maintained on Purina Lab Chow and tap water *ad libitum* until three to five days before injection of ^{125}I-IUdR. At this time the drinking water was replaced with a 0.1 percent solution of potassium iodide and the mice were maintained on this until sacrifice. When enough data had been collected to establish reliable growth curves, the mice were injected intraperitoneally with 10 μCi (0.001–20 mg IUdR/mouse) of ^{125}I-IUdR and after various times (2–120 hours) the mice were killed by cervical dislocation. Then the tumors were quickly extirpated, dropped into preweighed beakers containing ice-cold 5 percent citric acid, minced, and weighed. The skin overlying each tumor was also dropped into preweighed beakers, weighed, and the sample saved for radioactivity determinations. Next the tumors were homogenized for 2–5 minutes in a Sorval Omni-mixer with 15 volumes of ice-cold 5 percent citric acid, and the various tissue fractions were extracted from samples (0.5 ml) of the tumor homogenates by the technique of Scott *et al.* (33) as modified for macro-amounts of tissue (21).

The amount of DNA in a sample of the DNA fraction was estimated by measuring the U.V. absorption at 260 mμ with either a Beckman DK or a Cary Recording Spectrophotometer. The instruments were calibrated by measuring the absorption in known amounts of calf thymus DNA (Sigma Chemical Company) which was digested by the same procedure as the tumor DNA. The absorption spectrum was routinely observed between 240 and 290 mμ to check for possible protein contamination. When duplicate samples of the tumor homogenates were analyzed, the replication error for the DNA content was 3.8 percent.

The radioactivity in samples of the tumor homogenates, in the various tumor fractions and in the skin was determined at 60 percent efficiency in a well type

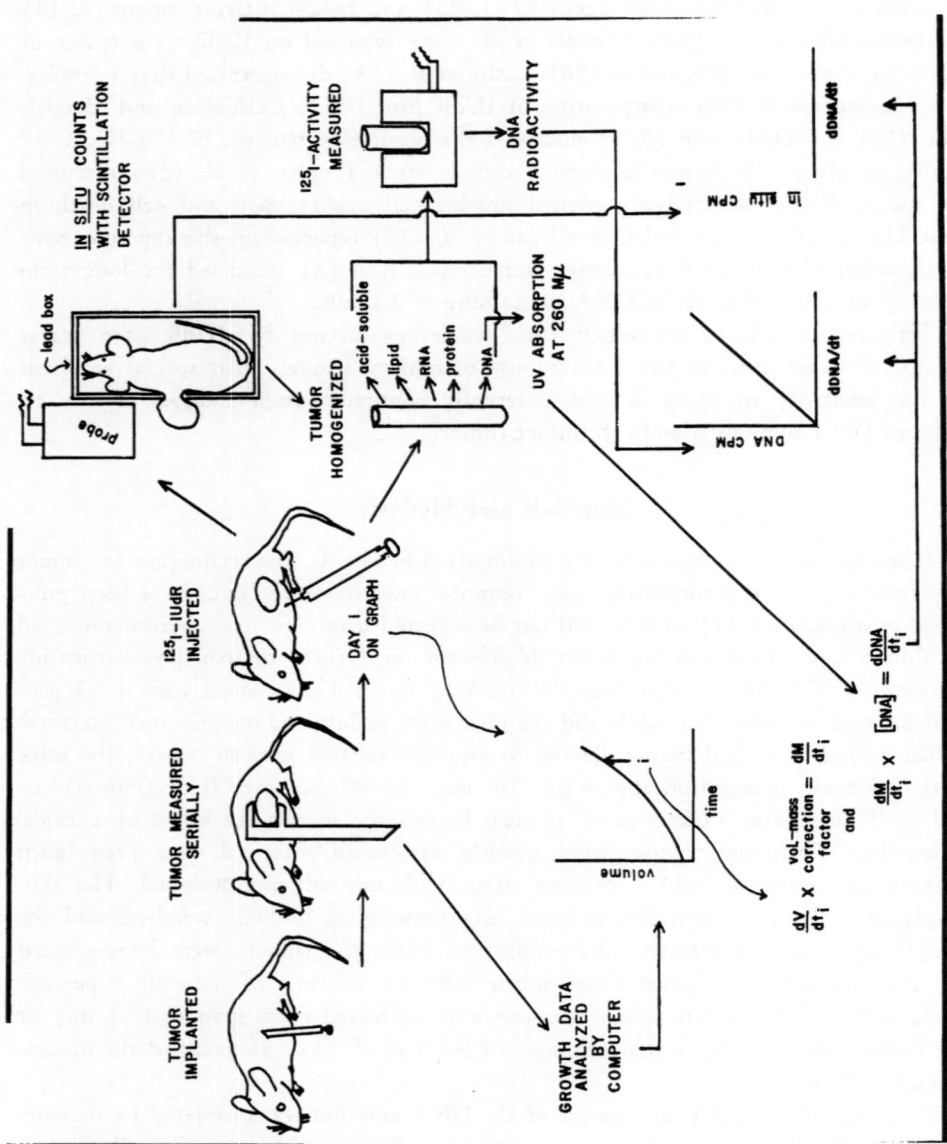

Fig. 1. Flow-chart for the experimental protocol. Tumor fragments were implanted and the ensuing tumors were measured until adequate growth curves were obtained. The mice were then injected with ^{125}I-IUdR (day i), and depending on the experiment, either the ^{125}I-activity in the tumor was counted *in situ* followed by sacrifice of the mouse and the tumor analyzed as shown, or the *in situ* step was omitted. The U.V. data were combined with the growth data to give the volumetric estimate for rate of DNA accumulation, and the radioactivity in the DNA or the *in situ* tumor radioactivity was the radioisotopic index used for comparison with the volumetric data.

scintillation detector with a sodium iodide crystal and pulse height spectrometer. Samples of the tumor homogenates (0.5 ml) and the total skin were adjusted to 3 ml of 5 percent citric acid for radioactivity measurements, and the various tumor fractions were adjusted to 3 ml, if necessary, with the respective solvents before counting. Because the low energy of the ^{125}I-photons allows appreciable internal absorption, it was necessary to correct for the chemical content of the solvent (1). Thus, all counts are reported after normalization to 5 percent citric acid and after correction for physical decay back to the day of ^{125}I-IUdR injection in the mouse. Radioactivity determined on duplicate samples of the tumor homogenates were reproducible to within 2 percent, while radioactivity in DNA extracted from duplicate samples of the homogenate had a replication error of 7 percent.

The *in situ* tumor ^{125}I-activity was determined by the specially constructed apparatus shown in Figs. 2 and 3. The peaks of the ^{125}Iodine spectrum from the two photomultiplier tubes were matched by adjusting the independent high-voltage sources for the photomultiplier tubes, and the tube outputs were summed and

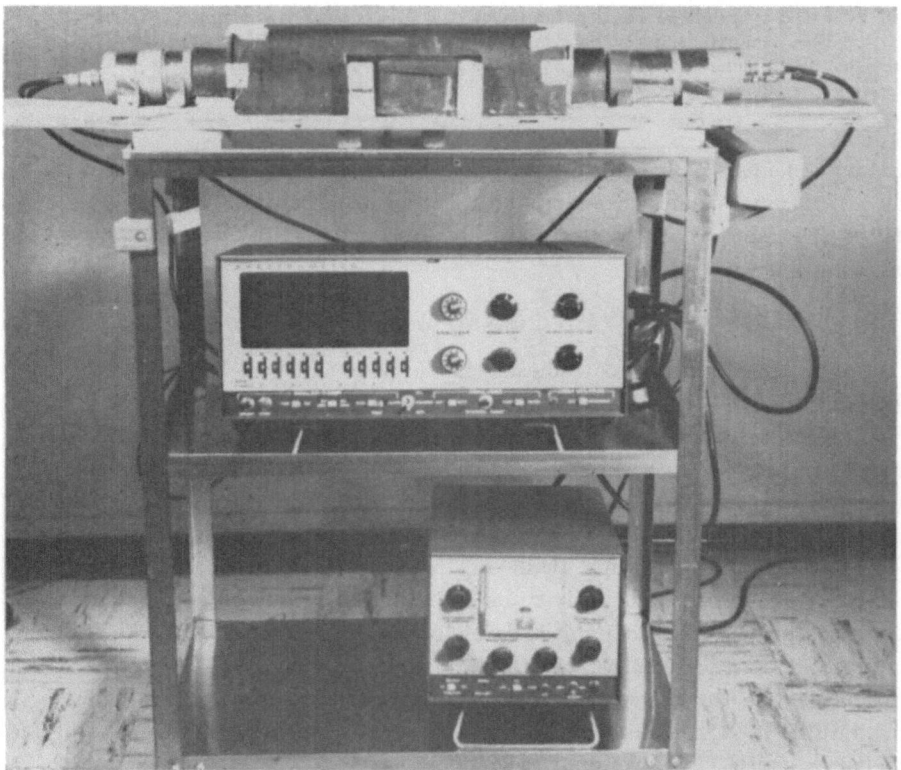

Fig. 2. *In situ* Counting Apparatus. The windows of the two photomultiplier tubes are inside the lead shield, directly opposite one another, and 20 cm apart. The two ^{125}I-spectrums are matched by adjusting the independent high-voltage supply of each photomultiplier tube while the outputs are summed and analyzed by the pulse-height spectrometer. The small lead box, located in the center cutout of the outside lead shield, holds the mouse while the radioactivity in the tumor is being determined.

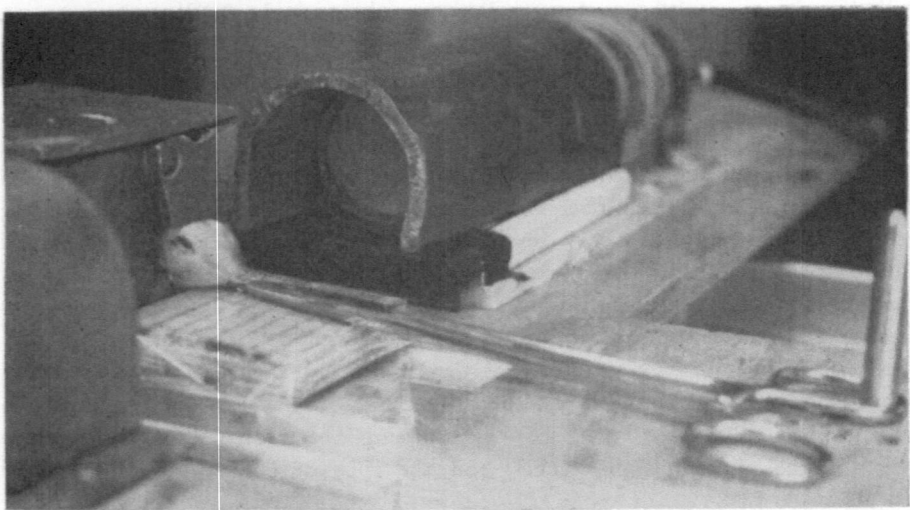

Fig. 3. C3H mammary tumor in position for radioactivity determinations. The outside shield seen in Figure 2 has been removed, and the photomultiplier tubes are seen in the rounded lead shields on either side of the tumor. The mouse is anesthetized, and a metallic wound clip is placed in the skin overlying the tumor. The clip is grasped with forceps to gently stretch the skin and maintain the tumor outside the lead box.

analyzed by the pulse-height spectrometer. The overall efficiency was about 3 percent, and the *in situ* tumor counts were reproducible to within 5 percent.

The *in situ* radioactivity was corrected for internal absorption in the tumors by the following equation: *

$$I_0 = I/[1 - \tfrac{3}{4}\mu R(1 - \tfrac{8}{15}R/a) + \tfrac{2}{5}\mu^2 R^2(1 - \tfrac{5}{6}R/a)].   \qquad [1]$$

I_0 is the corrected estimate for radioactivity in the tumor; I is the radioactivity actually measured; μ is the effective linear absorption coefficient ($\mu = 0.418$ cm^{-1} for ^{125}I in water); R is the radius of the tumor in centimeters and a is the distance in centimeters between the center of the tumor and the scintillation crystals (a = 10 cm in these experiments). After the *in situ* measurements were taken, the mouse was immediately killed and the tumor was prepared as described above.

The IUdR incorporation (mg IUdR/mg newly accumulated DNA) was calculated from the known specific activity of administered ^{125}I-IUdR and the measured DNA radioactivity (CPM/μCi injected/mg newly accumulated DNA). The mass of newly accumulated DNA was used instead of total tumor DNA because of the need to correct for the different growth rates of these tumors.

The rate of DNA accumulation was calculated from the computer-analyzed growth curves and U.V. absorption data as follows:

---

* Professor Robley D. Evans, Massachusetts Institute of Technology, Boston, Massachusetts, personal communications; R. D. Evans, The Atomic Nucleus. McGraw-Hill, New York, 1955, pp. 736–738 (14).

$$\frac{dV}{dt_i} \times \left(\frac{\text{volume} - \text{mass}}{\text{correction factor}} \right) = \frac{dM}{dt_i} \qquad [2]$$

and

$$\frac{dM}{dt_i} \times [\text{DNA}] = \frac{d\,\text{DNA}}{dt_i}, \qquad [3]$$

where dV/dt_i is the growth rate in mm^3/30 minutes on the day of ^{125}I-IUdR injection, and the volume mass correction factor is the ratio of measured mass to smoothed volume on day of sacrifice. Thus, the volumetric growth rate was converted to mass unit (*i.e.*, dM/dt_i is the growth rate in mg/30 minutes). The DNA concentration (μg DNA/mg tumor) was calculated from the U.V. absorption data and measured tumor mass; thus, d DNA/dt_i is the estimated rate of DNA accumulation (μg DNA/30 minutes) at the time of injection. The newly accumulated DNA was calculated for a period of 30 minutes at the time of ^{125}I-IUdR injection, since 30 minutes is the approximate time that intraperitoneally administered IUdR is available for incorporation into DNA (22).

The data reported here came from a select population of first-generation implants. First, the tumors were picked for the experiments on the following basis: 1. the hosts were males, 2. the tumors arose as single nodules in the midabdominal region, 3. no tumor exceeded 5000 mm^3 at the time of injection, and 4. they were smooth and hemi-ellipsoidal in shape. Then, after the experiment was finished, the data were discarded if computer analysis of the growth curves showed that: 1. the sampling error (the coefficient of variation of the mean volume) > 20 percent, 2. the 95 percent confidence interval of b $\geqq$ 1.0, or 3. the chosen b $\geqq$ 1.40. Sixteen mice, out of the 200 injected for these experiments, were discarded because of inadequate growth curves.

Results

The incorporation of IUdR into mammary tumor DNA (mg IUdR/mg newly accumulated DNA) as a function of IUdR administered (mg IUdR/mouse) is shown in Fig. 4. The slope of the regression line on this log-log plot is not significantly different from one; thus, indicating that the incorporation was proportional to administered dose from 0.001 to 5 mg IUdR/mouse. However, the mean incorporation at the 10 and 20 mg doses is significantly less than predicted from the regression line. The two observed means for 10 mg doses were 0.136 and 0.205 mg IUdR/mg newly accumulated DNA, and the mean incorporation at 20 mg was 0.347; but the predicted means with their 95 percent confidence limits are 0.546 (0.304 — 0.981) and 1.082 (0.564 — 2.074) respectively. Note also that a fortyfold excess of thymidine (59-fold molar excess) administered ten minutes before the ^{125}I-IUdR resulted in a significant reduction of IUdR incorporation. This dose of thymidine was not toxic to the host and showed no perturbing effects on tumor growth.

An injection dose of 0.1 mg (10 μCi) of ^{125}I-IUdR/mouse was selected for further studies on: 1. the distribution of radioactivity among the various tumor

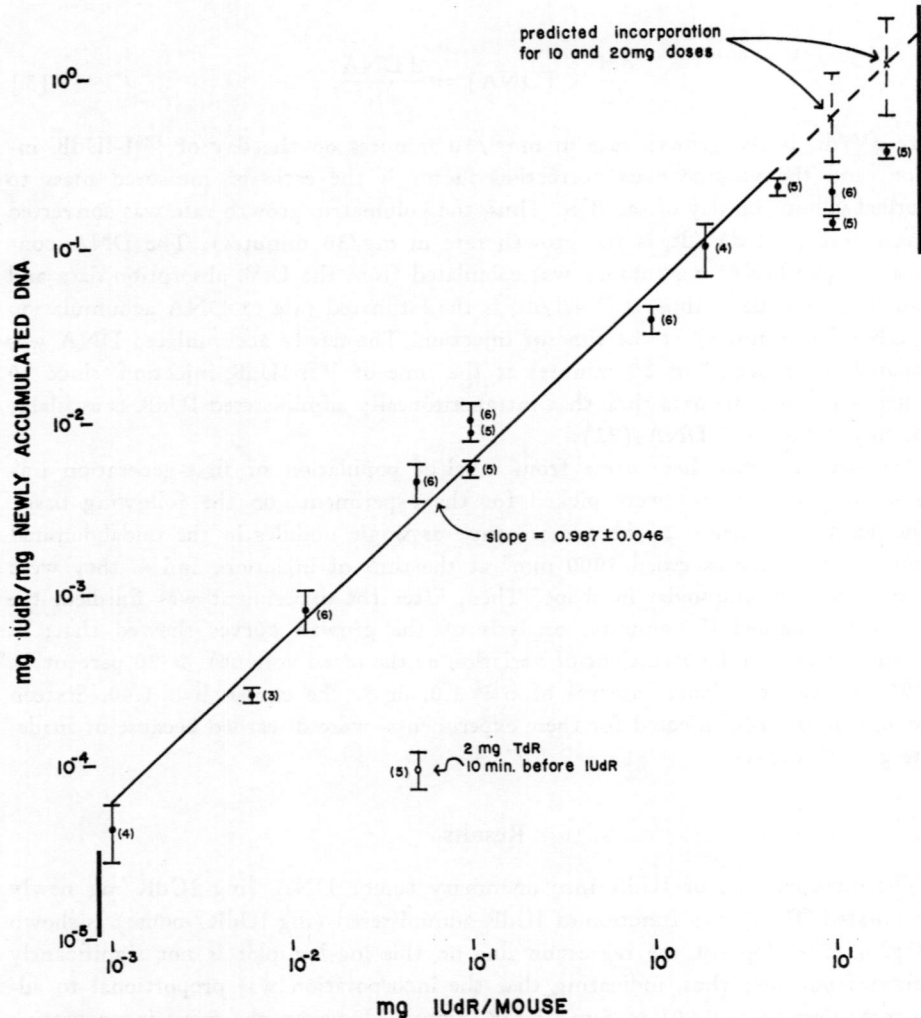

Fig. 4. Incorporation of IUdR into tumor DNA. The solid dots show the mg of IUdR incorporated per mg of newly accumulated DNA as a function of the mg of IUdR injected per mouse. The data are the group means ± the standard deviation of the means, and the numbers in parentheses indicate the number of mice per group. Note the repeat experiments at the 0.1 and 10 mg level. It was assumed that the IUdR is available for 30 minutes of incorporation (22). The two variables are highly correlated (r = 0.991, P < 0.01) for the data from 0.001 to 5.0 mg IUdR/mouse, and the slope of 0.987 ± 0.046 is not significantly different from one. The x's represent the predicted mean incorporation ± the 95 percent confidence limits for the 10 and 20 mg doses, and these are significantly greater than the observed data. The open dot shows the mean incorporation in an experiment where 2 mg thymidine/mouse was given 10 minutes before 0.05 mg (10 μCi) of ^{125}I-IUdR.

fractions, 2. the stability of tumor DNA containing ^{125}I-IUdR, and 3. the comparison of the two independent methods (*i.e.*, radioisotopic and volumetric) for estimating the rate of DNA accumulation. It was anticipated that such a dose would not have any perturbing effects on cell proliferation, but would be large enough to avoid the pitfalls associated with high specific-activity radiotracers (26).

The distribution of radioactivity among the acid-soluble, lipid, RNA, DNA, and protein fractions of the tumor tissue at various times following the injection of ^{125}I-IUdR is shown in Fig. 5. The radioactivity in the acid-soluble fraction dropped very rapidly from 86 percent of the total tumor radioactivity at 2 hours to about 9 percent by 24 hours, and then it continued to be lost at a considerably lower rate. In contrast, the radioactivity in the DNA fraction represented the majority of tumor radioactivity by 24 hours, and reached a plateau of about 70 percent of the total tumor radioactivity by 48 hours. The curves for radioactivity in the protein and lipid as well as the RNA fractions were essentially the same shape as the curve

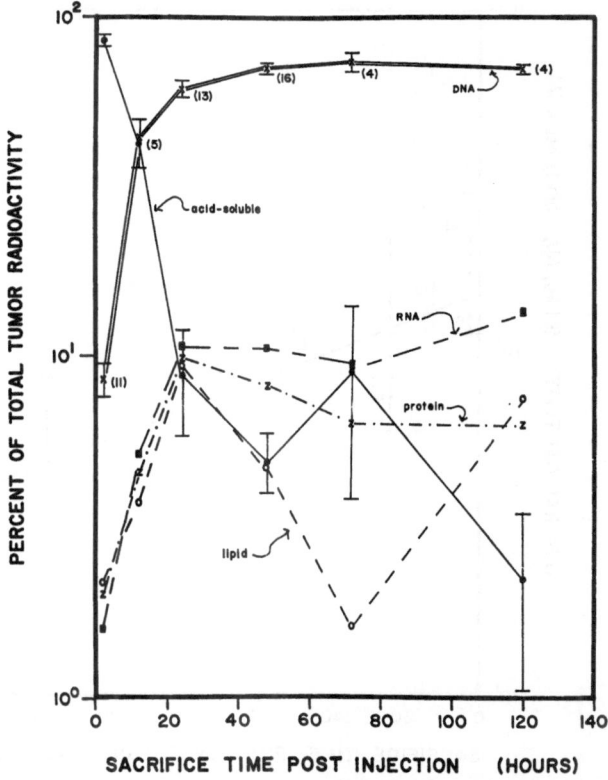

Fig. 5. Distribution of tumor ^{125}I-activity as a function of time. The log (percent of total tumor radioactivity) in the acid-soluble, lipid, RNA, DNA, and protein fractions is shown as a function of time post injection. The total tumor radioactivity is the sum of the radioactivity in all the above fractions. The respective group means are plotted, and the standard deviation of the means are shown for the DNA and acid-soluble fractions. The numbers in parentheses indicate the number of mice sacrificed at the various times.

for radioactivity in the DNA fraction. Other experiments using IUdR-6-^{3}H showed that the radioactivity in these fractions was proportional to the radioactivity in the DNA, and suggested that the majority of the radioactivity in these three fractions was due to residual DNA (manuscript in preparation). Thus, by 48 hours about 90 percent of the tumor radioactivity was associated with the DNA fraction, and the acid-soluble fraction contained about 5 percent of the total tumor radioactivity. These percentages were approximately the same from 48 to 120 hours post injection.

If the incorporated IUdR, *per se*, is not causing cell death or breakdown of DNA, and is not reutilized, then any loss of radioactivity from the DNA may be a measure of cell loss in both unperturbed and perturbed tumors. No loss of radioactivity with time would suggest either no tumor cell loss or efficient reutilization of the ^{125}I-label. The effect of time on radioactivity in the DNA is shown in Fig. 6. The radioactivity in the DNA (CPM/μCi injected/μg newly accumulated DNA) is shown as a function of sacrifice-time after ^{125}I-IUdR injection. The negative regres-

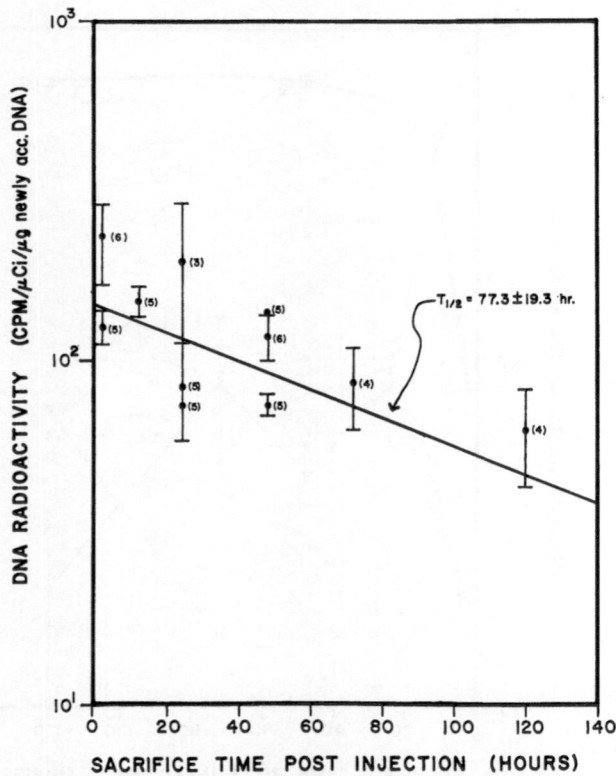

Fig. 6. Log DNA radioactivity as a function of time. The data (CPM/μCi injected/μg DNA accumulated in 30 minutes) are shown as the group means $\pm$ the standard deviation of the means, and the numbers in parentheses indicate the number of mice per experimental group. Note the repeat experiments at 2, 24, and 48 hours. The radioactivity in the DNA was normalized by the respective rates of DNA accumulation in these tumors, and this period of DNA accumulation was arbitrarily taken as 30 minutes. The negative slope of this regression line is highly significant (slope = -0.0089, F = 12.89, P < 0.005).

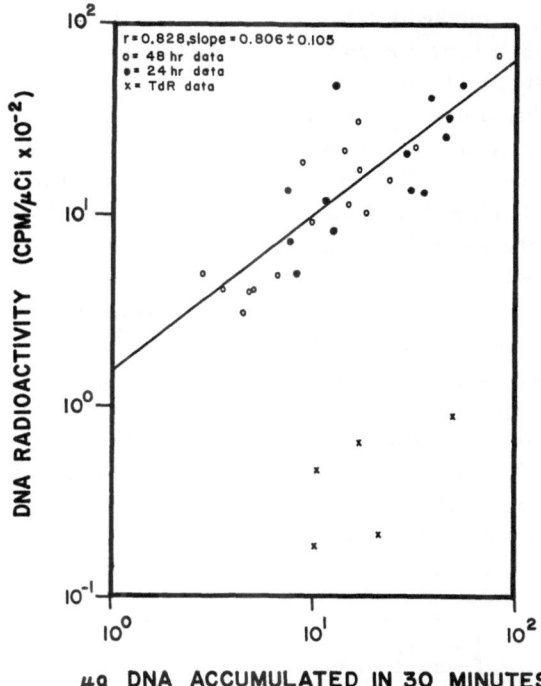

μg DNA ACCUMULATED IN 30 MINUTES

Fig. 7. A comparison of the volumetric and radioisotopic indices for estimating the rate of DNA accumulation. This log-log graph shows the radioactivity in the DNA (CPM/μCi injected $\times 10^{-2}$) plotted as a function of the volumetric estimate for the rate of DNA accumulation (μg DNA accumulated in 30 minutes). The solid dots represent the mice sacrificed at 24 hours following the injection of 0.1 mg (10 μCi) of ^{125}I-IUdR per mouse, and the open dots represent the 48 hour data. The period of DNA accumulation, though arbitrarily calculated for 30 minutes, was based on the rapid *in vivo* catabolism of IUdR (22). An analysis on the pooled 24 and 48 hour data showed that the indices are highly correlated (r = 0.828, P < 0.01), and the regression slope of 0.806 ± 0.105 is not significantly different from a hypothetical slope of one. The x's represent the data from an experiment in which thymidine (2 mg/mouse) was administered 10 minutes before the ^{125}I-IUdR (0.05 mg, 10 μCi/mouse).

sion-slope on this semi-log plot is highly significant, and the estimated biological half-life is 77.3 ± 19.3 hours.

In spite of the rapid loss of radioactivity from the DNA fraction, it still seemed valuable to examine the relationship between the radioactivity in the DNA at some fixed sacrifice time, and the volumetric estimate for rate of DNA accumulation. Correlation and regression analyses between the volumetric and radioisotopic indices for DNA accumulation were done on the 24 hour (r = 0.656, slope = 0.658 ± 0.228) and 48 hour data (r = 0.893, slope = 0.884 ± 0.119); then when no differences were found, a correlation and regression analysis was done on the pooled data. As shown in Fig. 7 the pooled correlation coefficient is highly significant and the slope is not significantly different from one. An independent analysis done on the data from the mice sacrificed at 2 hours gave similar results (r = 0.833, P < 0.01, slope = 0.736 ± 0.163). The data for the mice receiving 2 mg of thymidine ten minutes before ^{125}I-IUdR is also included in Fig. 7, and the radioactivity in this DNA is markedly below the data from the mice which received no thymidine. These data suggest the possibility of using the volumetric and radioisotopic methods simultaneously to study minor and transitory effects which antimetabolic or chemotherapeutic agents may have on DNA metabolism *in vivo,* even when this effect is not manifested at the level of tumor growth inhibition.

The high correlation of radioactivity in the DNA with the rate of DNA accumulation, and the finding that about 90 percent of the total tumor radioactivity was associated with the DNA by 48 hours suggested that *in situ* measurements at 48 hours may be a reasonable index for the rate of DNA accumulation. First, however, an evaluation of the *in situ* counting apparatus was in order. The *in situ* system could have been evaluated by using various sized tumor models containing known amounts of ^{125}Iodine. But it was considered more appropriate to validate the *in situ* system directly against the radioactivity of the extirpated and fractionated tumors as measured in the well-counting system (hereafter called *in vitro* to distinguish this system from the *in situ* apparatus). Such a comparison will not only evaluate the two systems of counting, but will also test the various procedures, normalizations, and assumptions used in the respective methods. As summarized in Fig. 8, the results indicate that the two independent estimates of ^{125}I-activity are

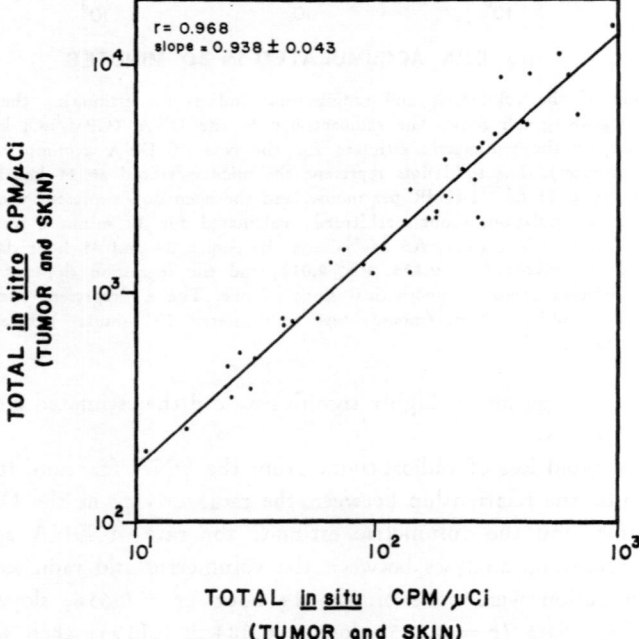

Fig. 8. An evaluation of the *in situ* counting apparatus. This log-log plot shows the well-counter determined radioactivity (*in vitro*) plotted against the *in situ* determined radioactivity. The *in vitro* radioactivity is the sum of all tumor fractions plus skin counted in the well-type scintillation detector, normalized to a standard in 3.0 ml of 5 percent citric acid, and corrected for physical decay back to the day of injection. The *in situ* radioactivity is that of the tumor and overlying skin as determined by the apparatus shown in Figures 2 and 3. This radioactivity was corrected for internal absorption of the ^{125}I-photons in the tumor (text equation 1) and physical decay back to the day of injection. The results for the two procedures are highly correlated (r = 0.968, P < 0.01), and the slope of 0.938 ± 0.043 is not significantly different from one.

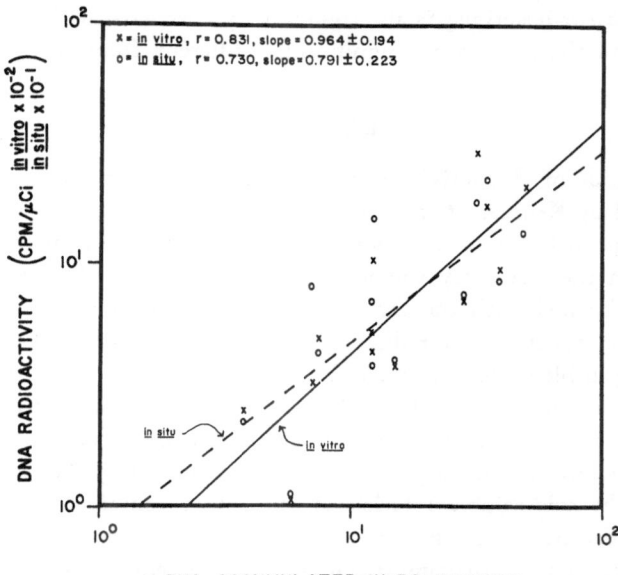

Fig. 9. A comparison of both radioactive indices (*in vitro* and *in situ*) with the volumetric estimate for rate of DNA accumulation. The data plotted here are from the mice which received 0.001, 0.006, and 1.0 mk (10 μCi) of ^{125}I-IUdR. The x's represent the *in vitro* radioactivity, and the results of a correlation and regression analysis (r = 0.831, P < 0.01, slope = 0.964 ± 0.194) are very similar to those discussed in Figure 7. The o's represent corrected *in situ* radioactivity. The *in situ* radioactivity in the tumor and overlying skin was reduced by the percent of the total tumor and skin radioactivity that was found to be in the skin as determined in the well-counter (see text). This corrected *in situ* radioactivity is also correlated with the volumetric rate of DNA accumulation (r = 0.730, P < 0.01, slope = 0.791 ± 0.223).

highly correlated. Moreover, the constant in the regression equation on the log-log plot gives an estimate of 20.6 ± 4.1 for the ratio (*in vitro* CPM/μCi/*in situ* CPM/μCi), and this is not significantly different from the value of 17.4 which was determined directly from the calibration of the respective equipment. Thus, it was concluded that the *in situ* system is reliable and the various correction and normalization factors are reasonably accurate.

The data for the following *in situ* study came from the mice which received 0.001, 0.006, or 1.0 mg IUdR. The radioactivity in the tumors was counted in the *in situ* apparatus at 48 hours post injection, then the mice were immediately sacrificed, and the tumors handled as described previously. The *in vitro* determined radioactivity in the DNA was compared to the volumetrically determined rate of DNA accumulation as discussed earlier (see Fig. 7). These data are plotted in Fig. 9 as the x's, and again the correlation between the volumetric and radioisotopic indices is highly significant. Next the *in situ* tumor radioactivity was corrected for skin radioactivity and the corrected radioactivity plotted in Fig. 9 as the o's. The skin correction factor was calculated from the *in vitro* determinations where the radioactivity in the skin overlying the tumor was expressed as a percent of the total radioactivity found in the tumor and skin. This percent, which averaged about 10 percent of the total radioactivity, was subtracted from the *in situ* measurements. Note that the "corrected" *in situ* radioactivity is also significantly correlated with the rate of DNA accumulation and the slope is not significantly different from one.

Discussion

The distribution of ^{125}I-activity in the mouse mammary tumor tissue was similar to that reported by Krueger *et al.* (24) and Hughes *et al.* (22) for normal murine tissues. They reported that by 24 hours essentially all the residual radioactivity was in the DNA. In the mammary tumor, about 90 percent of the total tumor radioactivity was associated with the DNA by 48 hours post injection. The difference may be due to a slower loss of radioactivity from the acid-soluble fraction because of a more sluggish blood flow in the tumor. Fox and Prusoff (16) upon using four injections over two days (3 μmoles, 1.92 μCi ^{125}I-IUdR/mouse/injection) reported similar findings for the radioactivity in the acid-soluble fractions of the mouse spleen and small intestine as compared to the Hepatoma-129. At one day after the last injection, the acid-soluble fraction of the spleen contained 10 percent of the total spleen radioactivity. This figure for the small intestine was 9 percent while the acid-soluble fraction from the tumor contained 38 percent of the total tumor radioactivity. Three days after the last injection, these figures were 3, 2, and 8 percent respectively. Thus it appears that one must wait at least 48 hours before the vast majority of the tumor radioactivity can be considered in the DNA fraction.

Since, in the context reported here, IUdR was used as a radiotracer, it was encouraging to observe that incorporation was proportional to the administered dose from 0.001 to 5.0 mg IUdR/mouse, and in another set of experiments (unpublished) there was no evidence for tumor growth inhibition from single intraperitoneal injections of IUdR until 5 mg IUdR/mouse was administered. Then the inhibiting effect was roughly the same for doses of 5, 10, 20, and 40 mg IUdR/mouse. Thus, the dose range for tumor growth inhibition roughly coincided with the doses at which IUdR incorporation no longer increased in proportion to dose injected.

The 10 mg dose corresponds to about 300 mg/kg of body weight, which on a per dose basis, is about twice that used in the multiple doses (100–150 mg/kg/day for six days) of Jaffee and Prusoff (23). They reported growth inhibition in the Sarcoma 180, and lymphomas L1210 and L5178-Y; also Calabresi *et al.* (3) used 2–3 hour daily infusions (100–120 mg/kg) for 5–6 days in humans and reported evidence for modest tumor inhibition. Morris and Cramer (28) reported that there is an apparent correlation between cell death and replacement of cellular DNA-thymidine with IUdR; but as they also pointed out, the causal relationship between the two has not been unequivocally demonstrated (29, 36). The data reported here, though preliminary, suggest that there may be an "all-or-none" principle relating the amount of IUdR incorporated to the chemotherapeutic effect.

The rapid loss of tumor DNA labeled with ^{125}I-IUdR (Fig. 6) was quite surprising since Commerford (6) had reported that the ^{125}I-label was not lost independently from DNA degradation, and as shown here, a dose of 0.1 mg IUdR/mouse is well below the lowest dose (5 mg) which showed any deleterious effects upon tumor growth. In an attempt to check on possible cellular effects, and well realizing the limitations of the technique for this, the percent of DNA-thymidine replaced by IUdR was calculated after the manner of Clifton et al. (5). If one assumes that all the ^{125}I-IUdR was incorporated into 30 minutes' work of DNA synthesis, as estimated from the growth curves, then a 0.1 mg dose results in approximately 2 percent IUdR replacement of DNA-thymidine. Combining the data of Cheong et al. (4) and Hampton et al. (19) one finds that about 10 percent continuous substitution of IUdR (seven days was the observed end point) gave a 30 percent growth inhibition of H.Ep.1 cells in tissue culture. If this can be applied to mammary tumor cells in vivo, then one may assume that the relatively rapid loss ($T_{1/2} = 77.3$ hours) of ^{125}I-activity was not due to IUdR killing the cells. Subsequently, we have demonstrated that the unperturbed mammary tumor has a high rate of cell turnover (26), and the half-life for ^{125}I-IUdR may well be a direct reflection of tumor cell death in situ. In addition to the possible cytotoxic effect of IUdR, interpretation of the half-life is clouded by the possibility of IUdR reutilization. In comparable studies with tritiated thymidine, Steel (34) found a progressive increase in the radioactivity of tumor DNA over several days, and he interpreted this as reutilization. Earlier Hughes et al. (22) and Feinendegen et al. (15) reported no reutilization of IUdR when tracer doses were administered; however, Mendelsohn and Dethlefsen (27) have shown that reutilization of IUdR-6-^{3}H did occur when growth-inhibiting doses (10 mg IUdR/mouse) were administered.

The high correlation found between the radioactivity in the DNA and the volumetric estimate for the rate of DNA accumulation suggests that the radioisotopic and volumetric methods are both reasonable indices for estimating DNA accumulation in unperturbed tumors. The data also suggest that the radioisotopic index can be measured in situ. However, one must point out that the radioisotopic method has only been tested on tumors ranging between 300 and 5000 mm^3. This is only part of the growth cycle of mouse mammary tumors and, indeed, a very small fraction of tumor growth in general. In addition, a combination of autoradiographic and volumetric data now indicates that cell turnover is quite rapid in these tumors (26). The radioisotopic method estimates the total increase in DNA as a function of time while the volumetric method only estimates the net increase in DNA. Therefore, in light of the cell loss and the high proportionality demonstrated between the volumetric and radioisotopic indices, one might assume that cell loss is proportional to cell birth in these tumors.

In conclusion, the radioisotopic measurements are a reliable index for the rate of DNA accumulation, and these measurements can be made in situ. It also appears that the simultaneous use of the volumetric and radioisotopic methods will be a fruitful procedure for many studies, and using these methods in conjunction with autoradiography will permit one to get more insight into the biology of solid tumors. However, much more work is required to evaluate these procedures as methods for studying DNA metabolism in perturbed tumors, and the success of the radioisotopic method for measuring tumor cell loss in situ remains to be confirmed.

References

1. BAKHLE, Y. S., PRUSOFF, W. H., and McCREA, J. F.: Precaution in the use of iodine-125 as a radioactive tracer. Science **143**, 799 (1964).
2. BERRY, R. J., and ANDREWS, J. R.: Modification of the radiation effect on the reproductive capacity of tumor cells *in vivo* with pharmacological agents. Rad. Res. **16**, 84 (1962).
3. CALABRESI, P., CARDOSO, S. S., FINCH, S. C., KLIGERMAN, M. M., VON ESSEN, C. F., CHU, M. Y., and WELCH, A. D.: Initial clinical studies with 5-iodo-2'-deoxyuridine. Cancer Res. **21**, 550 (1961).
4. CHEONG, L., RICH, M. A., and EIDINOFF, M. L.: Introduction of the 5-halogenated uracil moiety into deoxyribonucleic acid of mammalian cells in culture. J. Biol. Chem. **235**, 1441 (1960).
5. CLIFTON, K. H., SZYBALSKI, W., HEIDELBERGER, C., GOLLIN, F. F., ANSFIELD, F. J., and VERMUND, H.: Incorporation of I^{125}-labeled iododeoxyuridine into the deoxyribonucleic acid of murine and human tissues following therapeutic doses. Cancer Res. **23**, 1715 (1963).
6. COMMERFORD, S. L.: Biological stability of 5-Iodo-2'-deoxyuridine labeled with iodine-125 after its incorporation into the deoxyribonucleic acid of the mouse. Nature **206**, 949 (1965).
7. DELAMORE, I. W., and PRUSOFF, W. H.: Effect of 5-Iodo-2'-deoxyuridine on the biosynthesis of phosphorylated derivatives of thymidine. Biochem. Pharmacol. **11**, 101 (1962).
8. DETHLEFSEN, L. A.: *In vivo* volumetric and isotopic studies of the rate of tumor DNA synthesis. Fed. Proc. **26**, 817 (1967).
9. DETHLEFSEN, L. A.: Volumetric and isotopic studies of tumor growth. Ph.D. dissertation, University of Pennsylvania, Philadelphia (1966).
10. DETHLEFSEN, L. A., and MENDELSOHN, M. L.: Uptake of labeled 5-iodo-2'-deoxyuridine (I^{125}UdR) as an index of tumor growth. Rad. Res. **22**, 182 (1964).
11. DETHLEFSEN, L. A., PREWITT, J. M. S., and MENDELSOHN, M. L.: Analysis of tumor growth curves. J. Natl. Cancer Inst. **40**, 389 (1968).
12. EIDINOFF, M. L., CHEONG, L., and RICH, M. A.: Incorporation of unnatural pyrimidine bases into deoxyribonucleic acid of mammalian cells. Science **129**, 1550 (1959).
13. ERIKSON, R. L., and SZYBALSKI, W.: Molecular radiobiology of human cell lines III. Radiation-sensitizing properties of 5-iododeoxyuridine. Cancer Res. **23**, 122 (1963).
14. EVANS, R. D.: The Atomic Nucleus. McGraw-Hill, New York (1955).
15. FEINENDEGEN, L. E., BOND, V. P., and HUGHES, W. L.: ^{125}I-DU (5-Iodo-2'-deoxyuridine) in autoradiographic studies of cell proliferation. Exp. Cell Res. **43**, 107 (1966).
16. FOX, B. W., and PRUSOFF, W. H.: The comparative uptake of I^{125}-labeled 5-Iodo-2'-deoxyuridine and thymidine-H3 into tissues of mice bearing hepatoma-129. Cancer Res. **25**, 234 (1965).
17. FRINDEL, E., MALAISE, E. P., ALPEN, E., and TUBIANA, M.: Kinetics of cell proliferation of an experimental tumor. Cancer Res. **27**, 1122 (1967).
18. GITLIN, D., COMMERFORD, S. L., AMSTERDAM, E., and HUGHES, W. L.: X-rays affect the incorporation of 5-Iododeoxyuridine into deoxyribonucleic acid. Science **133**, 1074 (1961).
19. HAMPTON, E. G., RICH, M. A., and EIDINOFF, M. L.: Introduction of the 5-iodouracil moiety into deoxyribonucleic acid of mammalian cells. J. Biol. Chem. **235**, 3562 (1960).

20. HELL, E., BERRY, R. J., and LAJTHA, L. G.: A pitfall in high specific activity tracer studies. Nature **185**, 47 (1960).

21. HINRICHS, H. R., PETERSEN, R. O., and BASERGA, R.: Incorporation of thymidine into DNA of mouse organs. Arch. Path. **78**, 245 (1964).

22. HUGHES, W. L., COMMERFORD, S. L., GITLIN, D., KRUEGER, R. C., SCHULTZE, B., SHAH, V., and REILLY, P.: Deoxyribonucleic acid metabolism *in vivo*: I. Cell proliferation and death as measured by incorporation and elimination of iododeoxyuridine. Fed. Proc. **23**, 640 (1964).

23. JAFFEE, J. J., and PRUSOFF, W. H.: The effects of 5-iododeoxyuridine upon the growth of some transplantable rodent tumors. Cancer Res. **20**, 1383 (1960).

24. KRUEGER, R. C., GITLIN, D., COMMERFORD, S. L., STEIN, J., and HUGHES, W. L.: Iododeoxyuridine (IDU) as a tracer of DNA metabolism *in vivo*. Fed. Proc. **19**, 307 (1960).

25. MATHIAS, A. P., and FISCHER, G. A.: The metabolism of thymidine by murine leukemic lymphoblasts (L5178-Y). Biochem. Pharmacol. **11**, 57 (1962).

26. MENDELSOHN, M. L., and DETHLEFSEN, L. A.: Cell proliferation and volumetric growth of fast line, slow line, and spontaneous C3H mammary tumors. Proc. Am. Assoc. for Cancer Res. (in press) (1968).

27. MENDELSOHN, M. L., and DETHLEFSEN, L. A.: Tumor growth and cellular kinetics. *In:* The proliferation and spread of neoplastic cells. The University of Texas Press, Houston (in press) (1968).

28. MORRIS, N. R., and CRAMER, J. W.: DNA synthesis by mammalian cells inhibited in culture by 5-Iodo-2'-deoxyuridine. Mol. Pharm. **2**, 1 (1966).

29. PRUSOFF, W. H.: A review of some aspects of 5-iododeoxyuridine and azauridine. Cancer Res. **23**, 1246 (1963).

30. PRUSOFF, W. H.: Incorporation of Iododeoxyuridine into the Deoxyribonucleic Acid of Mouse Ehrlich-Ascites-Tumor Cells *in vivo*. Biochim. Biophys. Acta **39**, 327 (1960).

31. PRUSOFF, W. H.: Synthesis and Biological Activities of Iododeoxyuridine, an Analogue of Thymidine. Biochim. Biophys. Acta **32**, 295 (1959).

32. PRUSOFF, W. H., JAFFEE, J. J., and GÜNTHER, H.: Studies in the mouse of the pharmacology of 5-iododeoxyuridine, an analogue of thymidine. Biochem. Pharmacol. **3**, 110 (1960).

33. SCOTT, J. F., FRACCASTORO, A. P., and TAFT, E. G.: Studies in histochemistry: I. Determination of nucleic acids in microgram amounts of tissue. J. Histochem. and Cytochem. **4**, 1 (1956).

34. STEEL, G. G.: Delayed uptake by tumours of tritium from thymidine. Nature **210**, 806 (1966).

35. STEEL, G. G., ADAMS, K., and BARRETT, J. C.: Analysis of the cell population kinetics of transplanted tumours of widely-differing growth rate. Brit. J. Cancer **20**, 784 (1966).

36. WELCH, A. D., and PRUSOFF, W. H.: A synopsis of recent investigations of 5-Iodo-2'-deoxyuridine. Cancer Chem. Reports **6**, 29 (1960).

In Vivo Cell Kinetics of Human Cancers

M. Tubiana, E. Frindel, E. Malaise

Department of Radiation
Institute Gustave-Roussy
Villejuif, France

The kinetics of cancer cell proliferation is probably one of the main factors which determines its sensitivity to physical or chemical agents. It is well known that most of the drugs do not act the same way on quiescent and proliferating cells. The demonstration of variability of cell radiosensitivity as a function of the cellular cycle's (28, 25, 30) stage, is one of the important advances made in radiobiology during recent years.

The radiosensitivity of a cell population depends on the radiosensitivity of each phase of the cycle and on the proportion of the cells in each of these phases at the time of irradiation. If two tissues differ in their population structure, that is in the proportion of cells in each phase of the cell cycle, the effect of a single session of irradiation may be different, even though the radiosensitivity of the cells of the two tissues studied *in vitro* is the same. This demonstrates the need for a full appreciation of the types of information mentioned above in order to compare the radiosensitivity of different tumors. The presence of resting cells in G_0 must also be taken into account, although there is very little information about their radiosensitivity.

Breur (4) has shown the existence of a significant correlation between the rate of growth of human cancers and their radiosensitivity. The knowledge of the parameters of a human cancer's cell proliferation may therefore have a practical impact from a therapeutic point of view.

Unfortunately, there is very little information on the cellular kinetics of human tumors.

Four methods have been used for these studies:

1. The Measurement of the Labeling Index. It can be performed *in vivo* or *in vitro*. *In vivo*, it necessitates an intravascular injection of a relatively large amount of radioactive thymidine prior to a biopsy or surgical procedure. In view of the hazards involved in the use of tritiated thymidine (^{3}H-th) in human beings (3, 22), this procedure should be limited to patients with a short life expectancy. Some authors (17) have injected ^{3}H-th in the artery which irrigates the tumor. With this technique, 1 mCi of ^{3}H-th, is sufficient but there is a small risk of an heterogeneous distribution of the radioactive precursor within the tumor.

The labeling index has also been measured *in vitro*. The specimen is, immediately after surgery, incubated at 37°C in a medium containing radioactive thymidine.

The risk of this technique is that the radioactive precursor or some nutrients may not reach the cells located at the center of the specimen. Furthermore, some authors (27) claim that anoxic cells may not be able to synthesize DNA even if the precursor reaches these cells. This results in heterogeneous labeling and in artefacts in the measurement of the labeling index. In order to decrease this risk, only small specimens should be studied. Steel has also proposed to incubate the tissue under high pressure oxygen in order to obtain good oxygenation of all the cells (27).

The labeling index found in human tumors varies widely (2, 5, 7, 8, 14–17, 19, 23, 27, 29, 31). In some tumors, it is as low as 0.1 percent, in others it reaches 38 percent (7).

Even when measured under good conditions, the labeling index is difficult to interpret. The labeling index furnishes an indication of the relative length of the phase of DNA synthesis in relation to the average duration of the entire cell cycle, assuming that all the cells of the population are dividing. But it is impossible to assume a constant duration of the S phase for all the tumor cells as now it is known that this duration can vary by a large factor, at least, from 10 to 60 hours in human cells. Furthermore, all the cells of a tumor or tissue may not be engaged in active proliferation at the same time and a significant fraction of the cells may be in a quiescent state. One must therefore take into account the "growth fraction" (G.F.) concept which was introduced by Mendelsohn. The growth fraction varies widely from one tumor to another (20, 6). If one does not consider the growth fraction and the overall length of the cell cycle or the duration of the S phase, the labeling index alone furnishes an inadequate picture of growth kinetics, and cannot be used without great caution, for calculating a potential doubling time.

2. Determination by Microdensitometry of DNA Content of the Cells. The DNA content of a cell may be estimated by measuring the light absorption of the Feulgen stained nuclei. A histogram showing the distribution of DNA contents in tumor cell nuclei is obtained.

The cells can be grouped in 3 classes according to their DNA content: $G_0 + G_1$ cells which have a diploid mode, G_2 cells which have a tetraploid mode, and cells with a DNA content which indicates that they are engaged in DNA synthesis.

If the tissue has been incubated *in vitro* with ^{3}H-th, one can perform an autoradiography on the same Feulgen stained slide. The cells which are synthetising DNA are located and this gives further information about the distribution of cells in the various compartments of interphase.

This technique has been used by Cooper (7). He studied Burkitt tumors and malignant lymphoma and was able to measure the proportion of cells in each phase of the cell cycle.

If one of these phases had a known duration it would be possible to evaluate the transit time through all the phases. Unfortunately, none of them has a constant value and this is impossible.

This method has 2 advantages: 1. It provides good information on the cell phase distribution. This parameter seems to be linked to radiosensitivity or drug sensitivity and may be of great interest. 2. Artefacts may occur during the measurement of the labeling index *in vitro*. The results of the labeling index determinations are checked by the measurement of the DNA content in this method. A wide discrepancy between the estimation of S cells by the 2 methods indicates that the incubation may have not been performed in good conditions. On the other hand, aneuploidy may be important in tumor cells. In this case, the interpretation of the cytophotometric data would be difficult without autoradiography.

We have studied a few human tumors with this technique. The results of a patient with a reticulosarcoma will illustrate its possibility (Table I and Fig. 1). The labeling index is low, and most of the cells are in $(G_0 + G_1)$ phase.

3. The Mitotic Index. It was thought for a long time that the mitotic index was a reliable method for measuring the rate of cell proliferation in a tissue. This was based on the assumption that the mitotic duration remained relatively constant in each cell type. This assumption does not now seem valid and the mitotic index is not sufficient by itself.

To measure the mitotic rate, some authors have proposed a stathmokinetic method using for instance colchicine or Vinca-alcaloid. O. H. Iversen (13) has used this method in patients. A biopsy is first performed and the mitotic index measured in 1000 tumor cells. Then 10 mg of colcemid are injected intravenously. Four hours later a specimen is taken. The calculation of the mitotic rate is based on the increase of the mitotic count, assuming that all the cells which have entered into mitosis during these 4 hours have been arrested. The relationship between the mitotic count, the mitotic rate and duration is as follows: mitotic count (without colcemid) = mitotic rate (with colcemid) $\times$ mitotic duration.

With this method Refsum and Bendal (24) have measured the rate of cell proliferation in 61 patients with malignant tumours. They have found 1 percent of arrested mitoses per hour in carcinoma *in situ* and infiltrating carcinoma. The variation of the mitotic rate in different areas of the tissue was much greater in tumors than in normal epithelium. Most of the carcinoma proliferate at a somewhat faster speed

TABLE I

| | Microdensitometry | | M.I. before incubation | Incubation (1 hour) | | | |
| | | | | in O_2 10 atm. | | in air | |
				M.I.	L.I.	M.I.	L.I.
Smear	$N_{G_1 + G_0}$	89%					
	N_s	7%		0.2%	7.2%	0.03%	2.4%
	N_{G_2}	3%					
Sections			0.4%	0.4%	5.5%	0.4%	6.5

Human reticulosarcoma. Distribution of cell phases as determined on a smear by microdensitometry. The labeling index was measured after one hour of incubation *in vitro* with ^{3}H-thymidine (in atmospheric air or in oxygen under a pressure of 10 atmospheres). The mitotic index and the labeling index seem to be lower on the smear of the specimen incubated in air.

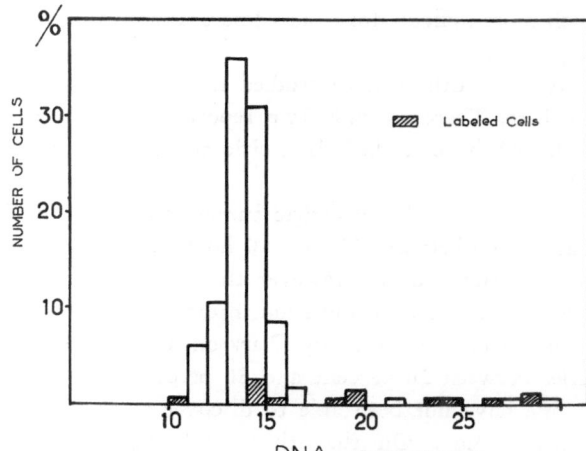

Fig. 1. Histogram of distribution of DNA contents of Reticulosarcoma cells (Patient). The cells in S phase were labeled by *in vitro* incubation with tritiated thymidine.

than normal epithelium. The mitotic rate seems to be greater than the growth rate of the tumor if all the cells remained within the tumor.

This technique has 2 problems: 1. The injection of colcemid may be harmful in young patients. 2. There is some uncertainty involved in the choice of the colchicine dosage.

4. *In Vivo* Study of the Labeled Mitoses Curve. A complete study of the cell proliferation kinetics of a tissue necessitates the measurement of the duration of each phase of the cell cycle and of the growth fraction. An evaluation of cell loss is also an important parameter. In order to get these data with the present techniques, an injection of ³H-th is necessary.

Many techniques such as grain halving time after a single injection of ³H-th or several samplings throughout continuous labeling, can be used for measuring the duration of the cell cycle but the labeled mitoses curve seems to be the most accurate. Furthermore, it has the advantage of enabling the measurement of all the phases of the cell cycle.

During recent years, these parameters have been measured in a few experimental tumors, but human data are still very rare. This is easy to understand when one considers the ethical and technical problems involved:

A. Late risks of an intravenous injection of ³H-th. They must be considered from 2 points of view: Genetic hazards and carcinogenesis (3, 22). In order to eliminate genetic risks only old patients should be considered for such studies.

The late somatic risks due to concentrations of the order of 0.1 to 0.5 mCi of ³H-th per kg are probably small but this is difficult to ascertain. In any case, it is safer to restrict the study to patients with a short life expectancy.

B. In order to be able to get a good labeled mitoses curve, the mitotic index of the tumor should be high enough. This introduces a bias, as patients with tumors with a low mitotic index cannot be studied.

C. A large number of specimens are necessary after the injection of ³H-th. In the case of a malignant hemopathy or of an ascitic tumor, this is relatively easy. It is much more difficult for solid tumors. Practically, it is possible only when the biopsies are painless.

A few authors have studied malignant hemopathies. This problem is discussed elsewhere. There are only two reports in the literature on human tumors. Clarkson *et al.* (6) have studied six ascitic tumors and we have studied 5 solid tumors (20, 10).

Clarkson results in ascitic tumors are shown in Table II. The duration of the S phase varies between 17 and 60 hours and the duration of the whole cell cycle between 3 and 5 days. However the 60 hour duration for S phase was probably abnormally long due to radiation injury from an excessive dose of tritiated thymidine. With the data obtained by Clarkson, the G.F. of these tumors can be estimated. It varies between 20 percent and 80 percent.

We have not been able to discover in the literature any study concerning solid human tumors. On the other hand, we have found in experimental work that neoplastic cells may behave differently in ascitic tumors and in solid tumors (11, 12, 9). For these reasons, we have recently taken advantage of the hospitalization of five unusual patients to study the cell cycles in their tumors. The results concerning these patients have been recently reported (20, 10), and will be summarized here.

TABLE II

Percent of Free Cancer Cells Labeled with H^3 Thymidine, Their Mitotic Index and the Mean

Diagnosis	Cancer cells labeled after single injection H^3-thymidine %	Mitotic index cancer cells	T_c (days)	Mitotic (M) phase (hours)	Post-mitotic (G_1) phase (days)	DNA Synthesis (S) phase (hours)	Pre-mitotic (G_2) phase (hours)
Carcinoma Endometrium	11	0.8	4.6	1	2	60?	4
Carcinoma ovary	18	0.8	5?	1	3.5	28	8
Carcinoma stomach	28	1.0	3	1	2	20	3
Carcinoma stomach	27	1.0	4.6	1.1	3	32?	5
Lymphosarcoma	4.5	0.2	3.8	1	3	17	2
Carcinoma ovary	20	1.2	5?	1.4?	3?	34	6

Neoplastic effusions in man. Labeling index, mitotic index and mean duration of the cell cycle and its phases (from Clarkson, 20).

Methods and Materials

Choice of Tumors and Technique. All tumors were large in size, approximately 10 cm in diameter or more. The mitotic indices were relatively high. The tumors were well vascularized and the biopsies were painless. Three types of skin tumor were examined: two cases of basal cell carcinoma, two cases of epidermoid epithelioma, and one spindle cell epithelioma.

During the three days prior to the biopsies and during the duration of the study, the tumors were washed twice daily with saline containing 100 U of penicillin and 250 micrograms of streptomycin per ml. The tumors were covered with sterile gauze and oily ointment, care being taken that the dressing did not compress the tumor. Twenty mg of vitamin K were injected daily in the patients during investigation.

Twenty mCi of radioactive thymidine, 3 H-th (specific activity 8,5 Ci/mM), dissolved in 5 ml of sterile saline solution were injected intravenously.

In each patient, 7 to 17 biopsies were performed at different time intervals after the injection. The biopsies were carried out with sharp pointed scissors to avoid lacerating the tumor. Each biopsy was at least 1 cm away from the previous one. In one of the patients, two biopsies were done at each time interval: one in the infero-exterior region and one on the super-interior portion of the tumor in order to compare the labeled mitotic indices in different zones of the tumor.

The specimens were fixed in Carnoy fixative and prepared for autoradiographic studies.

Histological sections 4 microns thick were prepared on thin glass slides and autoradiographs were made by the dipping method using Ilford K2 emulsion. After four weeks of exposure at 4°C, in light tight boxes containing a desiccator, the slides were developed in Kodak D 19 solution at 18°C and stained with phloxine hemalun stains.

Determination of the Cell Cycle. Twenty-five to 800 mitoses were counted in each fragment to determine the percentage of labeled mitoses and 1,000 to 11,000 cells were counted to determine the labeling index (L.I.). The mitotic index (M.I.) was determined on 36 to 169 mitoses.

The background being low, cells containing 3 grains or more were considered as positive.

The duration of the cell cycle was studied by the method of labeled mitoses curves. The number of labeled mitoses per 100 total mitoses was plotted against time after a single injection of ^{3}H-th. The duration of the cell cycle (T_G) was determined by taking the interval between the 50 percent values on the ascending curves of 2 successive waves of labeled mitoses. The minimum duration of G2 was determined by the time between the injection and the appearance of the first labeled mitoses. The average duration of G2 + M ($T_{G2 + M}$) is the time between administration of ^{3}H-th and when 50 percent of the mitoses are labeled. The duration of the DNA synthesis (T_s) is determined by the time between the 50 percent labeled mitoses on the ascending and descending portions of the curve. T_{G1} is calculated as the difference between the total generation time and the sum of the three other phases of the cell cycle $[T_c - (T_s + T_{G_2} + T_M)]$.

When a second wave of labeled mitoses was not observed, the length of the cell cycle was calculated by the following formula:

$$T_c = \frac{\text{Duration of DNA synthesis} \times \text{Growth fraction}}{\text{Labeling index}} \qquad [1]$$

The growth fraction is equal to the proportion of the diving cells in a cell population. It was measured by Mendelsohn's method 120 hours after the pulse label with ^{3}H-th and is the ratio of the percentage of labeled cells to the percentage of labeled mitoses (21).

Results

Basal Cell Carcinoma

CASE 1: Patient M was an 80 year old man with multiple tumors located on the thorax, abdomen and legs. The tumors were growing progressively for about 20 years. The tumor chosen was situated on the supero-interior region of the inferior limb. Its clinical doubling time was approximately 10 months. The study was performed in April 1965 and the patient died in August 1965 from uremia.

The cell cycle as described above was studied. The curve of percent labeled mitoses is shown in Fig. 2 and tabulated in Table III. The peak of labeled mitoses occurred 24 hours after the injection of ^{3}H-th and reached 80 percent. No second peak was observed during the study.

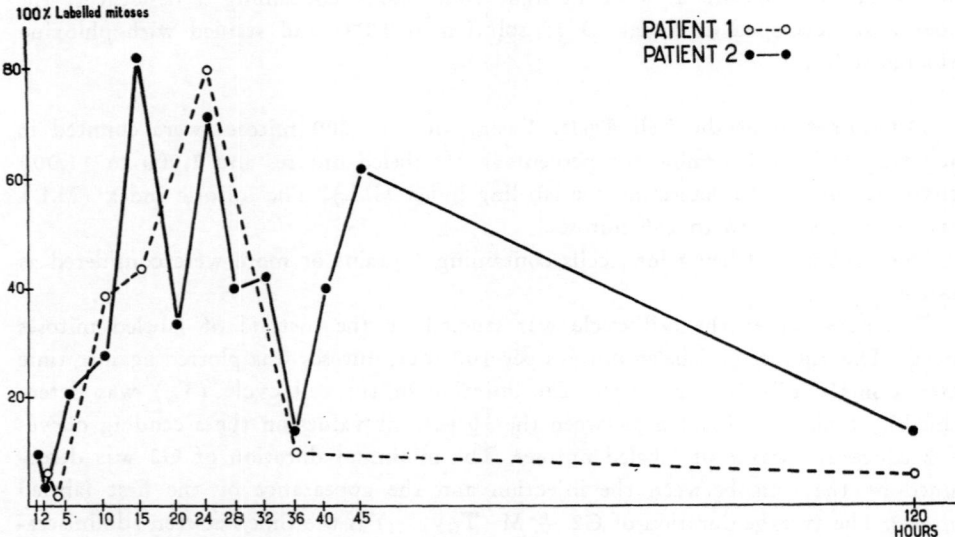

Fig. 2. Fraction of mitoses labeled after a single injection of ^{3}H-thymidine in 2 human Basal cell carcinoma of the skin.

TABLE III

PARAMETER OF CELL PROLIFERATION IN FIVE HUMAN SOLID TUMORS (21, 24)

	Pathologic type	M.I.	L.I.	T_{G_1} (hours)	T_S (hours)	T_{G_2+M} (hours)	T_c (days) on 2 d labeled mitoses wave	T_c (days) Based on G.F.	G.F.
PAT. 1	Basal cell	0.7%	6%	66	19	16		4	29%
PAT. 2	Basal cell	0.4–1%	5–20%	6–25	19	12	1.5	2.5	39%
PAT. 3	Epidermoid epith.	1.4%	18%	9–15	11	4.5	1	1.2	40%
PAT. 4	Epidermoid epith.	1.25	11%	31	12	6.1		2	40%
PAT. 5	Spindle cell carc.	1.4	7	?	21?			10?	82?

Solid tumors in man. Labeling index mitotic index, growth fraction, duration of the cell cycle and its phases (21, 24).

The labeling index (percent labeled cells) remained stable throughout the study, fluctuating between 5 percent and 8 percent. The mitotic index was 0.72 percent.

The generation time, T_c, calculated by the formula [1] is about 97 hours. T_{G1} evaluated by difference is about 66 hours.

Case 2: Patient Ph was a 74 year old woman. She had a single tumor in the trochanteric region; the tumor had been slowly growing for about 20 years. The study was performed in December 1965.

The results are given in Fig. 2 and Table III. The L.I. varied from 4.9 percent to 19.7 percent on the different specimens taken during the study. The labeled mitosis curve shows two waves: the first begins 15 hours after the injection and the percentage of labeled mitoses reaches a value of 82 percent; the second wave occurs at 40 hours. It should be mentioned that the percentage of labeled mitosis at 20 hours is only 34 percent. Without taking into account this point, which seems to be aberrant, and corresponds to a specimen with specially low L.I., the duration of phases can be determined graphically. The duration of the cell cycle T_c is about 36 hours.

The G.F. is equal to 39 percent T_c evaluated by the equation [1] is equal to 67 hours. The discrepancy between this value and the graphical measurement underlines the possible inaccuracy of this method.

Epidermoid Epithelioma

Case 3: Patient P was an 81 year old man. He had a small skin nodule on his right cheek, which was slowly but progressively growing for about 15 years. About a year before the study, the tumor size began to increase rapidly. In 9 months, it grew from about 1 gram to about 200 grams. The clinical doubling time was a little over 1 month.

The study was carried out on two opposing regions of the tumor for each time interval. The results are shown in Fig. 3 and Table III.

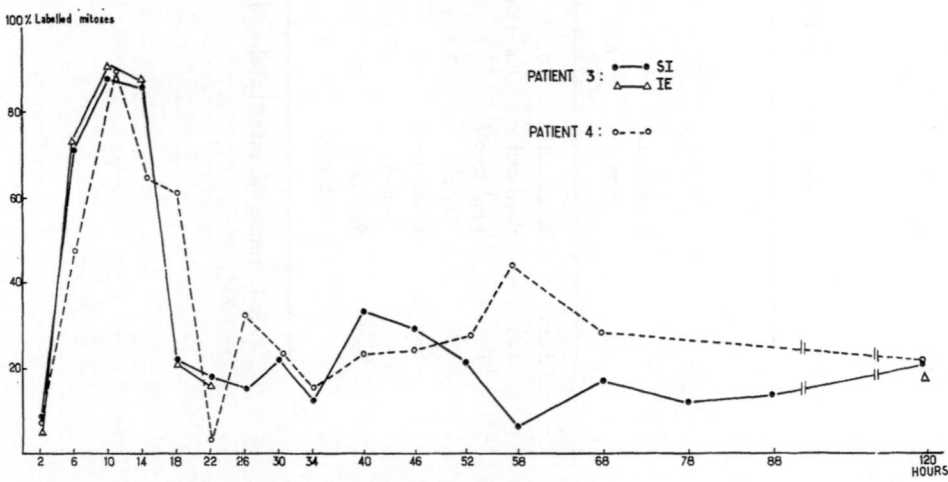

Fig. 3. Fraction of mitoses labeled after a single injection of ³H-thymidine in 2 human epidermoid carcinoma of the skin. For patient 3, two biopsies were performed at each time interval in order to compare different regions of the tumor.

The peak of labeled mitoses was observed 10 hours after the injection of ^{3}H-th and reached a value of 90 percent. A second peak was reached at about 40 hours when 32 percent of the mitoses were labeled.

T_c calculated by the equation [1] was found to be about 25 hours and it was of about 30 hours when measured graphically. The results of the two sets of specimens taken at each time interval were very similar (Fig. 3).

CASE 4: Patient L was a 79 year old woman who had an ulcerated tumor on the forehead just above the nose. The tumor first appeared 20 years ago and grew slowly without any treatment. It had been ulcerated for many years when the patient was first seen. At this time, the cancer was about 9 cm in diameter.

Figure 3 and Table III give the results of the percentages of labeled mitoses curves. The peak of labeled mitoses reaches 90 percent, 11 hours after the injection of ^{3}H-th.

Spindle Cell Epithelioma

CASE 5: Patient B is a 67 year old man. A lesion on his left cheek was first discovered in 1962. Various treatments were performed: electrocoagulation in 1963, radium implantation in 1964, surgery in February 1965, Cobalt beam therapy in July–October 1965 (33 sessions), surgery again in December 1965 and intra-arterial perfusion of cyclophosphamid and 5 F.U. in April 1966.

The study was performed in December 1966, a recurrence having been observed (Fig. 4). The peak of labeled mitoses was observed 12 hours after the injection of ^{3}H-th but only 50 percent of the mitoses were labeled. The duration of the dif-

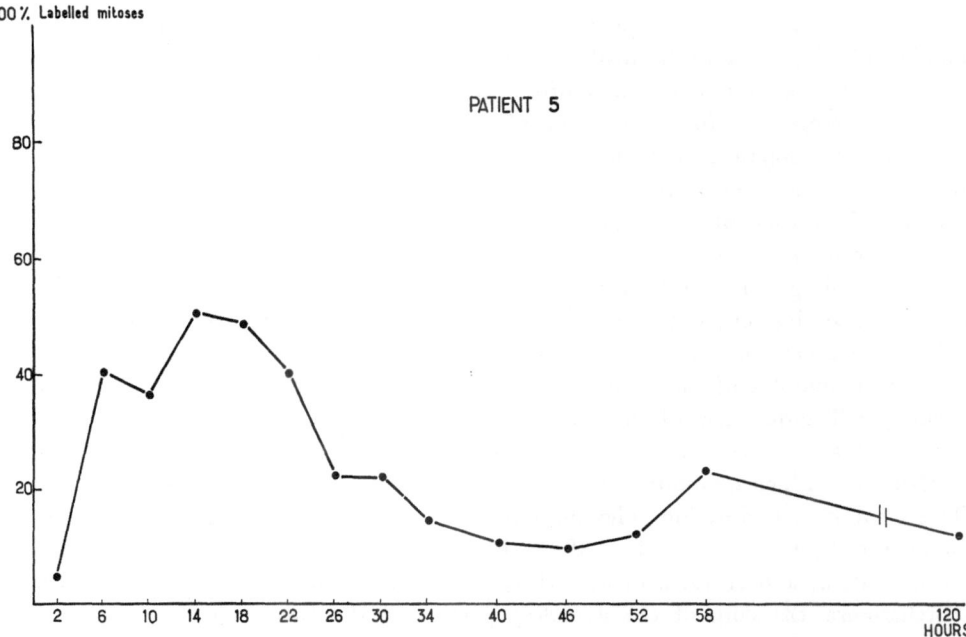

Fig. 4. Fraction of mitoses labeled after a single injection of ^{3}H-thymidine in one spindle-cell carcinoma of the skin.

ferent phases of the cell cycle is therefore difficult to evaluate and all values must be considered as tentative. The duration of S phase seems to be of the order of 20 hours. The G.F. measured at five days was 82 percent.

Discussion

In spite of the technical and ethical problems involved in establishing a labeled mitoses curve for a human tumor, it seemed to us that the knowledge of the cell proliferation kinetics of a human tumor justifies the multiple biopsies necessary for such a study in a few selected cases. In order to minimize the late risks of an intravenous injection of ^{3}H-th, we chose patients with a short life expectancy. In order to be able to perform multiple biopsies, we selected patients with large painless tumors. In order to be able to get a good labeled mitoses curve, we eliminated patients whose tumors had a low mitotic index. In 2 years, among many thousands of patients, five were finally found suitable for the study. It should be recognized that these patients may not be a representative sample of skin tumors.

High specific activity labeled thymidine may exert a lethal effect on mammalian cells or temporarily inhibit mitoses. We have injected 0.2 microcuries per gram of body weight. It is generally considered that this concentration does not have an immediate radiobiological effect (1). This seems to be confirmed by the study of the M.I. and the L.I., at different time intervals after the injection. In one patient, we compared the M.I. at 2 different time intervals and found them identical. In four of the patients we did not observe any significant variation of the L.I. throughout the study.

To obtain a labeled mitosis curve with reasonable accuracy, a relatively large number of biopsies must be made. For solid human tumor studies, this is a drawback not only because of the discomfort for the patient, but also because the tumor may be heterogenous. In consideration of the latter possibility, we have taken specimens on two opposing parts of the tumor for each time interval in one of the patients. The average duration of the cell cycle and its components were very similar in both parts of the tumor in this patient.

Furthermore, one can argue that each biopsy may influence the mitotic cycle of the surrounding cells. We have no human data concerning the influence of a biopsy on the remaining tumor. However, the shape of the curve suggests that little or no influence is exerted on the cells by previous biopsies.

The results of 4 of the patients are similar and give weight to the validity of the technique. The durations of the various phases of the cell cycle are nearly identical in patients 1 and 2, who have cancers of the same type. The duration of $(G_2 + M)$ is about 12 h. The minimum value of G_2 seems to be on the order of a few hours. This is an average duration. The duration of $(G_2 + M)$ may be considerably longer in some cells as the peak values of the labeled mitosis curve were reached at 24 h. in one patient and at 19 h. in the other, and moreover, does not exceed 80 percent. Furthermore, the slope of the ascending portion of the curve is not very steep indicating large fluctuations around the mean value. The duration of T_s is about 20 h. for these 2 patients. The fluctuation of T_s in different cells around this value does not seem to be very large as the slope of the descending part of the curve seems about equal to the slope of the ascending part.

These first 2 patients have a cycle which is longer than the T_c of about 1 day observed by Lipkin (18) for human rectal epithelial cells. But Clarkson (6) observed in some of his 6 patients with neoplastic effusions, durations of the same order.

Patients 3 and 4 whose cancers were of another type have shorter G_2 and S phases. These durations are analogous to what Lipkin (18) found in normal human cells. T_{G_1} is a little longer in patient 4 than in patient 3 but the difference is not very large. The peak value of the curve is of the order of 90 percent, the slope of the ascending and descending portions of the curves is steep indicating that the fluctuations to $T_{G_2} + M$ and of T_s are probably not very large.

For these 4 patients, the growth fraction is very similar varying between 29 percent and 41 percent. The duration of the cell cycle calculated on the basis of the G.F. varies from 25 to 97 hours.

The duration of the whole cell cycle was measured by a graphical method in only 2 patients (patient 2: 36 hr. and patient 3: 30 hr.). For patient 3, the calculation based on the G.F. gave a duration nearly identical, but for patient 2, the evaluated Tc is about two times greater than the measured one. This discrepancy is probably due to the inaccuracy of the measurement of the G.F. or to the inadequacy in this case of the concept or of the method used. It is possible that for this patient, the ratio of M^x/M has not yet reached its asymptotic value at the 5th day. It should be pointed out that for this patient, 5 days is only equal to 2 or 3 times the duration of the cell cycle. Furthermore Mendelsohn (21) has pointed out that when the duration of Tc varies widely among the cells, his method of measurement of G.F. is valid only if T_M and T_s are proportional to T_c for all growing cells in the population. This may not be the case in some tumors. Computed Tc should therefore be considered only as an order of magnitude.

In spite of this uncertainty it seems probable that the variations of T_c between patients are larger than the variations of T_s.

The interpretation of the results of patient 5 is much more difficult. The peak value of the labeled mitosis curve reaches only about 50 percent. This is probably due to large fluctuations of the durations of $T_{G_2} + M$ and of T_s, or the ^{3}H-th may not have reached some parts of the tumor. In order to investigate a possible block of cells in G_2, we used Cooper's method and determined by microdensitometry, on a squash preparation, the DNA content of the cells. The results are difficult to interpret because we did not study the caryotype. However, there does not seem to be an accumulation of the cells in a zone corresponding to the G_2 phase. Instead, there is a large number of cells with a DNA content corresponding to the post-mitotic G_1 phase which would confirm the possibility of a very long G_1. The G.F. is surprisingly high. This may be due to an artefact; for instance, the labeled mitosis may be widely divergent for the growing cells of the population. The evaluation of the duration of the cell cycle is based on the G.F. and should be considered with great caution. The labeled mitosis curve suggests large fluctuations on the duration of T_c within the tumor cell population and on the average a long T_c and therefore a long T_{G_1}. All these facts may be, at least in part, due to the many treatments received by this tumor.

An interesting point to emphasize is the comparison between the clinical doubling time of the tumors and the potential doubling time calculated on the hypothesis that all the mitosis give birth to 2 viable cells which remain in the tumor. The results of these comparisons are shown in Table IV. Taking patient 1 as an example, the cell cycle of the tumor cells is 4 days and the growth fraction 30 percent. The potential doubling time is therefore about 10 days. In fact, it took 20 years for the tumor to reach 200–300 grams; that is 3×10^{11} cells, which corresponds to a clinical doubling time of about 10 months. Since the actual doubling time is about 30 times greater than the potential, one must admit that the large majority of the cells die or migrate out of the tumor. The same discrepancy is observed in all the patients. It is probable that in the case of skin neoplasm, exfoliation has been a major factor of cell loss. However, it should be stressed that we have already observed for an experimental tumor, a fibrosarcoma, such a discrepancy when the tumor is growing as a solid tumor (9) as well as when it is growing as an ascitic tumor (11, 12). In both instances the extent of cell loss increases by a large factor when the growth rate is slowing down. Furthermore, the indirect data recently reviewed by Steel (26) and Iversen (13) support the hypothesis of cell loss in the majority of human tumors. In interpreting these data it should be pointed out that cell death is a normal phenomenon and that in a normal tissue, in steady state, the extent of cell loss is 100 percent. However, it is interesting to note that in many tumors a small increase in cell death would result in stabilizing their volume.

In conclusion these studies have: 1. suggested a similarity in cell kinetics of tumors of the same pathological type; 2. shown that in human as well as in animal tumors, the cell cycle may be of about the same length as that in normal tissue or slightly longer. The duration of S phase varied between 10 and 20 h. and the cell cycle between 1 and 4 days. In spite of the heterogeneity of a tumor there does not seem to be a great variation of cell cycle within the tumor; 3. shown that the extent of cell loss is a prominent parameter of human tumor growth rate.

It is obvious that for clinical practice, the labeled mitoses curve is highly inadequate. Which method can give such data if they are to be useful for therapy?

TABLE IV

	Patient 1 (Basal Cell Ca)	Patient 2 (Basal Cell Ca)	Patient 3 (Epidermoid Ca)
Clinical doubling time $T_{1/2}$	10 months	4–6 months	1 month
Potential doubling time $T_p = T_c/GF$	10 days	5–12 days	2–5 days
Extent of cell loss = $1 - \dfrac{T_p}{T_{1/2}}$	97%	90 to 97%	92%

Extent of cell loss in 3 solid tumors (patients with carcinoma of the skin).

Multiple biopsies after injection of IUDR labeled with radioactive iodine may be one of the possibilities.

Another one could be the association of an intravenous injection of IUDR and *in vitro* incubation of a specimen with tritiated thymidine.

A third possibility is prolonged incubation of organotypic tissue in culture. It should be pointed out that by using double labeling, the time required for getting the necessary parameters could be reduced to a few hours. Furthermore microdensitometry could help interpreting the data.

We are now investigating this last possibility. It can be reasonably hoped that within the next few years, one of these methods will be found suitable for routine investigations.

Summary

Four methods have been used for studying the in vivo cell kinetics of human cancers: 1. labeling index—the data are difficult to interpret when the growth fraction and the duration of the S phase are unknown; 2. labeling index, associated with a determination by microdensitometry of the DNA content of the cells. This technique enables a computation of the mean transit time of a cell through $G_0 + G_1$, S and G_2 phases but cannot, by itself, evaluate the duration of these phases or of the growth fraction; 3. mitotic index and estathmokinetic methods; 4. labeled mitoses curve—this method necessitates a large number of biopsies and is therefore limited to a few types of human cancer. On the other hand, its information content is much greater as it furnishes data on all the fundamental parameters of cell kinetics. It has been used by Clarkson *et al.* for studying cases of human ascitic tumors and by Frindel, Malaise and Tubiana for studying five cases of human solid tumors. In 4 of these cases, good data were obtained, T_s varied between 7 and 19 hours and T_c between 1 day and 4 days. In 2 of the patients, the shape of the curve suggests large fluctuations of the durations of the various phases of the cell cycle. For the 5th patient, the peak of the labeled mitosis curve never exceeds 50 percent; this large spread of the durations of the phases of the cell cycle within the tumor cell population may be due to the previous treatments received in this tumor.

There is a large discrepancy between the clinical doubling time and the potential doubling time computed on the basis of T_c and G.F. and assuming no cell loss. This discrepancy seems to indicate that the extent of cell loss is a major parameter of the growth rate of human tumors.

References

1. BASERGA, R.: The relationship of the cell cycle in tumor growth and control of cell diffusion, a review. Cancer Res. 25, 581 (1965).
2. BASERGA, R., HENEGAR, G. C., KISIELESKI, W. E. and LISCO, H.: Uptake of tritiated thymidine by human tumors *in vivo*. Lab. Invest. 11, 360 (1962).
3. BASERGA, R., LISCO, H. and KISIELESKI, W. E.: Tumor induction by radioactive thymidine. Rad. Res. 29, 583 (1966).

4. Breur, K.: Growth rate and radiosensitivity of human tumors. I. Growth rate of human tumors. Europ. J. Cancer 2, 157 (1966).
5. Chone, B. and Frischbier, H. J.: *In vivo* studies mit ³H-thymidine bei Peritoneal-karzinose. Nuclear Medizin, 240 (1962).
6. Clarkson, B., Ota, K., Okhita, T. and O'Connor, A.: Kinetics of proliferation of cancer cells in neoplastic effusions in men. Cancer 18, 1189 (1965).
7. Cooper, E. H., Frank, G. L. and Wright, D. H.: Cell proliferation in Burkitt tumors. Europ. J. Cancer 2, 377 (1966).
8. Dormer, P., Tulinus, H. and Oehlert, W.: Untersuchungen über die Generationszeit DNS-Synthesezeit und Mitosedauer von Zellen der Hyperplastischen Epidermis und des Plattenepithelcarcinoms der Maus nach Methylcholanthrenpinselung. Z. Krebsforsch. 38, 437 (1964).
9. Frindel, E., Malaise, E., Alpen, E. and Tubiana, M.: Kinetics of cell proliferation of an experimental tumor. Cancer Res. 27, 1122 (1967).
10. Frindel, E., Malaise, E. and Tubiana, M.: Cell proliferation kinetics in five solid human tumors. Cancer 22, 611 (1968).
11. Frindel, E. and Tubiana, M.: Durée du cycle cellulaire au cours dela crosance d'une ascite experimentale de la souris C^3H. Compt. Rend. Acad. Sci. (Paris) 265D, 829 (1967).
12. Frindel, E., Vassort, F. and Tubiana, M.: Proliferation kinetics of an experimental ascites tumor of the mouse. Cell and Tissue Kinetics. (In press.)
13. Iversen, O. H.: Kinetics of cellular proliferation and cell loss in human carcinomas. Europ. J. Cancer 3, 389 (1967).
14. Johnson, H. A. and Bond, V. P.: A method of labeling tissue with tritiated thymidine *in vitro* and its use in comparing rates of cell proliferation in duct epithelium fibro adenoma and carcinoma of the human breast. Cancer 14, 639 (1961).
15. Johnson, H. A., Haymaker, W. E., Rubini, J. R., Fliedner, T. M., Bond, V. P., Cronkite, E. P. and Hughes, W. L.: A radioautographic study of a human brain and glioblastoma multiforme after the *in vivo* uptake of tritiated thymidine. Cancer 13, 636 (1960).
16. Johnson, H. A., Rubini, J. R., Cronkite, E. P. and Bond, V. P.: Labeling of human tumor cells *in vivo* by tritiated thymidine. Lab. Invest. 9, 460 (1960).
17. Kissel, P., Duprez, A., Schmitt, J. and Dollander, A.: Autohistoradiographie des cancers digestifs humains *in vivo*. Compt. Rend. Soc. Biol. [Paris] 159, 1400 (1965).
18. Lipkin, M., Bell, B. and Cherlock, P.: Cell proliferation kinetics in the gastro-intestinal tract of man. I. Cell removal in rectum and colon. J. Clin. Invest. 42, 767 (1963).
19. Lieb, L. M. and Lisco, H.: *In vitro* uptake of tritiated thymidine by carcinoma of the human colon. Cancer Res. 26, 733 (1966).
20. Malaise, E., Frindel, E. and Tubiana, M.: Cinetique de la proliferation cellulaire de deux tumeurs humaines etudiee grace a l'injection de thymidine tritiee. Compt. Rend. Acad. Sci. (Paris) 264D, 1104 (1967).
21. Mendelsohn, M. L.: Autoradiographic analysis of cell proliferation in spontaneous breast cancer of C3H mouse. III. The growth fraction. J. Natl. Cancer Inst. 28, 1015 (1962).
22. Mewissen, D. J.: Induction de leucemies chez la souris C 57 B1, au moyens de thymidine tritiee. Compt. Rend. Soc. Biol. (Paris) 159, 1005 (1965).
23. Rajewsky, M. F.: Zell Proliferation in normalen und malignen Gewben: ³H-thymidin einbau *in vitro* unter Standardbedingungen. Biophysik. 3, 65 (1966).

24. REFSUM, S. B. and BENDAL, P.: Cell loss in malignant tumors in man. Europ. J. Cancer 3, 235 (1967).
25. SINCLAIR, W. K. and MORTON, R. A.: X-ray sensitivity during the cell generation cycle of cultured Chinese hamster cells. Rad. Res. 29, 450 (1966).
26. STEELE, G. G.: Cell loss as a factor in the growth rate of human tumors. Europ. J. Cancer 3, 381 (1967).
27. STEELE, G. G. and BENSTED, J. D. L.: *In vitro* studies of cell proliferation in tumors. Europ. J. Cancer 1, 275 (1965).
28. TERASIMA, T. and TOLMACH, L. J.: Variation in several responses of HeLa cells to x-irradiation during the division cycle. Biophys. J. 3, 11 (1963).
29. TITUS, J. L. and SHORTER, R. G.: Labeling of human tumors with tritiated thymidine. Arch. Path. 79, 324 (1965).
30. WHITMORE, G. F., GULYAS, S. and BOTOND, J.: Radiation sensitivity throughout the cycle and its relationship to recovery. *In:* Cellular Radiation Biology. Williams and Wilkins, Baltimore, 423 (1965).
31. WOLBERG, W. H. and BROWN, R. R.: Autoradiographic studies of *in vitro* incorporation of uridine and thymidine by human tumor tissue. Cancer Research 22, 1113 (1962).

Summary of Symposium on
Normal and Malignant Cell Growth *

HARVEY M. PATT

Laboratory of Radiobiology
University of California
San Francisco, California

In this Symposium, we have come to grips with the nature of cancer growth, cytokinetic variables and controls that may be operative during tumor development. One face of the Symposium has been turned toward normal growth, another toward abnormal growth. But, in the fashion of Janus, the two faces are really quite alike in many respects even if they appear to be turned in opposite directions. Although it is my purpose in these concluding remarks to weave together information and ideas that have been presented here, it is not my intention to cover all that has been put forth even if I could do so. Because of this limitation, I ask the indulgence of the authors and the audience. I wish rather to focus mainly on the cytokinetic basis of tumor growth and to do so in relation to the behavior of normal cell systems. Lamerton really summarized the essence of this Symposium in his introductory lecture when he reminded us that the behavior of cells in organized populations, as well as that of individuals in a society, is determined by properties of the organization as well as by characteristics of the components.

Throughout this Symposium, growth has been used primarily in the context of an increase in cell number, not in cell size. Thus, in growing systems the birth of cells must exceed the loss of cells, whereas in typical cell renewal systems such as bone marrow and intestines in the adult organism, the two must be equivalent. Cell renewal systems are often referred to as steady state systems and while this is appropriate, it is important to recognize that growing systems may, theoretically, also reflect a steady state. In point of fact, however, the growth of cell populations rarely, if ever, follows a constant course. The growth rate usually shifts in a characteristic fashion with times appropriate to the particular population: from rapid growth to slow growth to no growth and even on occasion to negative growth. This general pattern is seen in the growth of a fetus or a liver or a tumor. The more or less progressive decrease in growth rate with time has been described by Laird (1), McCredie et al. (2) and others as a Gompertzian function. The Gompertz equation expresses exponential growth when a population is small; it expresses an

---

* Personal studies noted here were performed under the auspices of the U.S. Atomic Energy Commission.

exponentially increasing growth retardation as a population enlarges. Other mathematical formulations, reviewed recently by Mendelsohn (3), may also be appropriate,
but it is doubtful whether any unitary growth function accurately reflects the dynamics of growth throughout the history of a normal or tumor system. The temporary
regression of a tumor is a case in point.

Whether we are concerned with an *in vivo* population that is growing or merely
being replaced, it is essential to recognize that the population does not represent an
isolated class of cells. Rather, it represents a system with heterogeneity, cell interactions, and a certain probability of transition from one cell class to another. Unlike
a normal cell renewal system, a tumor system is not subject to the constraints of
the steady state; moreover, there are fewer restrictions of possible transitions from
one functional state to another and across the boundary of the system. Accordingly,
more parameters are required to describe a tumor system, or for that matter any
growing system, than a similarly constituted renewal system.

All of the speakers have referred in one way or another to the compartmentaliza-
tion of cell systems or the proliferation process itself. Apropos of the former, it is
agreed that every system consists of progenitor elements or stem cells. In the termi-
nology of Lajtha, stem cells are responsive to "self" with proliferation balancing the
outflow for differentiation. Since this concept makes it necessary to postulate a very
large number of stem cell generations in order to satisfy the lifetime requirements
of rapidly turning-over systems, an alternative possibility based on clonal succession
has been proposed by Kay (4). Because of the exponential nature of the clonal succession hypothesis, many fewer generations would satisfy the requirements for differentiation. This would, of course, be consistent with the inference by Hayflick (5)
that all normal mammalian cells, unlike tumor cells, have a limited proliferative
capacity.

Be that as it may, our concepts of the unseen stem cell have broadened considerably in recent years and we are now confronted with degrees of "stemness." Lajtha has pointed out that stem cells, at least of the hematopoietic variety,
may represent a heterogeneous population with unipotential as well as pluripotential
components and with variable proliferative capacity. Assays of the presumptive stem
cells often lead to different results. It is of more than passing interest that repeated
irradiation results in a greater depression of colony-forming capacity than of the
erythropoietin response. Does the colony-forming cell lead to the erythropoietin sensitive cell which represents a secondary stem cell? Is the colony-forming cell involved
in normal hemopoiesis? What is the significance of the erythropoietin response?
Curiously, according to Brambel and Brecher (6), continuously irradiated rats may
respond normally to bleeding and hypoxia at a time when they apparently respond
very poorly to large doses of erythropoietin.

Bond noted that there is a rapid and extensive efflux of colony-forming cells from
a shielded site. Some CFU are presumably always circulating but the magnitude of
this early effect surprises me. The normal renewal of marrow seems to be subject
more to a pull from the periphery than to a push owing to proliferation. There is
certainly no deficit of differentiating and functional cells within a half hour of
irradiation. He indicated also that there are late changes in CFU in heavily exposed

areas and stressed the importance of the microenvironment, *e.g.*, stroma, blood vessels, as well as the matter of cell kinetics in the overall response. I shall return to this point later.

Apropos of the CFU, it has been estimated that there are some 2×10^5 CFU in the marrow of a mouse. But with a very low turnover rate of CFU (10^{-2} cells per cell per hour), this number is at least a hundred-fold less than the number needed to maintain peripheral erythrocyte and granulocyte levels (7). Of course, we can save the situation if we postulate that there is an intermediate stem cell as well. The fact is that we just do not know.

It may be important to recall that virtually all assays of stem-type cells are performed under conditions that tend to promote maximum proliferation of a population with a presumably low steady state proliferation rate. The picture may be somewhat analogous to evaluation of the proliferative capacity of an irradiated liver after partial hepatectomy. The point is that the recognizable effect of small radiation doses on the progenitor pool may be less than anticipated unless such doses also promote greatly increased stem cell turnover.

The integrity of a tumor also depends on a stem-type cell, that is a cell with long term reproductive capacity. Hauschka (8) suggested many years ago that only a fraction of a tumor cell population was capable of normal and regular mitosis. The constancy of a certain chromosomal modality or "germ line" through many transplant generations was adduced as supportive evidence for the existence of tumor stem cells. More recent chromosomal studies by Ford (9) suggest that there may be a sequence of stem cell lines during the growth of reticular neoplasms. Hence, even in a tumor cell population there may be more than one germ line with the possibility of clonal succession complicating interpretation of the growth kinetics.

In a cell renewal system, the induction of differentiation which leads to the formation of functional cells is usually followed by one or more mitoses. The mean number of proliferative steps differs in the different renewal systems. There may be 2 to 3 divisions on the average in the intestinal crypts and 4 to 6 in the bone marrow with a consequent difference in stem cell amplification or clone size. It is important to note that not all the cells that are capable of proliferation may in fact divide. On the other hand, the cells that divide may do so at a very rapid rate, the cell cycle for intestinal and bone marrow cells in the rodent being about 10 hours. Cancer cells in the rodent rarely proliferate more rapidly than this. Indeed, we might recall the suggestion put forth by Rowley that antibody-forming cells may have a cell cycle of only 5 to 8 hours.

Once the capacity for proliferation seems to be lost, the completion of differentiation is a rather straightforward process in normal systems. It should be pointed out that proliferation and differentiation are not necessarily bound together; in other words, a given number of divisions is not a requirement for differentiation to a functional state. Prescott suggested that differentiation was characterized not only by development of a functional state but also by a progressive decrease in proliferation rate, *i.e.*, lengthening of the cell cycle. I do not believe that the picture in gut and bone marrow is indicative of the latter. In these tissues, there is a rather sharp transition from a proliferative to a non-proliferative state.

Studies of tumor growth kinetics as presented here by Baserga, Bertalanffy, Mauer, Clarkson and Tubiana are consistent with the concept that the malignant transformation leads to an anomalous cell development in which enhanced proliferative capacity is incidental to a basic impairment of differentiation, or loss of differentiation, along with a failure of growth control. It is now recognized, and amply documented here, that the cancer cell as such does not necessarily proliferate at a particularly rapid rate. Thus, the expansive growth that is characteristic of cancer may reflect mainly an accumulation of proliferating cells rather than an increase in cell proliferation rate.

What are the normal stimuli for differentiation? Why do tumor cells more closely resemble embryonic or undifferentiated or dedifferentiated cells? One does not really know the answers, but Siminovitch and Axelrad (10) have reviewed this problem recently and have concluded that the process of differentiation and the maintenance of differentiation are indeed intimately related to cell-cell interactions. Although there are many examples of the importance of the spatial configuration of cells and of the flow of information among cells, we know very little about the nature of the interactions. If the *in situ* configuration of tumor cells and normal cells can be duplicated in the sponge matrix culture described by Leighton, or in the plasma clot system of Sanford, these techniques should be useful in the exploration under controlled conditions of the role of associative factors, and of the microenvironment generally, in cancer growth.

Aside from the social behavior of cells as a factor in differentiation, are there any clues in the biochemical events during the proliferative cell cycle? In normal cells DNA, RNA and protein synthesis are closely correlated in time. According to Seed (11, 12), there is an uncoupling of DNA and protein synthesis in malignant cells but the significance of this is not clear. Factors that may control the orderly progress of the various biosynthetic reactions have been alluded to by Prescott. It would appear that the crucial decision to recycle, to decycle or to differentiate is probably taken soon after mitosis, at least in cells with a fairly short G_1. There is, I think, a good example of this in the work of Okazaki and Holtzer (13), in which the presumptive myogenic cells withdrew from the cell cycle and began to translate for myosin a short time after mitosis. Studies in our laboratory by Lala (14) indicate that suspension of the cycle in ascites tumor cells also occurs upon completion of mitosis, not during S or G_2. Such cells can re-enter the cycle almost immediately after retransplantation. Decycling has been reported to occur in G_2 in some normal tissues (15); however, the evidence for this could also be indicative of G_2 variability rather than of overt decycling. In this connection, we may recall Baserga's observation that the G_2 period in Ehrlich ascites tumor cells is more sensitive to caloric restriction than other phases of the cycle. It seems reasonable to assume that recycling (G_1 to S) or decycling (G_1 to G_0) depends upon the presence or absence of an "initiator" soon after completion of the mitotic process. The induction of differentiation would require a separate mechanism so that a cell could recycle or decycle as is, or recycle or decycle with differentiation. Apparently the cancer cell has a greater probability of recycling and a lesser probability of differentiating to a non-proliferative state. Why this is so is another matter. Approaches to carcinogenic

mechanisms in relation to the cell cycle, as described by Reiskin, may perhaps shed
some light on this crucial question.

Mauer has considered the transitions between proliferating and non-proliferating
cells in acute lymphoblastic leukemia. Of particular interest is the suggestion that
small non-proliferative leukemic cells, derived from the larger proliferative variety,
may re-enter the cell cycle and serve as a nidus for continued growth.

The question of decycling and recycling is, of course, germane to the question of
whether or not there is a G_0 state. I agree that the distinction between G_0 and a
long G_1 is difficult to demonstrate. But it is important conceptually and should not
be dismissed as a matter of semantics. My colleague, Lala (16), has shown that ascites
tumor cells apparently do leave the cycle in a readily reversible way. He showed this
by blocking cells with colcemide, then labeling first with $C^{14}TdR$ and then at intervals with H^3TdR. If decrease in growth fraction were due to a lengthening of
G_1, which is ordinarily very brief in these cells, there should have been a continued
influx of cells into S, demonstrable with double labeling. There was none over a
period of a few hours, which we can interpret as evidence for a G_0 state.

Bertalanffy has pointed out that neoplasms can proliferate faster than the corresponding tissue of origin, but that normal renewal systems may show an even
greater proliferative capacity than tumors during certain physiologic or regenerative
states. To understand how this may occur, it is necessary to consider the system
aspects of normal and tumor cell populations. In respect to its kinetic behavior, a
tumor system may be taken to consist of proliferating and non-proliferating compartments. Cells may flow in either direction, i.e., proliferating cells may become
non-proliferating and vice versa, and cells may be lost at any point in the system.
The growth fraction, that is, the proportion of the total population that is proliferating, may vary from place to place at a given time, for example, from
periphery to center of a solid tumor, and from time to time at a given place. Because of the impairment of differentiation to a mature functional state, it is expected that the growth fraction would be greater in a hepatoma than in normal
liver, or in an intestinal neoplasm than in normal intestinal mucosa, or in an acute
leukemia than in normal marrow. Unless the increased growth fraction was out-
weighed by a lengthened proliferative cycle of the cancer cell relative to the normal
cell, it is easy to see why such neoplasms would manifest a greater cell birth rate
than the normal tissue. But, as discussed by Bertalanffy, this may not obtain in those
instances where increased demands are placed upon a normal system. I would like to
suggest, parenthetically, that we use the term "birth rate" to designate the cell flux
and "proliferation rate" to signify the rate at which a cell that is in cycle is dividing,
the latter being given by the reciprocal of the cell cycle time.

Lesher's paper on intestine and Grisham's and Bucher's on liver provide good
examples of the compensatory ability of normal and conditional renewal systems.
During recovery from radiation damage, a very high rate of cell production can be
achieved in the intestine mainly by a reduced rate of withdrawal of crypt cells and
an increase in growth fraction, although an increase in proliferation rate is con-

tributory. Indeed, the histological appearance of the disorganized hyperplastic crypts during the regenerative phase may be suggestive of neoplasia.

Lipkin noted that the so called cut-off region for proliferation in crypts changed in disease states. With precancerous lesions, there was an increase in the proliferative zone, which is, of course, consistent with the general notion of an increase in growth fraction.

It is well known that the growth rate of tumors is not unyielding. With transplantable tumors particularly, there is with time a quite characteristic decrease in growth rate. There is good reason to think that the growth rate at any instant is strongly dependent upon the size of the tumor cell population or tumor mass. Several studies with ascites tumors and solid tumors indicate that the growth fraction decreases as the tumor mass increases. But this *per se* is insufficient to account for the entire growth deceleration and it is thought that a decrease in proliferation rate (*i.e.*, a lengthening of the cell cycle), and an increase in rate of cell loss may be contributing factors.

A progressive decrease in proliferation rate has been shown to occur in an ascites tumor and it is possible that the same events may influence both the cell cycle prolongation and cell cycle suspension (17). It is of interest that the probability of recycling in an ascites tumor declines with an increase in the cell cycle time. Whether a similar effect on the cell cycle occurs in a solid tumor is open to question, as reported by Tubiana and his colleagues, although they also find prolongation of the cell cycle in the ascites form of the same tumor. Apropos of this, it should be noted that a gradual prolongation of the cell cycle time and its components, associated with a decrease in growth fraction, has been seen in liver cells in growing rats and also in cultured Chinese hamster cells (18, 19).

The possible difference in cell cycle lengthening between an ascites tumor and a solid tumor may be a reflection of a difference in the organization of these two forms of tumor tissue. An ascites tumor is, of course, more homogeneous than a solid tumor and, because of the continuous mixing of the ascites, any given area should be representative of all areas. There is much greater variability in a solid tumor where proliferating cells are located mainly in the periphery, presumably because of better vascularization. As a solid tumor enlarges, the number of peripheral cells decreases relative to the total number. A meaningful comparison is possible only if the sample that is studied is representative of the tumor as a whole. Representative sampling may be difficult to achieve in a solid tumor even when several randomly selected sections are analyzed. It is conceivable that the peripheral cells may show little, if any, change in cell cycle, or even in growth fraction, until there is a general deterioration of the physiological milieu. In this connection, it is noteworthy that there is also little change in the growth kinetics of an ascites tumor when the ascites is aspirated at frequent intervals. While it is tempting to suggest a parallelism between the repeatedly aspirated ascites tumor and the peripherally located cells of a solid tumor, I have been told by Lamerton of the work of Tannock which indicates that there seems to be little change in distribution of cell cycle times with distance from blood vessels in a mouse tumor. The growth fraction, however, decreased markedly with distance. The same picture occurs in regenerating liver, as described by Grisham.

The ^{125}I-IUdR method described by Dethlefson will not resolve the question of the relative significance of a change in growth fraction and perhaps in cell cycle time as a solid tumor enlarges. It should, however, provide a useful *in situ* method for evaluation of DNA (*i.e.*, cell) accumulation and loss during the course of tumor growth. Change in rate of cell loss appears to be relatively unimportant in the Ehrlich ascites tumor but it is known to be a factor of considerable consequence in a solid tumor. The importance of cell loss in human tumors has been emphasized by Tubiana; this follows from the apparent discrepancy between theoretical and actual doubling times. This is borne out also in recent analyses by others.

An intimate knowledge of the growth pattern is pertinent to the application of various therapeutic procedures. For example, are cycling cells more or less sensitive than non-cycling cells to radiation and chemotherapeutic agents? The papers by Philips and Whitmore suggest that the former may be so, but not necessarily. Then there is also the apparent enigma of the small lymphocyte. This cell is very sensitive but when it is transformed by a mitogen and enters the cell cycle, it is apparently less sensitive. Why this is so is not known.

If we irradiate a tumor or apply a chemotherapeutic agent, will surviving cells manifest a more rapid growth by analogy to the behavior of an ascites tumor with repeated aspiration? If there is a faster regrowth of the residual tumor mass, will a progressive shortening of the intervals between application of therapeutic agents lead to a greater effect? These are some of the practical questions that have emerged from the more recent studies of cancer cell kinetics.

Finally, I should say a word about regulatory mechanisms. We have, I think, touched on this topic only in a rather cursory way. Perhaps this is appropriate because there is really little that can be said about the way in which the initiation of proliferation and differentiation in mammalian cells is regulated. Aside from the molecular aspects of regulation at the cellular level, there is also the question of system aspects of regulation. Do crypt cells proliferate because cells fall off of the villus? And if so, what is the nature of the feedback? We know a little more about the bone marrow, mainly because of erythropoietin, but even here we have only a glimmer about the control mechanisms. This applies also to antibody-forming cells, as described by Talmage. Experience with liver regeneration points to the importance of a humoral mechanism but one which is still not very well defined even though it has been many years since the possibility was put forth.

Before the advent of DNA labels and our present kinetic bent, we were inclined to view normal systems and tumor systems in terms of micro-structure and function. With our increasing sophistication in the handling of mammalian cells, as seen for example in the methods for synchronizing cells described by Sinclair, we have become increasingly preoccupied with cell kinetics. And there is a tendency to think of events at the tissue and organismal level as first-order effects of events at the cellular level. It is clear, however, that we have a lot to learn about the interactions of cells and about the influence of their environment in the regulation of growth.

References

1. LAIRD, A. K.: Dynamics of tumor growth. Brit. J. Cancer 18, 490 (1964).

2. McCREDIE, J. A., INCH, W. R., KRUUV, J., and WATSON, T. A.: The rate of tumor growth in animals. Growth 29, 331 (1965).

3. MENDELSOHN, M. L.: Cell Proliferation. L. F. Lamerton and R. J. M. Fry (eds.), Blackwell, Oxford (1963).

4. KAY, H. E. M.: How many cell-generations? Lancet II, 418 (1965).

5. HAYFLICK, L.: The limited *in vitro* lifetime of human diploid cell strains. Exp. Cell Res. 37, 614 (1965).

6. BRAMBEL, C. and BRECHER, G.: Personal communication, 1968.

7. PATT, H. M.: The radiobiology of cell renewal systems. *In:* Effects of Radiation on Cellular Proliferation and Differentiation, IAEA, Monaco (in press).

8. HAUSCHKA, T. S.: Cell population studies on mouse ascites tumors. Trans. N.Y. Acad. Sci. 16, 64 (1953).

9. FORD, C. E. and CLARKE, C. M.: Cytogenetic evidence of clonal proliferation in primary reticular neoplasms. Canadian Cancer Res. Conf. 5, 129 (1963).

10. SIMINOVITCH, L. and AXELRAD, A. A.: Cell-cell interactions *in vitro:* Their relation to differentiation and carcinogenesis. Canadian Cancer Res. Conf. 5, 149 (1963).

11. SEED, J.: The synthesis of DNA, RNA, and nuclear protein in normal and tumor strain cells III. Mouse ascites tumor cells. J. Cell Biol. 28, 257 (1966).

12. SEED, J.: The synthesis of DNA, RNA, and nuclear protein in normal and tumor strain cells IV. HeLa tumor strain cells. J. Cell Biol. 28, 263 (1966).

13. OKAZAKI, K., and HOLTZER, H.: Myogenesis: fusion, myosin synthesis, and the mitotic cycle. Proc. Nat. Acad. Sci. (USA) 56, 1484 (1966).

14. LALA, P. K., and PATT, H. M.: Cell turnover and mammalian radiosensitivity. Cell and Tissue Kinetics 1, 81 (1968).

15. GELFANT, S.: Methods in Cell Physiology. D. Prescott (ed.), Academic Press, New York, Vol. 2, 359 (1966).

16. LALA, P. K.: Cytokinetic control mechanisms in Ehrlich ascites tumour growth. *In:* Effects of Radiation on Cellular Proliferation and Differentiation, IAEA, Monaco (in press).

17. LALA, P. K. and PATT, H. M.: Cytokinetic analysis of tumor growth. Proc. Nat. Acad. Sci. (USA) 56, 1735 (1966).

18. POST, J., and HOFFMAN, J.: Changes in the replication times and patterns of the liver cell during the life of the rat. Exptl. Cell Res. 36, 111 (1964).

19. HAHN, G.: Personal communication (1968).

Round-Table Discussion

Symposium on Normal and Malignant Cell Growth

DR. SWIFT: If there is to be a discussion and I consider my part to be largely one of a catalyst trying to get people discussing among themselves, it has to deal with several problems raised in this symposium. The obvious thing that most of us have talked about so far is the mitotic cycle. Dr. Prescott, who is always a good place to start because he likes to make dogmatic statements, thinks there is no such thing as a prolonged G_2 in the mitotic cycle; that is, if cells stop in the cycle, they are arrested in the G_1 period. Then, there is the question which was mentioned by Dr. Lamerton, whether there is a G_0 or not.

I would say from my experience that there can be a prolonged G_2, at least in some plant tissues where we know very well that there are tissues that have a 4C amount of DNA so that you can say that they are tetraploid although you can't see their chromosomes to count them. When you stimulate them to divide by wounding, they divide into two diploid cells without any intervening period of DNA synthesis. This has been shown by E. Rasch, for example, in our laboratory with plant tissues, and S. Gelfant showed very much the same thing in mouse epidermis. Did he not, David?

DR. PRESCOTT: What a challenging way you put it. I am very much aware of Gelfant's work, and I accept his conclusions that there is a population in the epithelium that stays in G_2 for a relatively long time, according to Gelfant for as long as 48 hours. But this is true for a relatively small part of the population, and there are apparently fairly strict limits on how long these cells can stay in G_2. They can linger on in G_2 for many hours, but nothing like as long as is possible with G_1. We did some work ourselves on G_2 cells in the esophagus and confirmed Gelfant's extended G_2. But I don't think the fact that you have a longer G_2 period interferes with the generality that I made that the normal arrest of the cell cycle takes place in G_1. I would like to exclude any mention of such dramatic or traumatic things as toxic substances. I know that you can arrest cells in other parts of the cycle with poisons of one sort or another, but I would exclude these because they are not normal.

DR. LESHER: How about after irradiation? Isn't it usually thought that cells are blocked in G_2 for periods of time depending upon the dose level? Cells which are in mitosis either die or they struggle on through in three-quarters of an hour to an hour, and then there are no mitotic figures for a varying period. After 300 R, the block is for about 4 hours. This is true for the intestine. After 1000 R, the block is between 10 and 12 hours. After irradiation, if you study the generation cycle by the labeled mitosis method, you seldom, even at low doses, get a 100 percent plateau so there always are unlabeled cells in mitosis. The cells labeled immediately before irradiation break out from the G_2 block at approximately the same time as the unlabeled ones so even after 300 R you have 50 percent labeled and 50 percent non-labeled cells. I think this indicates the block is in G_2 cells.

DR. PRESCOTT: Yes, I would put these in the drastic-treatment category.

DR. LESHER: Well, how about low temperature? You can make G_2 hours or days long.

DR. PRESCOTT: Yes, but you also extend the other periods proportionally if you lower the temperature. I would like to mention certain plant embryos. I took more than my allotted time so I didn't have time to cite the work of Davidson who is now at Case Western Reserve who says that up to 1 percent of the cells in the plant embryo appears to be arrested in G_2. The other 99 percent of the cells in the plant embryo are in G_1 using thymidine labeling followed by labeled mitosis as the criterion. One would have to concede that there are some possibilities of expanding G_2 and arresting cells in G_2. Certainly it is much easier for a cell to be arrested in G_1.

DR. SWIFT: Is there a G_0?

DR. PRESCOTT: G_0 is mysterious and if you add the two mysteries do you still have two mysteries or do you now have just one mystery?

DR. SWIFT: We are going back to the holy grail now.

DR. PRESCOTT: I myself have not yet been compelled to use G_0 although I appreciate the concept.

DR. LAJTHA: If you arrest cells in a late G_1 and later increase proliferation, there should be an immediate increase in labeling index or in DNA specific activity. If you have a set amount of time which has to elapse before the cells can get into an S period, which means that they have been arrested in early G_1 or G_0, whichever the case may be, they have to go through a minimum G_1 before they can enter S. Of course there are exceptions, but in most systems that I know of there is this period of 6–15 hours, depending upon the system, before DNA specific activity can increase. I am referring primarily to systems where the majority of the cells are in this inhibited state. And, in fact, this is really what gave the idea that G_0 might exist in the regenerating liver even allowing for the very intensive RNA synthesis occurring about 2 hours after partial hepatectomy. You still have to wait some times 10–12 hours before you get an increase in DNA synthesis.

DR. LAMERTON: I think it is very interesting, but if you take the conditional renewal systems in the liver, thyroid, and salivary gland and stimulate them in various ways, it always takes about 18 hours before you start DNA synthesis. This is very much Dr. Baserga's field, but I think in these cases you really have got a G_1.

DR. PRESCOTT: You mean you really have G_0?

DR. LAMERTON: No. In these particular cells, as far as we know, the interval between successive mitoses may be hundreds of days. If you stimulte proliferation by partial hepatectomy, then some 15–20 hours later the cells begin to go into synthesis. Something must be happening during those 15 hours which I would have called a true G_1.

DR. LAJTHA: Are you trying to imply that before they were in G_0 and after hepatectomy the cells enter G_1?

DR. LAMERTON: If you say that of liver cells, why not of more rapidly dividing cells? Dr. Prescott, did you mean that you regard the interval between mitosis and synthesis, except for a very short time just before synthesis, as essentially a G_0 with cells waiting to be triggered into G_1?

DR. PRESCOTT: No. I don't accept the concept of G_0. I have not felt compelled to use it. Since G_1 is a mystery, I'm satisfied to call that period G_1 for the moment. When cells are arrested for some time, for example, in small lymphocytes arrested in a pre-DNA synthesis, it takes 15–18 hours after stimulation before you can get them back into DNA synthesis. But if you let these small lymphocytes which turn into blast cells go through one period of DNA synthesis and come around to G_1 again, then the G_1 period is only 6 hours or so. Why is this G_1 period 6 hours when the first G_1 period was 18 hours? So something extra had to be done in the initial rescue or reversal of these cells that does not have to be done in subsequent cycles.

DR. SWIFT: Not only that but haven't Drs. Hecht and Potter shown that there is a suppression of DNA synthesis during this 18-hour period? I think that the early period of liver regeneration is very different from a normal G_1 and the cell of a normal tissue is perhaps something different, as Dr. Bucher has studied. Would either of you like to talk about the preparatory steps, Dr. Bucher?

DR. BUCHER: I don't really want to talk about the preparatory steps because I don't think we know enough about them. RNA synthesis in liver is very active all the time; and when you turn on regeneration, it goes up by 50 or 100 percent which really isn't much in terms of what happens with DNA synthesis, for example, and many other changes must occur. But I wonder if this isn't a slightly semantic argument and if we knew what the biochemistry was, we wouldn't have to worry about what was G_1 or G_0. We would just say that this happens and then that happens. It seems to me that this is really the crux of the matter.

DR. GRISHAM: I would like to add that many of the things that happen in the hepatocyte between the time of partial hepatectomy and the time DNA synthesis occurs may actually be non-sequitur as far as the cell at the periphery is concerned. We studied the incorporation of orotic acid into RNA in the isolated perfused livers, and by perfusing intact liver at a high perfusion pressure, a pressure double that occurs normally, you can induce a burst of RNA synthesis and increased incorporation of orotic acid in RNA and that approximates the values obtained following hepatectomy. Yet, from other experiments we know that this is not correlated with DNA synthesis. If you keep the tissue perfusion level at the normal level, the 2-hour RNA synthesis does not go up. I think many of the events that occur during the early time after partial hepatectomy can be mimicked by other manipulations in the liver.

DR. PRESCOTT: It is always easier for me to explain things to myself if I can draw a picture. Part of the problem of bringing the cell out of retirement and back into the cell cycle hinges on the fact that when it gave up the cell cycle it also gave up a number of things that it would have kept. For example, we know from the work of Littlefield and other people and some of our own work that enzymes, like DNA polymerase, thymidylic synthetase and thymidine kinase are kept in G_1 in a cell that is constantly cycling. The synthesis of these enzymes does not form the basis of G_1 because it is not living in G_1 in order to make enzymes that are necessary to make DNA. When the cell leaves the cycle and wanders off down some other trail like a small lymphocyte, does it lose thymidine kinase, thymidylic synthetase and DNA polymerase? Now it is called back, and it would have to retrace this step in order to get back on the track and proceed; maybe that's G_0.

DR. SWIFT: Are there any other comments on this subject? It really doesn't matter what you call it as long as you know what it is, and we don't yet. This brings up another crucial point that everyone talked about; namely, the initiation of DNA synthesis. It certainly is a unique thing about this system that you can stop it in G_1. As Dr. Lesher said, you can stop cells in G_2 in the case of radiation and many mitotic inhibitors, but stopping this process during the S period is extremely difficult. I only know of perhaps one case which is in a polyploid nucleus of protozoa where one could possibly stop a cell in the process of DNA synthesis. I suspect that once the beginning of the S period is reached many cells proceed on through.

What about the initiation of DNA synthesis? Of course, this is the crux of a lot of problems. I think we can say that certain factors in the initiation are cytoplasmic in origin because in almost all multinucleate or syncytial cells the DNA synthesis in all nuclei goes on almost simultaneously. This is true, for example, in the slime mold *Physarium* and in binucleate cells of the liver. On the other hand, there are the examples which Dr. Prescott mentioned, where DNA synthesis is known to be under precise chromosomal control. For example, Stubblefield showed three kinds of chromosome regions, euchromatin, autosome heterochromatin and sex heterochromatin where DNA initiation is early, intermediate and late. So there must be factors associated with the chromosome itself, in addition to those in the cytoplasm, which control the initiation of DNA synthesis. Does anyone have comments on this point? If you look at a slime mold, as studied by Dr. Rusch, for example, you can see 2,000 nuclei all dividing at once.

DR. LAJTHA: That is quite true. I think there is perhaps a very good reason why the interruption of the cycle cannot occur in S and that is that you are duplicating the genome at that time and at any stage a certain part of the genome is not double. Obviously, there is a time sequence of genome duplication and from the various examples in the mammalian systems where we know the time sequence of chromosome duplication. It is the most logical conclusion to think that in evolution there was a sequence in which it was possible to duplicate gene number one before gene number two, and I can't magine that halfway through this process the cell could be held up with half its genome duplicated. It is a very vulnerable situation.

DR. LIPKIN: I would like to add a few comments to what Dr. Lajtha has just said. I think he touched on the question of why interruption in S can be so disastrous to cells. I think he gave a genetic explanation, but I wonder if this isn't the same kind of problem that Dr. Bucher was talking about. It seems to me that we simply don't know enough about the enzymatic organization of the replicating system to be able to know whether the death is due to an imbalance in genetic factors or whether it is due to a change in the actual mechanics of the replication. A slight interruption in time of events may release certain very dangerous enzymes out of kilter. I think we should remember that the nucleus is filled with enzymes that would kill us all promptly if they weren't kept in check. The cytoplasm is also filled with hydrolases of RNA. One wonders why they are there; there is much speculation and some good information. Nevertheless, one could intuitively feel that they probably play some sort of a role in the replicative process and that during the course of the replication things are in a very unstable state without having to assume that the imbalance is necessarily on a genetic basis. I simply think we don't understand why, for example, crypt cells will die so quickly and other cells will take a little longer to die, but I think this is certainly worthy of exploration. Do you?

DR. PHILIPS: I should defer to Dr. Lesher's more expert knowledge of the proliferative field but if you compare the response of rapidly dividing cells in tissue culture to agents, like hydroxyurea and cystosine arabinoside or methotrexate, it is quite clear that there are many examples of cells which will live for many hours with DNA synthesis completely arrested. If you don't wait too long, you can get these cells back to the division state again just by taking away the offending agent. Some will go as long as a full generation time before they will lose reproductive capacity. It is also quite clear, *in vivo*, that the response of different proliferating cells varies to the same type of insult. For instance, it is very difficult to demonstrate death of cells in the middle of liver regeneration with doses that produce such a long block of DNA synthesis as the one in the intestine. Obviously, there must be something different about stability of the regenerating liver cell to be able to withstand such a long period of DNA synthesis inhibition. There is a stability which is not present in the crypt cells. It plays a role in determining the susceptibility of different proliferative cells to the same biochemical inhibition.

DR. SWIFT: Now, could we add the spleen to the intestine and the liver, Dr. Talmage?

DR. TALMAGE: I don't have any answers; I just want to ask a related question. Do you have any idea why the small lymphocyte, which is partly or completely a resting cell, is probably the most sensitive cell in the body to x-radiation?

DR. PHILIPS: The small lymphocyte doesn't seem to break down after giving agents like hydroxyurea so that an inhibitor of DNA synthesis is not likely to damage the small lymphocyte. At least we did not see it in our rats and mice.

DR. PRESCOTT: Let me refer back to the replicon of my hypothesis of organization. It is true in bacteria, and evidently in DNA viruses, that the chromosome is one replicon and once it is initiated to replicate, it continues to the end unless you do something very drastic to interrupt it, and it doesn't require RNA or protein to continue. But of course that is quite different from something like a mammalian cell which has many replicons which start at different times during S and so you constantly need protein synthesis during S. I'm not satisfied with any of the explanations of why a cell, like a mammalian cell, cannot stop in S. Let us say that you stopped protein synthesis during S in the mammalian cell and all that would happen would be that the replicons that are in replication would finish and no new ones would start, and I can't see how that would be uncomfortable except on the basis of genetic dosage that you have any balance in genetic dosage. Unless there is something susceptible about DNA when it presents itself for replication, it changes its molecular configuration by exchanging off some of its proteins and adopting new proteins or it opens up at points so that replication can begin. It changes somehow into a delicate condition, and it is therefore very susceptible to accidental damage. But this isn't very satisfactory. Again, we don't know enough to say anything very intelligent.

DR. SWIFT: Yes, I think this is probably our theme song for the moment: The control of DNA synthesis is certainly going to turn out to be an extremely complicated thing which cannot lie, as I said before, exclusively in the DNA molecule itself. One of the most beautiful examples of what one might call environmental control of DNA synthesis has to do with late replicating heterochromatin of the X chromosome, which is late replicating in all of the cells of the body, except the spermatogonial cells where it replicates with the autosomes as shown very clearly now by Nicklas and Jacqua.

DR. PRESCOTT: Well, to observe a cell in cleavage where both X's replicate in synchrony relatively early, but about the time that the cells go into G_1 one of the X's becomes heterochromatic and changes its period of DNA synthesis. We know it is the same DNA; it is the same cell and there are 2 changes that come along, the G_1 and one of the X's goes dead. So it is more complicated than just saying that an initiator protein will interact with replicons and start replication. Why is the heterochromatin late and yet the exact same DNA in the other X chromosome is still early?

DR. SINCLAIR: I would like to say something about the inhibition of protein synthesis during S. With inhibitors like cyclohexamide you can stop the cell in S by arresting protein synthesis, of course DNA synthesis stops too. The cell really doesn't mind this a bit, even for quite an extensive period. If you do the same thing in G_1, it minds it a great deal more. There is a progression in G_1 in the extent of toxicity of cyclohexamide which indicates that there is some sequence of events going on and the cell is sensitive to interruptions in these cells. But certainly during S inhibition of protein synthesis does not upset the cell.

DR. PHILIPS: How long can you keep a cell arrested in S and rescue it?

DR. SINCLAIR: For a few hours.

DR. SWIFT: And the DNA of an individual cell has gone halfway through and then stopped?

DR. SINCLAIR: Of course there is no essential effect on DNA synthesis then because it is presumably over, but the cell can be arrested in G_2 by stopping protein synthesis, and it survives quite well.

DR. PRESCOTT: Where do you rescue the S-phase cells? DNA synthesis starts up where it left off presumably?

DR. SWIFT: I think that is a very interesting observation. Thank you. Are there some other remarks on this point? Again, I wanted to take issue with a statement made by Dr. Prescott. I feel that some control of DNA synthesis can go on in tissue cultures, and yet you said that there is no regulation in cultured cells. The experiments on contact inhibition indicate for certain strains of epithelial cells, but not others, that when cells come in contact with one another DNA synthesis doesn't stop but the rate falls precipitously to much lower levels, and the RNA synthesis as well. The fact that a cell senses it has a neighbor inhibits DNA synthesis.

DR. PRESCOTT: Yes, I like the word inhibits. I said that phenomenon happens and it appears to happen in G_1. G_1 is the sensitive period of contact inhibition, and I don't think that inhibition is controlled or regulated. Again, we are in a semantic dilemma. I think regulation is something much more specific. I didn't even use the word "control." I stuck to two words, "inhibition" and "regulation." I think that when cells are stopped *in vitro*, that's inhibition. When they are stopped *in vivo*, that's regulation. The point really is that it may be the same. It is just a matter of degree *in vitro*; it is a generalized thing. Cells may stop because some amino acid has been depleted or gas exchange is inadequate. Some general deterioration of the environment stops the cells, whereas as *in vivo* it's an active, specific continuous regulation of cell reproduction. But these may be just different degrees of specificity of the same thing.

DR. SWIFT: Just in summary of what we have said, the cell cycle in all cells has many basic points in common, but I think we should also keep in mind the fact, should we not, that a liver cell undergoing its 16–18 hour preparation for DNA synthesis following hepatectomy, and a lymphocyte stimulated by phytohemagglutinin are really undergoing two quite different processes, and that DNA synthesis may be turned on initially by very different methods, even though the final outcome is the same. Also, DNA synthesis may be turned off again by contact inhibition in a very different way than is done in Dr. Philips' studies with hydroxyurea. Again, we must consider that each turn of the mitotic cycle involves a tremendous series of interdigitating events in which both the nucleus and cytoplasm interact. It seems to me that we have no other final conclusion, except that we should go back to the drawing board or to our microscopes and learn more of the details.

Monographs already published

SCHINDLER, R., Lausanne: Die tierische Zelle in Zellkultur (Volume 1).

Neuroblastomas—Biochemical Studies. Edited by C. BOHUON, Villejuif (Volume 2, Symposium).

HUEPER, W. C., Bethesda: Occupational and Environmental Cancers of the Respiratory System (Volume 3).

GOLDMAN, L., Cincinnati: Laser Cancer Research (Volume 4).

METCALF, D., Melbourne: The Thymus. Its Role in Immune Responses, Leukaemia Development and Carcinogenesis (Volume 5).

Malignant Transformation by Viruses. Edited by W. H. KIRSTEN, Chicago (Volume 6, Symposium).

MOERTEL, CH. G., Rochester: Multiple Primary Malignant Neoplasms. Their Incidence and Significance (Volume 7).

New Trends in the Treatment of Cancer. Edited by L. MANUILA, S. MOLES and P. RENTCHNICK, Genève (Volume 8).

LINDENMANN, J., Zürich/P. A. KLEIN, Gainesville, Florida: Immunological Aspects of Viral Oncolysis (Volume 9).

NELSON, R. S., Houston: Radioactive Phosphorus in the Diagnosis of Gastrointestinal Cancer (Volume 10).

FREEMANN, R. G., and J. M. KNOX, Houston: Treatment of Skin Cancer (Volume 11).

LYNCH, H. T., Houston: Hereditary Factors in Carcinoma (Vol. 12).

Tumours in Children. Edited by H. B. MARSDEN and J. K. STEWARD, Manchester (Vol. 13).

ODARTCHENKO, N., Lausanne: Prolifération cellulaire érythropoiétique (Vol. 14).

SOKOLOFF, B., Lakeland/Florida: Cancer and Serotonin (Vol. 15).

JACOBS, M. L., Duarte/California: Malignant Lymphomas and their Management (Vol. 16).

Normal and Malignant Cell Growth. Edited by W. H. KIRSTEN, Chicago (Vol. 17, Symposium).

In production

ANGLESIO, E., Torino: The Treatment of Hodgkin's Disease (Vol. 18).

BANNASCH, P., Würzburg: The Cytoplasm of Hepatocytes during Carcinogenesis (Vol. 19).

BERNARD, J., R. PAUL, M. BOIRON, C. JACQUILLAT, and R. MARAL, Milano: Rubidomycin—a new Agent against Leukemia (Vol. 20).

MATHÉ, G., Villejuif: Seminar on the Scientific Bases of Chemotherapy in the Treatment of Cancer in Man.

In preparation

ACKERMANN, N. B., Boston: Use of Radioisotopic Agents in the Diagnosis of Cancer.

BOIRON, M., Paris: Les Virus de groupe Leucémies-Sarcomes.

CAVALIERE, R., A. ROSSI-FANELLI, B. MONDOVI, and G. MORICCA, Roma: Selective Heat Sensitivity of Cancer Cells.

CHIAPPA, S., Milano: Endolymphatic Radiotherapy in Malignant Lymphomas.

DENOIX, P., Villejuif: Le traitement des cancers du sein.

FISHER, E. R., Pittsburgh: Ultrastructure of Human Normal and Neoplastic Prostate.

FUCHS, W. A., Bern: Lymphography in Cancer.

GRUNDMANN, E., Wuppertal-Elberfeld: Morphologie und Cytochemie der Carcinogenese.

HAYWARD, J. L., London: Hormonal Research in Human Breast Cancer.

IRLIN, I. S., Moskva: Mechanisms of Viral Carcinogenesis.

KOLDOVSKY, P., Praha: Tumor Specific Transplantation Antigen (TTSA).

LANGLEY, F. A., and A. C. CROMPTON, Manchester: Epithelial Abnormalities of the Cervix Uteri.

MEEK, E. S., Bristol: Antiviral and Antitumour Agents of Biological Origin.

MULLER, J. H., Zürich: Therapeutic Incorporations of Radiopharmaceuticals in Cancer and Allied Diseases.

NEWMAN, M. K., Detroit: Neuropathies and Myopathies Associated with Occult Malignancies.

OGAWA, K., Osaka: Ultrastructural Enzyme Cytochemistry of Azo-dye Carcinogenesis.

PACK, G. T., New York: Clinical Aspects of Cancer Immunity and Cancer Susceptibility.

PACK, G. T., and A. H. ISLAMI, New York: Tumors of the Liver.

PARKER, J. W., Los Angeles: Lymphocyte Transformation.

RITZMAN, S. E., and W. C. LEVIN, Galveston: The Syndrome of Macroglobulinemia.

ROY-BURMAN, P., Los Angeles: Biochemical Mechanisms Involved in the Inhibition of Metabolic Processes by Purine, Pyramidine, and Nucleoside Analogs.

Seminar of the Scientific Bases of Chemotherapy in the Treatment of Cancer in Man. Edited by G. MATHÉ, Villejuif.

WEIL, R., Lausanne: Biological and Structural Properties of Polyoma Virus and its DNA.

WILLIAMS, D. C., Caterham, Surrey: The Basis for Therapy of Hormone Sensitive Tumours.

WILLIAMS, D. C., Caterham, Surrey: The Biochemistry of Metastasis.

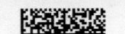